Lecture Notes in Computer Science 16377

The series Lecture Notes in Computer Science (LNCS), including its subseries Lecture Notes in Artificial Intelligence (LNAI) and Lecture Notes in Bioinformatics (LNBI), has established itself as a medium for the publication of new developments in computer science and information technology research, teaching, and education.

LNCS enjoys close cooperation with the computer science R & D community, the series counts many renowned academics among its volume editors and paper authors, and collaborates with prestigious societies. Its mission is to serve this international community by providing an invaluable service, mainly focused on the publication of conference and workshop proceedings and postproceedings. LNCS commenced publication in 1973.

Spyridon Bakas · Emily Dennis ·
Mehdi Astaraki · Ujjwal Baid ·
Gian Marco Conte · Martha Foltyn-Dumitru ·
Zhifan Jiang · Dominic Labella ·
Marie-Christin Metz · Udunna Anazodo ·
Maria Correia de Verdier · Florian Kofler ·
Hongwei Bran Li · Marius George Linguraru ·
Nazanin Maleki
Editors

Segmentation, Classification, and Synthesis for Brain Tumors and Traumatic Brain Injuries

MICCAI 2025 Challenges: BraTS-Lighthouse 2025 and AIMS-TBI 2025, Held in Conjunction with MICCAI 2025
Daejeon, South Korea, September 23, 2025
Proceedings, Part II

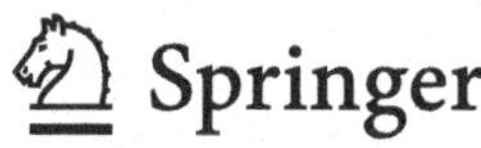

Editors
Spyridon Bakas
Indiana University School of Medicine
Indianapolis, IN, USA

Emily Dennis
University of Utah
Emerald Hills, CA, USA

Mehdi Astaraki
Karolinska Institutet
Huddinge, Sweden

Ujjwal Baid
Emory University School of Medicine
Atlanta, GA, USA

Gian Marco Conte
Mayo Clinic
Rochester, MN, USA

Martha Foltyn-Dumitru
University Hospital Bonn
Bonn, Germany

Zhifan Jiang
Children's National Hospital
Washington, D.C., USA

Dominic Labella
Duke University
Durham, NC, USA

Marie-Christin Metz
Klinikum rechts der Isar, TU Munich
Munich, Germany

Udunna Anazodo
McGill University
Montréal, QC, Canada

Maria Correia de Verdier
Uppsala University
Uppsala, Sweden

Florian Kofler
University of Tübingen
Tübingen, Germany

Hongwei Bran Li
NUS Medicine and Engineering
Singapore, Singapore

Marius George Linguraru
Children's National Hospital
Washington, D.C., USA

Nazanin Maleki
Children's Hospital of Philadelphia
Philadelphia, PA, USA

ISSN 0302-9743 ISSN 1611-3349 (electronic)
Lecture Notes in Computer Science
ISBN 978-3-032-16369-1 ISBN 978-3-032-16370-7 (eBook)
https://doi.org/10.1007/978-3-032-16370-7

This Springer imprint is published by the registered company Springer Nature Switzerland AG
The registered company address is: Gewerbestrasse 11, 6330 Cham, Switzerland

Preface

This volume contains papers accepted for the Brain TumorS (BraTS) 2025 Lighthouse Cluster of Challenges, and the Automated Identification of Moderate-Severe Traumatic Brain Injury Lesions (AIMS-TBI) 2025 Challenge. Both events were held in conjunction with the Medical Image Computing and Computer Assisted Intervention (MICCAI) conference on September 23–27, 2025 in Daejeon, Republic of Korea.

The presented manuscripts describe the latest research from computational scientists and clinical researchers working on adult and pediatric brain abnormalities, and specifically glioma, meningioma, metastases, and traumatic brain injuries. This compilation does not claim to provide a comprehensive understanding from all points of view; however, the authors present their latest advances in segmentation, detection, classification, and synthesis.

After the introductory chapter, My Model Is Better Than Yours! Statistically Aware Ranking for Fair Benchmarking of AI Models, the volume is divided into sections: The first through the seventh sections comprise a selection of accepted BraTS papers describing medical image segmentation methods for adult and pediatric brain glioblastoma, meningioma, and metastases. The eighth and ninth sections focus on accepted BraTS submissions showing advances in the field of image synthesis and inpainting for adult brain tumors. The tenth and eleventh sections focus on methods presented at the BraTS challenge, targeting the workload of classification for glioblastoma pathology sub-regions and disease progression. The twelfth section focuses on providing an overview of new medical image analysis advances from the AIMS-TBI challenge.

The focus of the first through the seventh sections is a selection of papers from the BraTS 2025 challenge participants developing the current state-of-the-art segmentation algorithms for routine, multi-institutional, clinically acquired multiparametric magnetic resonance imaging (mpMRI) scans towards addressing: Challenge 1, pre- and post-operative adult diffuse glioma (BraTS-GLI); Challenge 2, pre-treatment intracranial meningioma (BraTS-MEN); Challenge 3, pre-radiotherapy intracranial meningioma (BraTS-MEN-RT); Challenge 4, pre- and post-treatment brain metastases (BraTS-METS); Challenge 5, the underserved sub-Saharan African brain glioma patient population (BraTS-Africa); Challenge 6, pre-treatment pediatric high grade glioma patients (BraTS-PEDS); and Challenge 7, generalizability of segmentation methods across tumors (BraTS-GOAT). [Regarding the BraTS-GLI Challenge 1, Errol Colak, Adam Flanders, Felipe C. Kitamura and Luciano M. Prevedello were involved in the BraTS 2021 challenge, the data of which were used for training and validation in the 2023 and 2025 pre-treatment challenges, but they were not involved in the organization of the 2025 challenge.]

The eighth and ninth sections focus on generative artificial intelligence (AI). Challenge 8 addresses the synthesis of entire missing MRI sequences (BraTS-Synth), towards enabling the broader use of BraTS segmentation methods that mandate the availability of four structural MRI sequences (T1w, T1w with contrast, T2w, and T2-FLAIR) in clinical settings with limited imaging protocols or for the retrospective analysis of archival tumor datasets. Challenge 9 addresses the task of Local Inpainting of healthy tissue in brain tumor MRI scans (BraTS-Inpainting). Participants inpaint either brain tumor tissue or partially corrupted image regions. These forms of data corruption are often technical in nature, resulting from localized artifacts, an incomplete field of view, or missing or corrupted 2D slices. The objective is to develop algorithms that can locally synthesize missing image intensities within a predefined inpainting mask.

The tenth and eleventh sections focus on the computational workload of classification. Challenge 10 specifically includes papers representing the latest developments on AI models capable of assessing the heterogeneous histomorphologic landscape of glioblastoma by identifying nine distinct histopathologic tumor sub-regions on formalin-fixed paraffin-embedded (FFPE) H&E-stained tissue sections, acquired from standard clinical practice across 11 international sites (BraTS-Path). Challenge 11 then builds on longitudinal MRI sequences to present methods able to predict tumor progression during therapy (BraTS-PRO). Longitudinal properties are central to clinical practice, as defined by the Response Assessment in Neuro Oncology (RANO) criteria, which categorize treatment response into: complete response, partial response, stable disease, and progressive disease.

Challenge 12 focuses on the AIMS-TBI challenge, in which participants were tasked with developing new classification and segmentation algorithms for lesions due to traumatic brain injury. TBI-related lesions are highly heterogeneous and are not reliably identified by current methods focusing on other abnormalities (e.g., ischemic stroke, tumors). Our inability to accurately segment these lesions introduces significant bias in research, as lesions are either ignored, leading to methodological inaccuracies, or excluded, decreasing the generalizability of research.

Ninety papers were submitted and subsequently underwent a single-blind review process, with each receiving evaluation from a minimum of two independent reviewers. This process resulted in the acceptance of 80 papers which are presented across two volumes. We wholeheartedly hope that these two volumes will promote further exciting computational research on brain abnormalities.

October 2025

Spyridon Bakas
Emily Dennis
Mehdi Astaraki
Ujjwal Baid
Gian Marco Conte
Martha Foltyn-Dumitru
Zhifan Jiang
Dominic Labella
Marie-Christin Metz
Udunna Anazodo
Maria Correia de Verdier
Florian Kofler
Hongwei Bran Li
Marius George Linguraru
Nazanin Maleki

Organization

Challenge 1: BraTS-GLI

Leading Organizers

Organizing Committee

Rachit Saluja	Cornell University, Cornell Tech, Weill Cornell Medicine, USA
Russell T. Shinohara	University of Pennsylvania, USA
Arti Singh	Sage Bionetworks, USA
Nourel Hoda Tahon	University of Missouri, USA
Philip Vollmuth	Heidelberg University, Germany

Data Contributors

Pre-treatment

Christos Davatzikos	University of Pennsylvania, USA
Spyridon Bakas	Indiana University, USA
John Mongan	University of California, San Francisco, USA
Evan Calabrese	University of California, San Francisco, USA
Jeffrey D. Rudie	University of California, San Francisco, USA
Christopher Hess	University of California, San Francisco, USA
Soonmee Cha	University of California, San Francisco, USA
Javier Villanueva-Meyer	University of California, San Francisco, USA
John B. Freymann	National Institutes of Health (NIH), USA
Justin S. Kirby	National Institutes of Health (NIH), USA
Benedikt Wiestler	Technical University of Munich, Germany
Bjoern Menze	University of Zurich, Switzerland
Errol Colak	University of Toronto, Canada
Priscila Crivellaro	University of Toronto, Canada
Rivka R. Colen	MD Anderson Cancer Center, USA
Aikaterini Kotrotsou	MD Anderson Cancer Center, USA
Daniel Marcus	Washington University in St. Louis, USA
Mikhail Milchenko	Washington University in St. Louis, USA
Arash Nazeri	Washington University in St. Louis, USA
Hassan Fathallah-Shaykh	University of Alabama at Birmingham, USA
Roland Wiest	University of Bern, Switzerland
Andras Jakab	University of Debrecen, Hungary
Marc-Andre Weber	Heidelberg University, Germany
Abhishek Mahajan	Tata Memorial Centre, Mumbai, India
Ujjwal Baid	Emory University, USA

Post-treatment

Name	Affiliation
Evan Calabrese	Duke University, USA
Dominic LaBella	Duke University, USA
Jikai Zhang	Duke University, USA
Jeffrey D. Rudie	University of California, San Francisco, USA
Andreas Rauschecker	University of California, San Francisco, USA
Brandon Fields	University of California, San Francisco, USA
Javier Villanueva-Meyer	University of California, San Francisco, USA
Ayman Nada	University of Missouri, Columbia, USA
Nourel Hoda Tahon	University of Missouri, Columbia, USA
Talissa Altes	University of Missouri, Columbia, USA
Yaseen Dhemesh	University of Missouri, Columbia, USA
Filip Garrett	University of Missouri, Columbia, USA
Jaime Gass	University of Missouri, Columbia, USA
Edvin Isufi	University of Missouri, Columbia, USA
Lester J. Layfield	University of Missouri, Columbia, USA
Jason Sinclair	University of Missouri, Columbia, USA
Jonathan Thacker	University of Missouri, Columbia, USA
Jeffrey D. Rudie	University of California, San Diego, USA
Maria Correia de Verdier	University of California, San Diego, USA
Nikdokht Farid	University of California, San Diego, USA
Louis Gagnon	University of California, San Diego, USA
Jona Hattagandi Gluth	University of California, San Diego, USA
Paul Manning	University of California, San Diego, USA
Tyler Seibert	University of California, San Diego, USA
Sevcan Turk	University of Michigan, USA
Lubomir Hadjiiski	University of Michigan, USA
Sebastian Oliva	University of Michigan, USA
Patil Basavasagar	University of Michigan, USA
Ujjwal Baid	Emory University, USA
Spyridon Bakas	Indiana University, USA
Yuri S. Velichko	Northwestern University, USA

Challenge 2: BraTS-MEN

Leading Organizers

Name	Affiliation
Evan Calabrese	Duke University, USA
Dominic Labella	Duke University, USA

Organizing Committee

Mariam Aboian	Yale University, USA
Mehdi Astaraki	Karolinska Institutet, Sweden
Ujjwal Baid	Emory University, USA
Spyridon Bakas	Indiana University, USA
Sully Chen	Duke University, USA
Devon Godfrey	Duke University, USA
Collin Kent	Duke University, USA
Omaditya (Goldey) Khanna	Thomas Jefferson University, USA
John Kirkpatrick	Duke University, USA
Ryan McLean	Yale University, USA
Ayman Nada	Missouri University, USA
Arif Rashid	University of Pennsylvania, USA
Andreas Rauschecker	University of California, San Francisco, USA
Zachary Reitman	Duke University, USA
Jeffrey Rudie	University of California, San Diego, USA
Nourel Tahon	Missouri University, USA
Yury Velichko	Northwestern University, USA
Javier Villanueva-Meyer	University of California, San Francisco, USA
Chunhao Wang	Duke University, USA
Pranav Warman	Duke University, USA

Data Contributors

Mariam Aboian	Children's Hospital of Philadelphia, USA
Ryan McLean	Yale University, USA
Ujjwal Baid	Emory University, USA
Spyridon Bakas	Indiana University, USA
Evan Calabrese	Duke University, USA
Omaditya (Goldey) Khanna	Thomas Jefferson University, USA
Ayman Nada	Missouri University, USA
Nourel Tahon	Missouri University, USA
Andreas Rauschecker	University of California, San Francisco, USA
Javier Villanueva-Meyer	University of California, San Francisco, USA

Challenge 3: BraTS-MEN-RT

Leading Organizers

Evan Calabrese	Duke University, USA
Dominic Labella	Duke University, USA

Organizing Committee

Mariam Aboian	Children's Hospital of Philadelphia, USA
Mehdi Astaraki	Karolinska Institute, Sweden
Ujjwal Baid	Emory University, USA
Spyridon Bakas	Indiana University, USA
Gian Marco Conte	Mayo Clinic, USA
Maria Correia de Verdier	University of San Diego, USA
Nourel Hoda Tahon	University of Missouri, USA
Raymond Huang	Harvard Medical School, USA
Ayman Nada	University of Missouri, USA
Andreas M. Rauschecker	University of California, San Francisco, USA
Jeffrey Rudie	University of San Diego, USA
Benedikt Wiestler	Technical University of Munich, Germany

Data Contributors

Jeffrey Rudie	University of California, San Francisco, USA
Andreas Rauschecker	University of California, San Francisco, USA
Brandon Fields	University of California, San Francisco, USA
Javier Villanueva-Meyer	University of California, San Francisco, USA
Michael Mix	SUNY Upstate, USA
Katherine Schumacher	SUNY Upstate, USA
Peter Taylor	SUNY Upstate, USA
Lia Halasz	University of Washington, USA
Justin Leu	University of Washington, USA
Ayman Nada	University of Missouri, USA
Nourel Hoda Tahon	University of Missouri, USA
Evan Calabrese	Duke University, USA
Dominic LaBella	Duke University, USA
John Kirkpatrick	Duke University, USA
Scott Floyd	Duke University, USA
Zachary Reitman	Duke University, USA
Trey Mullikin	Duke University, USA

Jonathan Shapey	King's College London, UK
Tom Vercauteren	King's College London, UK
Jeffrey D. Rudie	University of California, San Diego, USA
Maria Correia de Verdier	University of California, San Diego, USA
Nikdokht Farid	University of California, San Diego, USA
Louis Gagnon	University of California, San Diego, USA
Jona Hattagandi Gluth	University of California, San Diego, USA
Tyler Seibert	University of California, San Diego, USA

Challenge 4: BraTS-METS

Leading Organizers

Mariam Aboian	Children's Hospital of Philadelphia, USA
Nazanin Maleki	Children's Hospital of Philadelphia, USA
Ahmed Moawad	Mercy Catholic Medical Center, USA

Organizing Committee

Raisa Amiruddin	Children's Hospital of Philadelphia, USA
Nikolay Yordanov	Medical University, Sofia, Bulgaria
Crystal Chukwurah	Yale School of Medicine, USA
Pascal Fehringer	Friedrich Schiller University, Germany
Athanasios Gkampenis	University of Tübingen, Germany
Fabian Umeh	Teesside University, UK

Data Contributors

Mariam Aboian	Children's Hospital of Philadelphia, USA
Satrajit Chakrabarty	Washington University, USA
Maria Correia de Verdier	University of California, San Diego, USA
Jeffrey Rudie	University of California, San Diego, USA
Devon Godfrey	Duke University, USA
Scott Floyd	Duke University, USA
Nourel Hoda Tahon	University of Missouri, USA
Ayman Nada	University of Missouri, USA
Yuri S. Velichko	Northwestern University, USA
Ayda Youssef	National Cancer Institute, USA

Data Annotators

Fatima Memon	Medical University of South Carolina, USA
Mohanad Ghonim	University of Pennsylvania, USA
Bojan D. Petrovic	University of Chicago, USA
Mohamed Ghonim	University of Pennsylvania, USA
Justin Cramer	Mayo Clinic (Arizona), USA
Sedra Mhana	University of Pennsylvania, USA
Mark Krycia	Carolina Radiology, USA
Albara Alotaibi	Jordan University of Science and Technology, Jordan
Elizabeth Brooke Shrickel	Ohio State University, USA
Nathan Page	Friedrich Schiller University of Jena, Germany
Ichiro Ikuta	Mayo Clinic (Arizona), USA
Amirreza Manteghinejad	Children's Hospital of Philadelphia, USA
Gerard Thompson	University of Edinburgh, UK
Prisha Bhatia	Mohammed Bin Rashid University of Medicine and Health Sciences, Dubai
Lorenna Vidal	Children's Hospital of Philadelphia, USA
Yasaman Sharifi	Iran University, Iran
Vilma Kosovic	General Hospital of Dubrovnik, Croatia
Marko Jakovljevic	Children's Hospital of Philadelphia, USA
Adam Goldman-Yassen	Emory University, USA
Nikolay Yordanov	Medical University, Sofia, Bulgaria
Virginia Hill	Northwestern University, USA
Salma Abosabie	Julius-Maximilians-Universität Würzburg, Germany
Tiffany So	Chinese University of Hong Kong, China
Sara Abosabie	Charité – Universitätsmedizin Berlin, Germany
Mark Krycia	Carolina Radiology, USA
Marko Jakovljevic	Children's Hospital of Philadelphia, USA
Melisa S. Guelen	Massachusetts General Hospital, USA
Basimah Albalooshy	Children's Hospital of Philadelphia, USA
Michael Veronesi	University of Wisconsin, USA
Raisa Amiruddin	Children's Hospital of Philadelphia, USA

Challenge 5: BraTS-Africa

Leading Organizers

Udunna Anazodo	McGill University, Canada and Medical Artificial Intelligence Laboratory (MAI Lab), Nigeria
Maruf Adewole	Medical Artificial Intelligence Laboratory (MAI Lab), Nigeria

Organizing Committee

Ujjwal Baid	Emory University, USA
Spyridon Bakas	Indiana University, USA
Bjoern Menze	University of Zurich, Switzerland

Clinical Evaluators

Jeff Rudie	Scripps Health and University of California, San Diego, USA
Farouk Dako	University of Pennsylvania, USA
Abiodun Fatade	Medical Artificial Intelligence Laboratory (MAI Lab) and Crestview Radiology, Nigeria
Oluyemisi Toyobo	Medical Artificial Intelligence Laboratory (MAI Lab) and Crestview Radiology, Nigeria

Data Contributors

Kenneth Aguh	Federal Medical Centre, Umuahia, Nigeria
Rachel Akinola	Lagos State University Teaching Hospital, Lagos, Nigeria
Feyisayo Daji	National Hospital, Abuja, Nigeria
Abiodun Fatade	Medical Artificial Intelligence Laboratory (MAI Lab) and Crestview Radiology, Nigeria
Chinasa Kalaiwo	National Hospital, Nigeria
Mayomi Onuwaje	Lily Hospital, Benin, Nigeria
Olubukola Omidiji	Lagos University Teaching Hospital, Lagos, Nigeria
Mohammad Abba Suwaid	NSIA-Kano Diagnostic Center, Kano, Nigeria

Data Annotators

Challenge 6: BraTS-PEDS

Leading Organizers

Organizing Committee

Data Contributors

Mariam Aboian	Children's Hospital of Philadelphia, USA
Miriam Bornhorst	Children's National Hospital, USA
Evan Calabrese	Duke University, USA
Ethan Castellino	Duke University, USA
Peter de Blank	Cincinnati Children's Hospital, USA
Michelle Deutsch	Nationwide Children's Hospital, USA
Maryam Fouladi	Nationwide Children's Hospital, USA
Lindsey Hoffman	Phoenix Children's Hospital, USA
Trent Hummel	Cincinnati Children's Hospital, USA
Benjamin Kann	Dana-Farber Brigham Cancer Center and Boston Children's Hospital, USA
Margot Lazow	Nationwide Children's Hospital, USA
Justin Low	Duke University, USA
Nazanin Maleki	Children's Hospital of Philadelphia, USA
Ali Nabavizadeh	University of Pennsylvania, USA
Avani Mangoli	Duke University, USA
Leonie Mikael	Nationwide Children's Hospital, USA
Roger Packer	Children's National Hospital, USA
Adam Resnick	Children's Hospital of Philadelphia, USA
Brian Rood	Children's National Hospital, USA
Tina Young Poussaint	FACR, Dana-Farber Brigham Cancer Center and Boston Children's Hospital, USA
Anna Zapaishchykova	Dana-Farber Brigham Cancer Center and Boston Children's Hospital, USA

Data Annotators

Debanjan Haldar	Thomas Jefferson University Hospital, USA
Shuvanjan Haldar	Children's Hospital of Philadelphia, USA
Nastaran Khalili	Children's Hospital of Philadelphia, USA
Neda Khalili	Children's Hospital of Philadelphia, USA
Hollie Lai	Children's Health Orange County, USA
Aaron McAllister	Nationwide Children's Hospital, USA
Khanak Nandolia	All India Institute of Medical Sciences, India
Sanjay Prabhu	Boston Children's Hospital, USA
Mariana Sánchez Montaño	Unidad de Patología Clínica, Mexico
Ibraheem Shaikh	Beth Israel Deaconess Medical Center, USA
Nakul Sheth	Weill Cornell Medicine and New York Presbyterian Hospital, USA
Wenxin Tu	University of Pennsylvania, USA

Bhavyasri Vunnava	Children's Hospital of Philadelphia, USA
Sanaz Varshochi	Children's Hospital of Philadelphia, USA

Data Approvers

Mariam Aboian	Children's Hospital of Philadelphia, USA
Ali Nabavizadeh	University of Pennsylvania, USA
Arastoo Vossough	Children's Hospital of Philadelphia, USA
Jeffrey B. Ware	University of Pennsylvania, USA

Challenge 7: BraTS-GOAT

Leading Organizers

Ujjwal Baid	Emory University, USA
Spyridon Bakas	Indiana University, USA
Gian Marco Conte	Mayo Clinic, USA

Data Contributors

Same data contributors as in Challenges 1, 2, 4, 5 and 6.

Challenge 8: BraTS-Synth

Leading Organizers

Hongwei Bran Li	Harvard Medical School, USA
Athinoula A. Martinos	Harvard Medical School, USA

Organizing Committee

Mariam Aboian	University of Pennsylvania, USA
Mehdi Astaraki	Karolinska Institute, Sweden
Ujjwal Baid	Emory University, USA
Spyridon Bakas	Indiana University, USA
Gian Marco Conte	Mayo Clinic, USA
Verena Chung	Sage Bionetworks, USA
Keyvan Farahani	National Institutes of Health (NIH), USA

Juan Eugenio Iglesias	Harvard Medical School, USA
Florian Kofler	Hertie AI, University of Tübingen, Germany
Marius George Linguraru	Children's National Hospital, USA
Bjoern Menze	University of Zurich, Switzerland
Matthew S. Rosen	Harvard Medical School, USA
Benedikt Wiestler	Klinikum rechts der Isar, Technical University of Munich, Germany

Data Contributors

Same data contributors as in Challenges 1, 2 and 4.

Challenge 9: BraTS-Inpainting

Leading Organizers

Florian Kofler	Hertie AI, University of Tübingen, Germany

Organizing Committee

Bjoern Menze	University of Zurich, Switzerland
Benedikt Wiestler	Klinikum rechts der Isar, Technical University of Munich, Germany
Ivan Ezhov	Technical University of Munich, Germany
Marie Piraud	Helmholtz AI, Germany

Data Contributors

Same data contributors as in Challenges 1 and 2.

Challenge 10: BraTS-Path

Leading Organizers

Spyridon Bakas	Indiana University, USA
Siddhesh Thakur	Indiana University, USA

Organizing Committee

Mehdi Astaraki	Karolinska Institute, Sweden
Ujjwal Baid	Emory University, USA
Robert Bell	Indiana University, USA
Verena Chung	Sage Bionetworks, USA
Lee A. D. Cooper	Northwestern University, USA
Jason Huse	Anderson Cancer Center, USA
Shahriar Faghani	Mayo Clinic, USA
Keyvan Farahani	National Institutes of Health (NIH), USA
Mana Moassefi	Mayo Clinic, USA

Clinical Annotators

Jose Javier Otero	Florida International University, USA
Jason Huse	Anderson Cancer Center, USA
C. J. Lucas	Johns Hopkins University, USA
Kenneth Aldape	National Cancer Institute, USA
Leo Y. Ballester	Anderson Cancer Center, USA
Aditya Raghunathan	Mayo Clinic, USA, USA
Michael L. Miller	Columbia University, USA
Valeria Barresi	University of Verona, Italy
Leonille Schweizer	University Hospital Frankfurt, Germany
Marwan M. Majeed	Indiana University, USA
Maria A. Gubbiotti	Anderson Cancer Center, USA
Michael Rodriguez	Macquarie University, Australia
Hrvoje Miletić	Haukeland University Hospital, Norway
Claire Delbridge	Technical University of Munich, Germany
Giselle Y. López	Duke University, USA
Tibor Hortobagyi	University Hospital Zurich, Switzerland
Regina Rose Reimann	University Hospital Zurich, Switzerland
Joanna J. Phillips	University of California, San Francisco, USA
MacLean P. Nasrallah	University of Pennsylvania, USA
Keith L. Ligon	Dana-Farber Cancer Institute, USA

Challenge 11: BraTS-PRO

Leading Organizers

Organizing Committee

Challenge 12: AIMS-TBI

Leading Organizers

Organizing Committee

Spyridon Bakas	Indiana University, USA
Matthew Pease	Indiana University, USA
Adrian Onicas	University of Utah, USA
Nicholas Tustison	University of Virginia, USA
Elisabeth Wilde	University of Utah, USA

Data Contributors

Robert Asarnow	University of California, Los Angeles, USA
Karen Caeyenberghs	Deakin University, Australia
Nancy Chiaravalloti	Kessler Foundation, USA
Brenda Bartnik-Olson	Loma Linda University, USA
Kristen Dams-O'Connor	Mount Sinai, USA
Ekaterina Dobryakova	Kessler Foundation, USA
Linda Ewing-Cobbs	University of Texas, Houston, USA
Helen Genova	Kessler Foundation, USA
Frank Hillary	Pennsylvania State University
Kristen Hoskinson	Nationwide Children's Hospital, USA
Nicholas Ryan	Murdoch Children's Research Institute, Australia
Stacy Suskauer	Kennedy Krieger Institute, USA
Lars Westlye	University of Oslo, Norway
Elisabeth Wilde	University of Utah, USA

Data Annotators

Emily Dennis	University of Utah, USA
Evelyn Deutscher	Deakin University, Australia
Morgan Hafen	Brigham Young University, USA
Elizabeth Hovenden	University of Utah, USA
Jamie Johnson	University of Utah, USA
Finian Keleher	University of Utah, USA
Hannah Lindsey	University of Utah, USA
Courtney McCabe	University of Utah, USA
Jake Mitchell	Monash University, Australia
Emma Read	University of Utah, USA
Madeleine Reading	Brigham Young University, USA
Emmanuella Sybrowsky	University of Utah, USA
Dayna Thayn	University of Utah, USA

Contents

Challenge 8 – BraTS-Synth

Unified Brain MRI Synthesis with Mixture of Multimodal Hierarchical VAEs (BraSyn 2025)

Reuben Dorent[1,2](✉)

[1] MIND Team, Inria Saclay, Université Paris-Saclay, Palaiseau, France
reuben.dorent@inria.fr
[2] Sorbonne Université, Institut du Cerveau - Paris Brain Institute - ICM, CNRS, Inria, Inserm, AP-HP, Hôpital de la Pitié Salpêtrière, 75013 Paris, France

Abstract. Unified synthesis of missing MRI sequences facilitates robust image analysis in brain tumor patients when imaging data are incomplete. We present a unified framework based on the Mixture of Multimodal Hierarchical Variational Autoencoders (MMHVAE), which performs cross-modal MRI synthesis with arbitrary missing sequences. MMHVAE leverages a hierarchical latent representation and a mixture of unimodal posteriors to flexibly model incomplete inputs. For the MICCAI 2025 BraSyn challenge, our approach synthesizes one randomly missing sequence from the remaining three, while addressing inter-center acquisition variability through contrast harmonization. On the BraSyn validation set, the method achieves high-quality synthesis with Structural Similarity Index Measures (SSIM) exceeding 99.7% in tumor regions and promising Dice scores in downstream tumor segmentation tasks. These results demonstrate the potential of MMHVAE as a unified solution for brain MRI synthesis in the presence of missing sequences.

Keywords: Hierarchical Variational Auto-Encoder · Image Synthesis · Brain Tumor

1 Introduction

Automated brain tumor segmentation from multi-sequence magnetic resonance imaging (MRI) is becoming increasingly integrated into clinical workflows, with deep learning methods now achieving levels of accuracy and robustness that support clinical decision-making. These methods typically rely on four MRI sequences: T1-weighted images with (ceT_1) and without (T_1) contrast enhancement, T2-weighted images (T_2), and FLAIR images. However, in real-world clinical practice, some sequences are often unavailable due to time or cost constraints or acquisition issues. This particularly limits their applicability in centers with less extensive imaging protocols or when analyzing retrospective datasets. Addressing this challenge, the Brain MR Image Synthesis Benchmark (BraSyn) [16], organized as part of the MICCAI 2025 conference, aims to evaluate image synthesis methods that can realistically generate missing MRI sequences from a set of available images.

S. Bakas et al. (Eds.): MICCAI 2025, LNCS 16377, pp. 3–14, 2026.
https://doi.org/10.1007/978-3-032-16370-7_1

Generating missing MRI sequences has attracted significant interest in recent years. In particular, unified cross-modal synthesis frameworks, where a single model handles arbitrary combinations of observed and missing sequences, have been proposed leveraging generative adversarial networks (GANs) [14,15,25] and Transformers [4]. These methods typically concatenate all available sequences and replace missing ones with zero tensors during training. While this approach can be effective, it neither models shared latent representations across sequences nor gracefully handles incomplete training data, as most assume full modality availability during development. More recent methods based on latent- or image-space diffusion models [11,18,19,29] have shown impressive synthesis quality but require large training sets and are computationally expensive, especially at inference time. Furthermore, most diffusion- and GAN-based unified methods lack dedicated mechanisms to manage missing data during training, limiting their practical use in clinical settings where incomplete data is the norm.

In this work, we address these limitations by building on our previously published hierarchical multimodal variational auto-encoder (MMHVAE) framework [5,6]. MMHVAE has been successfully used for unified cross-modal image synthesis using ultrasound and multiparametric brain MRI data from the ReMIND dataset [12], has been applied in downstream tasks such as patient-specific image segmentation [9], keypoint matching [22,23], or cross-modal domain adaptation [5,8]. For the BraSyn challenge, we apply exploit MMHVAE without significant modification. MMHVAE is designed specifically for unified cross-modal image synthesis in the presence of incomplete data. It learns a structured latent space capturing shared information across modalities while flexibly integrating missing modality scenarios during both training and inference. The key innovations of MMHVAE include: (i) a hierarchical latent architecture that supports unified synthesis with incomplete inputs; (ii) a variational posterior modeled as a mixture of Product-of-Experts, encouraging robust encoding of both observed and missing information; and (iii) an adversarial regularization strategy applied at the dataset level to handle non-observed modalities in incomplete training sets. In this paper, we describe the MMHVAE framework, detail its application to the BraSyn benchmark, and present preliminary qualitative results on the validation set of the BraSyn 2025 dataset.

2 MMHVAE: Mixture of Multimodal Hierarchical Variational Auto-encoders

In this section, we present the Mixture of Multimodal Hierarchical Variational Auto-Encoders (MMHVAE) framework, originally introduced in [5]. This framework is designed to address the challenges of synthesizing missing modalities from observed images in different modalities. The MMHVAE framework focuses on four key challenges: (i) creating complex latent representations of multimodal data, (ii) learning to fuse multimodal information in the context of missing data, (iii) estimating missing information for cross-modal image synthesis, and (iv) leveraging dataset-level information to handle incomplete datasets at training time. While challenge (iv) is central to MMHVAE's general design, it is less relevant in the context of the BraSyn 2025 challenge, where all the training samples are complete.

2.1 Hierarchical Latent Representation of Multimodal Images

The MMHVAE framework introduces a hierarchical latent representation of multimodal images. Let the random variable $\boldsymbol{X} = (X_1, \ldots, X_M) \in \mathbb{R}^{M \times \Omega}$ represent a complete set of paired multimodal images, where M is the total number of image modalities and Ω is the number of pixels. The images $\boldsymbol{X}$ are assumed to be conditionally independent given a latent random variable $\boldsymbol{Z}$. The conditional distribution $p_\theta(\boldsymbol{x}|\boldsymbol{z})$ parameterized by θ can be written as:

$$p_\theta(\boldsymbol{x}|\boldsymbol{z}) = \prod_{j=1}^{M} p_\theta(x_j|\boldsymbol{z}) \ . \tag{1}$$

To increase the expressiveness of the model and tackle the issue of blurry images typically produced by VAEs [13] and MVAEs [7,26,28], MMHVAE employs a hierarchical representation of the latent variable $\boldsymbol{Z}$. The latent variable $\boldsymbol{Z}$ is partitioned into disjoint groups, i.e., $\boldsymbol{Z} = (Z_1, \ldots, Z_L)$, where L is the number of groups. The prior $p(\boldsymbol{z})$ is then represented by:

$$p_\theta(\boldsymbol{z}) = p(z_L) \prod_{l=1}^{L-1} p_{\theta_l}(z_l|\boldsymbol{z}_{>l}) \ , \tag{2}$$

where $\boldsymbol{z}_{>l} = (z_k)_{k=l+1}^{L}$, $p(z_L) = \mathcal{N}(z_L; \mathbf{0}_{H_L}, I_{H_L})$ is an isotropic Normal prior distribution and the conditional prior distributions $p_{\theta_l}(z_l|\boldsymbol{z}_{>l})$ are Normal distributions with mean and diagonal covariance parameterized using neural networks, i.e. $p_{\theta_l}(z_l|\boldsymbol{z}_{>l}) = \mathcal{N}(z_l; \mu_{\theta_l}(\boldsymbol{z}_{>l}), D_{\theta_l}(\boldsymbol{z}_{>l}))$.

In MMHVAE, the finest latent representation z_1 carries all the information required to describe each image, i.e.:

$$p_\theta(\boldsymbol{x}|\boldsymbol{z}) = \prod_{j=1}^{M} p_{\theta_j}(x_j|z_1) \ , \tag{3}$$

where the image decoding distributions are modeled as Normal with a mean parametrized by a neural network and fixed variance σ, i.e. $p_{\theta_j}(x_j|z_1) = \mathcal{N}(x_j; \mu^x_{\theta_j}(z_1), \sigma I)$.

2.2 Marginal Log-Likelihood Objective with Incomplete Data

MMHVAE is designed to handle partially observed and fully observed data during both training and inference. Let $\boldsymbol{R}$ be a binary vector indicating observed modalities, with $R_j = 1$ if X_j is observed and 0 otherwise. The partially observed samples $\boldsymbol{X}$ can be divided into an observed component $\boldsymbol{X}_{\boldsymbol{R}}^{o} = \{\boldsymbol{X}_i,$ such that $R_i = 1\}$ and a missing one $\boldsymbol{X}_{\boldsymbol{R}}^{m} = \{\boldsymbol{X}_i,$ such that $R_i = 0\}$.

The overall objective is to maximize the expected observed marginal log-likelihood, i.e., $\mathbb{E}_{(\boldsymbol{x},\boldsymbol{r})\sim p_{\text{data}}}[\log p_\theta(\boldsymbol{x}_{\boldsymbol{r}}^{o})]]$. Since the true posterior is intractable, the expected value of a tractable lower bound is instead maximized by introducing a variational distribution $q_\phi(\boldsymbol{z}|\boldsymbol{x}_{\boldsymbol{r}}^{o})$ that approximates the posterior $p_\theta(\boldsymbol{z}|\boldsymbol{x}_{\boldsymbol{r}}^{o})$.

2.3 Modeling the Variational Posterior as a Mixture

The MMHVAE framework proposes modeling the variational posterior $p_\theta(\boldsymbol{z}|\boldsymbol{x}_{\boldsymbol{r}}^{o})$ as a mixture distribution, where each component approximates the true posterior with incomplete input data. Authors in [5] have shown that this encourages the mixture components to encode all available information and estimate the missing information needed for cross-modal image synthesis.

Let S be the set of all vectors of length M consisting solely of zeros and ones, with each vector having at least one non-zero entry. For any vector $\boldsymbol{r} \in S$, let $S_{\boldsymbol{r}}$ be the set that contains all subsets of the observed modalities in $\boldsymbol{r}$, i.e. $S_{\boldsymbol{r}} = \{\boldsymbol{r'} \in S, \text{ s.t.: } r'_i = 0 \text{ if } r_i = 0\}$ (e.g. $S_{[1,1,0,0]} = \{[1,1,0,0],[1,0,0,0],[0,1,0,0]\}$).

The variational distribution $q_\phi(\boldsymbol{z}|\boldsymbol{x}_{\boldsymbol{r}}^{o})$ is expressed as a mixture (convex combination) of distributions represented by:

$$q_\phi^{\text{MMHVAE}}(\boldsymbol{z}|\boldsymbol{x}_{\boldsymbol{r}}^{o}) = \sum_{\boldsymbol{r'}\in S_{\boldsymbol{r}}} \alpha_{\boldsymbol{r'}}^{(\boldsymbol{r})} q_\phi(\boldsymbol{z}|\boldsymbol{x}_{\boldsymbol{r'}}^{o}) \tag{4}$$

where the input data $\boldsymbol{x}_{\boldsymbol{r'}}^{o}$ is a subset of the observations $\boldsymbol{x}_{\boldsymbol{r}}^{o}$ and $\alpha_{\boldsymbol{r'}}^{(\boldsymbol{r})}$ are the mixture weights such that $\alpha_{\boldsymbol{r'}}^{(\boldsymbol{r})} \geq 0$ and $\sum_{\boldsymbol{r'}\in S_{\boldsymbol{r}}} \alpha_{\boldsymbol{r'}}^{(\boldsymbol{r})} = 1$. These weights are hyperparameters. The choice for α is discussed in Sect. 3.

2.4 Variational Parameterization for Fusing Incomplete Multimodal Inputs

The MMHVAE framework aims to construct a variational component for each non-empty subset of observed data that approximates the posterior distribution. Inspired by MVAEs [28], the framework proposes creating M unimodal encoding networks instead of handling $2^M - 1$ encoding networks. Importantly, a closed-form solution allows merging unimodal contributions from each available modality at each level l of the hierarchy. Specifically, the conditional variational distribution $q_{\phi_l,\theta_l}(z_l|\boldsymbol{x}_{\boldsymbol{r'}}^{o}, \boldsymbol{z}_{>l})$ is a Normal distribution with mean $\mu_{\phi_l,\theta_l}(\boldsymbol{x}_{\boldsymbol{r'}}^{o}, \boldsymbol{z}_{>l})$

and diagonal covariance $D_{\phi_l,\theta_l}(\boldsymbol{x}^o_{\boldsymbol{r}'}, \boldsymbol{z}_{>l})$ defined by:

$$\begin{cases} D_{\phi_l,\theta_l}(\boldsymbol{x}^o_{\boldsymbol{r}'}, \boldsymbol{z}_{>l}) = \left(D_{\theta_l}(\boldsymbol{z}_{>l})^{-1} + \sum_{\substack{j=1 \\ \text{s.t.} \\ r'_j=1}}^{M} D_{\phi_l^j}(x_j, \boldsymbol{z}_{>l})^{-1} \right)^{-1} \\ \mu_{\phi_l,\theta_l}(\boldsymbol{x}^o_{\boldsymbol{r}'}, \boldsymbol{z}_{>l}) = D_{\phi_l,\theta_l}(\boldsymbol{x}^o_{\boldsymbol{r}'}, \boldsymbol{z}_{>l})^{-1} \\ \qquad \left(D_{\theta_l}(\boldsymbol{z}_{>l})^{-1}\mu_{\theta_l}(\boldsymbol{z}_{>l}) + \sum_{\substack{j=1 \\ \text{s.t.} \\ r'_j=1}}^{M} D_{\phi_l^j}(x_j, \boldsymbol{z}_{>l})^{-1}\mu_{\phi_l^j}(x_j, \boldsymbol{z}_{>l}) \right) \end{cases} \tag{5}$$

Here, $(\mu_{\phi_l^j}(x_j, \boldsymbol{z}_{>l}), D\phi_l^j(x_j, \boldsymbol{z}_{>l}))$ denotes the unimodal encoding of modality j at level l, conditioned on the higher-level latent variables $\boldsymbol{z}_{>l}$. At the top level $l = L$, the prior is standard Normal with $D_{\theta_L}(\boldsymbol{z}_{>L}) = I_{H_L}$ and $\mu_{\theta_L}(\boldsymbol{z}_{>L}) = \mathbf{0}_{H_L}$.

3 MMHVAE for the BraSyn Challenge

In this section, we describe how the MMHVAE framework was adapted for the BraSyn Challenge.

3.1 Mixture Weights

In the BraSyn challenge, all $M = 4$ imaging sequences are available for every training sample, i.e., $\boldsymbol{r} = \mathbf{1} = [1, 1, 1, 1]$. For clarity, we denote the observed data $\boldsymbol{x}^o$ simply as $\boldsymbol{x}$ in the remainder of this work. The task involves synthesizing one randomly missing sequence from the remaining three, with each sequence being equally likely to be missing. Accordingly, we define the mixture weights as:

$$\forall \boldsymbol{r}' \in S_1, \quad \alpha_{\boldsymbol{r}'} = \begin{cases} \frac{1}{4} & \text{if } \boldsymbol{r}' \in \{[1,1,1,0], [1,1,0,1], [1,0,1,1], [0,1,1,1]\} \\ 0 & \text{otherwise.} \end{cases} \tag{6}$$

3.2 Training Procedure

We optimize model parameters by minimizing a total loss $\mathcal{L}^{\text{Total}}$ that combines reconstruction, hierarchical KullbackLeibler (KL) divergences, and an adversarial component to improve visual quality. The training procedure proceeds as follows: (1) A mini-batch of B fully observed training examples is sampled; (2) we sample $T = 1$ binary mask vector $\boldsymbol{r}' \in S_1$ with probability $\alpha_{\boldsymbol{r}'}$, simulating a missing-sequence configuration; (3) we compute and minimize the average total loss $\mathcal{L}^{\text{Total}}(\boldsymbol{x}, \boldsymbol{r}'; \theta, \phi)$ over the mini-batch. To estimate the expectations involved in KL divergences of the variational objective, we follow [17] and use a single

Monte Carlo sample per latent variable. Given a pair $(\boldsymbol{x}, \boldsymbol{r'})$, the total loss $\mathcal{L}^{Total}$ is defined as:

$$\begin{aligned} \mathcal{L}^{Total}(\boldsymbol{x}, \boldsymbol{r'}; \theta, \phi) = & \sum_{j=1}^{M} ||\mu_{\theta_j^x}(z_1) - x_j||^2 \\ & + \lambda_{KL} \sum_{l=1}^{L} \log \frac{q_{\phi_l, \theta_l}(z_l|\boldsymbol{x}_{\boldsymbol{r'}}, \boldsymbol{z}_{>l})}{p_{\theta_l}(z_l|\boldsymbol{z}_{>l})} \\ & + \lambda_{GAN} \sum_{j=1}^{M} d^j_{\psi_j}\left(\mu_{\theta_j^x}(z_1)\right) , \end{aligned} \tag{7}$$

where $\mu_{\theta_j^x}(z_1)$ is the reconstruction of sequence j, and $d^j_{\psi_j}$ is a discriminator network (with parameters ψ_j) trained to distinguish real sequence-j images from synthesized ones.

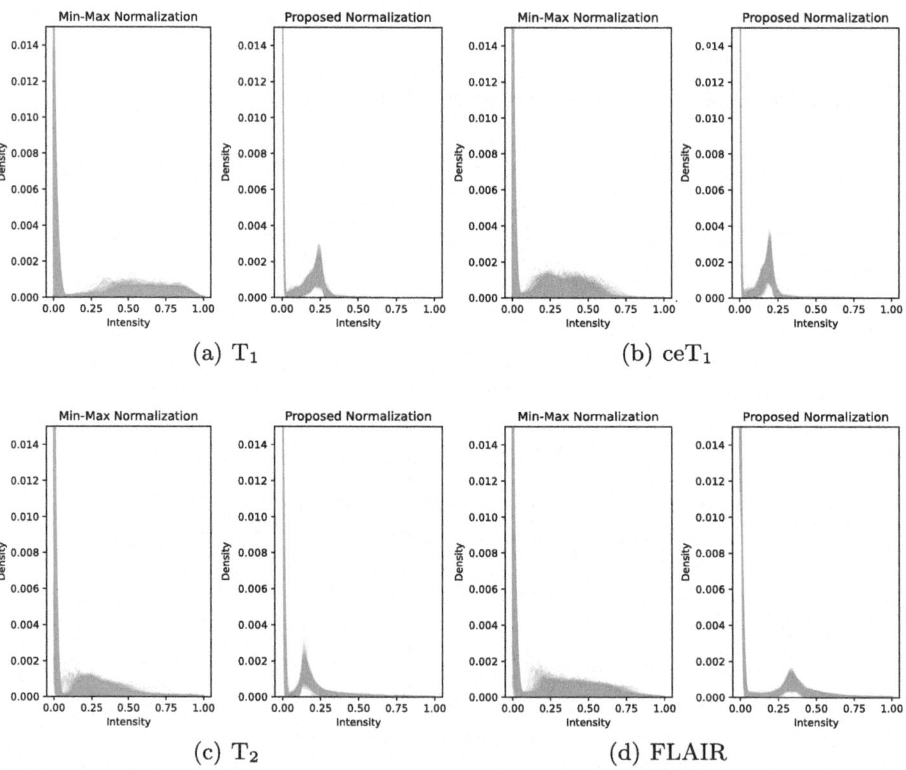

Fig. 1. Intensity distribution of (a) T_2; (b) ceT_1; (c) FLAIR images using either min-max normalization and the proposed harmonization technique.

3.3 Harmonized Cross-Modal Image Synthesis

The BraSyn dataset was acquired at different centers with varying imaging protocols (e.g., different scanners and acquisition parameters). Therefore, intra-sequence shifts can be observed, as shown in Fig. 1. This leads to an intrinsic one-to-many contrast mapping between input and target images. To address this issue, we performed data harmonization on the target data.

For data harmonization, we applied contrast linear normalization. We first shifted the minimum intensity value to 0. Then, we aligned the median intensity values within white matter, estimated using SynthSeg [3], to $\frac{1}{7}$, $\frac{1}{5}$ and $\frac{1}{3}$ for T_2, $ceT_1$and FLAIR respectively, As shown in Fig. 1, this method aligns well the intensity distribution when median values are obtained from the 3D volumes. Following prior work [5], this harmonization is applied only to the ground truth target images during training, not to the 2D input slices. Consequently, the model learns to (i) harmonize input slices when present, and (ii) synthesize harmonized versions when they are missing.

3.4 Network Implementation Details

The implementation leverages the publicly available code of MMHVAE available at https://github.com/ReubenDo/MMHVAE. We only modified the number of levels from 7 to 6 to accommodate the different image size of $(192, 224)$.

Network Architecture: The MMHVAE is based on a 2D U-Net architecture. The spatial resolution and feature dimension of the coarsest latent variable (z_L) were chosen as 1×1 and 256, respectively. The spatial and feature dimensions were successively doubled and halved after each level, resulting in a feature representation of dimension 8 for each pixel at group 1, denoted as $z_1 \in \mathbb{R}^{192 \times 224 \times 8}$. A total of $L = 6$ latent variable levels were used. The MMHVAE network architecture uses residual cells from MobileNetV2 [24] for the encoder and decoder, with Squeeze and Excitation [10] and Swish activation. The image decoders $(\mu_{\theta_j^x})_{j=1}^M$ correspond to 5 ResNet blocks. At inference, we lower the temperature of the parametric distributions to 0.5, as performed in other HVAEs [27].

Training Parameters: We used the same optimization hyperparameters as in the original MMHVAE framework. The model is trained for 1000 epochs with a batch size of $B = 16$. At each training iteration, $T = 1$ indicator vectors $\boldsymbol{r'}$ are drawn. The KL divergence is set to $\lambda_{KL} = 0.001$. The weight of the GAN loss is set to $\lambda_{\text{GAN}} = 0$ for the 800 first epochs and then to $\lambda_{\text{GAN}} = 0.025$ for the last 200 epochs. Models were trained on a H100 40GB GPU during 35 hours.

4 Experiments on the BraSyn 2025 Dataset

Dataset. We conducted experiments using the BraSyn 2025 dataset, which includes subjects with glioma [1,2,20] (N = 1,251 for training, N = 219 for validation) and brain metastasis [21] ($N = 238$ for training, $N = 31$ for validation). Each training subject is provided with four MR sequences (T1, T2, FLAIR, and T1ce) and corresponding tumor segmentation masks. The validation set contains the same four sequences but no segmentation masks. To enable quantitative evaluation on different brain regions and downstream tumor segmentation tasks, we generated bronze-standard segmentation masks for glioma subjects using the FeTS model. As a result, all reported metrics exclude metastasis subjects.

Data Processing. All images have a size of $240 \times 240 \times 155$ and have undergone skull-stripping and registration. The input data was normalized to the intensity range of $[-1, 1]$ using linear scaling, cropped to 192×224-sized axial slices were used as input, but those slices with no brain pixels were excluded from the training set to ensure the quality of the training data. At inference, the same processing is employed and reversed.

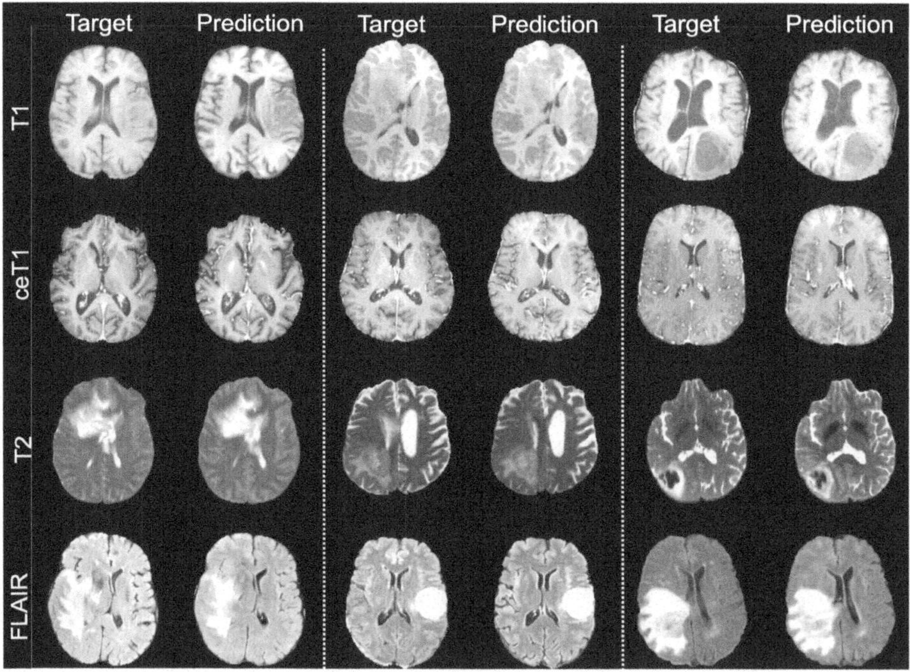

Fig. 2. Qualitative comparison of our method for synthesizing missing sequences: (a) T1-non-contrast (T_1); (b) T1-contrast-enhanced (ceT_1); (c) T2-weighted (T_2); and (d) T2-FLAIR (FLAIR), each synthesized from the remaining available sequences.

Evaluation. For each validation case, one MRI sequence was randomly selected as missing following the masking protocol provided by the challenge organizers[1].

[1] https://github.com/hongweilibran/BraSyn/blob/main/dropout_modality.py.

Table 1. Structural Similarity Index Measure (SSIM) scores for each modality, reported separately for tumor and non-tumor regions and Dice score for each subregion of the tumor. Means and standard deviations are reported.

Sequence	SSIM (%) ↑		Dice score (%) ↑		
	Tumor	Non-Tumor	Whole Tumor	Core Tumor	Enhanced Tumor
T_1	99.7 (0.0)	95.7 (2.1)	98.1 (1.6)	88.1 (20.0)	84.5 (24.9)
ceT_1	99.6 (0.2)	93.6 (2.8)	89.4 (19.0)	30.3 (27.1)	19.3 (22.2)
T_2	99.7 (0.0)	94.4 (3.2)	95.3 (6.4)	89.6 (22.2)	94.9 (12.4)
FLAIR	99.7 (0.1)	92.9 (2.5)	84.4 (21.5)	87.2 (26.1)	88.5 (23.9)
Average	99.7 (0.3)	94.1 (1.9)	91.4 (16.0)	71.1 (35.9)	68.7 (38.7)

Table 2. Segmentation and similarity results for different groups. Dice scores and Normalized Surface Dice (NSD) are reported for enhancing tumor (ET), tumor core (TC), and whole tumor (WT). Structural Similarity Index Measure (SSIM) is also reported. Means and standard deviations are shown.

	Dice score (%) ↑			NSD (0.5) (%) ↑			SSIM (%) ↑
	ET	TC	WT	ET	TC	WT	
Glioma	70.2 (33.1)	77.6 (29.4)	91.0 (9.7)	50.9 (30.6)	44.9 (30.3)	47.6 (19.2)	93.8 (5.0)
Meningioma	71.0 (39.3)	72.2 (38.0)	78.8 (32.1)	56.1 (34.7)	56.1 (35.0)	53.4 (28.0)	94.1 (1.5)
All	69.3 (35.5)	74.8 (33.0)	85.7 (22.2)	51.6 (31.9)	47.9 (32.1)	48.2 (22.9)	93.8 (4.1)

The missing sequence was then synthesized from the remaining three sequences, and the Structural Similarity Index Measure (SSIM) was computed between the synthesized and corresponding ground truth images. To evaluate the utility of the synthetic images for a downstream task, we performed brain tumor segmentation using the FeTS model, taking the synthesized MRIs as input. Segmentation outputs were compared to the bronze-standard reference labels using Dice scores computed over three tumor subregions: whole tumor, enhancing tumor, and tumor core.

Validation Results. Table 1 and Fig. 2 present the quantitative and qualitative results on the synthesis of missing MR sequences. Table 1 shows that MMH-VAE achieves near-perfect SSIM scores ($\geq$ 99.6%) in tumor regions across all sequences, indicating high similarity between the synthesized and ground truth images. Non-tumor SSIM values are slightly lower (averaging 94.1%), likely due to sequence-specific information of brain tissues and possible differences in image contrast across centers. Overall, the synthesized images shown in Fig. 2 are highly realistic. Dice scores for the downstream segmentation task are highest for synthesized T_2 and FLAIR sequences, with whole tumor Dice scores reaching 95.3% and 84.4%, respectively. The enhanced tumor Dice scores vary more significantly, with synthesized ceT1 yielding the lowest score (19.3%), suggesting that synthesizing this sequence is particularly challenging due to its high dependence on contrast agent dynamics and subtle enhancements that may be hard to infer from the other sequences.

Test Results. Table 2 reports the segmentation and synthesis performance across the glioma, meningioma, and combined test sets. For the glioma test set, automatic segmentations were generated by an ensemble of state-of-the-art algorithms from the BraTS-GLI 2023 challenges, while for the meningioma test set, an ensemble of the winning solutions from BraTS-Meningioma was employed. The evaluation was conducted on three tumor subregions: whole tumor (WT), tumor core (TC), and enhancing tumor (ET). The tumor core encompasses the enhancing, non-enhancing, and necrotic components that are typically resected during surgery, whereas the whole tumor includes both the tumor core and the surrounding edema or invasion. Segmentation quality was assessed using the Dice score and Normalized Surface Dice (NSD), while the Structural Similarity Index Measure (SSIM) was used to evaluate the quality of the synthetic images.

5 Conclusion

We demonstrated that MMHVAE, a mixture-based hierarchical VAE framework, effectively synthesizes missing brain MRI sequences with high structural fidelity and supports downstream segmentation tasks. Its ability to handle incomplete data and modality-specific challenges without hyperparameter finetuning showcases its robustness and versatility. These findings position MMHVAE as a strong candidate for integration into imaging pipelines where full multi-modal MRI acquisition is not feasible. Future work will focus on further improving synthesis quality, particularly for contrast-enhanced sequences.

Acknowledgents. R.D. received a Marie Skłodowska-Curie grant No 101154248 (project: SafeREG). This work was performed using HPC resources from GENCIIDRIS (Grant 2024-SafeREG, 2025-SafeREG).

References

1. Baid, U., et al.: THE RSNA-ASNR-MICCAI brats 2021 benchmark on brain tumor segmentation and radiogenomic classification. arXiv preprint arXiv:2107.02314 (2021)
2. Bakas, S., et al.: Advancing the cancer genome atlas glioma MRI collections with expert segmentation labels and radiomic features. Scientific Data **4**(1), 1–13 (2017)
3. Billot, B.: Synthseg: Segmentation of brain MRI scans of any contrast and resolution without retraining. Med. Image Anal. **86**, 102789 (2023)
4. Dalmaz, O., Yurt, M., Çukur, T.: Resvit: Residual vision transformers for multimodal medical image synthesis. IEEE Trans. Med. Imaging **41**(10), 2598–2614 (2022)
5. Dorent, R., et al.: Unified cross-modal medical image synthesis with hierarchical mixture of product-of-experts. IEEE Trans. Pattern Anal. Mach. Intell. (2024)

6. Dorent, R., et al.: Unified brain mr-ultrasound synthesis using multi-modal hierarchical representations. In: MICCAI 2023, pp. 448–458 (2023)
7. Dorent, R., Joutard, S., Modat, M., Ourselin, S., Vercauteren, T.: Hetero-Modal variational encoder-decoder for joint modality completion and segmentation. In: Shen, D., et al. (eds.) MICCAI 2019. LNCS, vol. 11765, pp. 74–82. Springer, Cham (2019). https://doi.org/10.1007/978-3-030-32245-8_9
8. Dorent, R., et al.: Crossmoda 2021 challenge: benchmark of cross-modality domain adaptation techniques for vestibular schwannoma and cochlea segmentation. Med. Image Anal. **83** (2023)
9. Dorent, R., et al.: Patient-specific real-time segmentation in trackerless brain ultrasound. In: MICCAI 2024, pp. 477–487. Springer (2024)
10. Hu, J., Shen, L., Sun, G.: Squeeze-and-excitation networks. In: CVPR (2018)
11. Jiang, L., Mao, Y., Wang, X., Chen, X., Li, C.: Cola-diff: Conditional latent diffusion model for multi-modal MRI synthesis. In: MICCAI 2023, pp. 398–408. Springer (2023)
12. Juvekar, P., et al.: ReMIND: The Brain Resection Multimodal Imaging Database. medRxiv (2023)
13. Kingma, D.P., Welling, M.: Auto-encoding variational Bayes. In: ICLR (2014)
14. Lee, D., Kim, J., Moon, W.J., Ye, J.C.: CollaGAN: Collaborative GAN for missing image data imputation. In: CVPR, pp. 2487–2496 (2019)
15. Li, H., et al.: DiamondGAN: unified multi-modal generative adversarial networks for MRI sequences synthesis. In: Shen, D., et al. (eds.) MICCAI 2019. LNCS, vol. 11767, pp. 795–803. Springer, Cham (2019). https://doi.org/10.1007/978-3-030-32251-9_87
16. Li, H.B., et al.: The brain tumor segmentation (brats) challenge 2023: Brain MR image synthesis for tumor segmentation (brasyn). ArXiv pp. arXiv–2305 (2024)
17. Maaløe, L., Fraccaro, M., Liévin, V., Winther, O.: BIVA: A Very Deep Hierarchy of Latent Variables for Generative Modeling. NeurIPS (2019)
18. Meng, X., et al.: A novel unified conditional score-based generative framework for multi-modal medical image completion. arXiv preprint arXiv:2207.03430 (2022)
19. Meng, X., Sun, K., Xu, J., He, X., Shen, D.: Multi-modal modality-masked diffusion network for brain MRI synthesis with random modality missing. IEEE Trans. Med. Imaging (2024)
20. Menze, B.H.: The multimodal brain tumor image segmentation benchmark (brats). IEEE Trans. Med. Imaging **34**(10), 1993–2024 (2014)
21. Moawad, A.W., et al.: The brain tumor segmentation-metastases (brats-mets) challenge 2023: Brain metastasis segmentation on pre-treatment MRI. ArXiv pp. arXiv–2306 (2024)
22. Morozov, D., Dorent, R., Haouchine, N.: A 3D Cross-modal Keypoint Descriptor for MR-US Matching and Registration. arXiv preprint arXiv:2507.18551 (2025)
23. Rasheed, H., et al.: Learning to match 2D keypoints across preoperative MR and intraoperative ultrasound. In: International Workshop on Advances in Simplifying Medical Ultrasound, pp. 78–87. Springer (2024)
24. Sandler, M., Howard, A., Zhu, M., Zhmoginov, A., Chen, L.C.: MobileNetV2: Inverted Residuals and Linear Bottlenecks. In: CVPR (2018)
25. Sharma, A., Hamarneh, G.: Missing MRI pulse sequence synthesis using multi-modal generative adversarial network. IEEE Trans. Med. Imaging **39**(4), 1170–1183 (2020)
26. Shi, Y., Paige, B., Torr, P., et al.: Variational mixture-of-experts autoencoders for multi-modal deep generative models. NeurIPS **32** (2019)

27. Vahdat, A., Kautz, J.: NVAE: a deep hierarchical variational autoencoder. NeurIPS **33** (2020)
28. Wu, M., Goodman, N.: Multimodal generative models for scalable weakly-supervised learning. NeurIPS **31** (2018)
29. Xiao, X., Hu, Q.V., Wang, G.: FgC2F-UDiff: Frequency-guided and coarse-to-fine unified diffusion model for multi-modality missing MRI synthesis. IEEE Trans. Comput. Imaging (2024)

No More Slice Wars: Towards Harmonized Brain MRI Synthesis for the BraSyn Challenge

Omar Carpentiero, Kevin Marchesini, Costantino Grana, and Federico Bolelli(✉)

University of Modena and Reggio Emilia, Modena, Italy
{omar.carpentiero,kevin.marchesini,costantino.grana, federico.bolelli}@unimore.it

Abstract. The synthesis of missing MRI modalities has emerged as a critical solution to address incomplete multi-parametric imaging in brain tumor diagnosis and treatment planning. While recent advances in generative models, especially GANs and diffusion-based approaches, have demonstrated promising results in cross-modality MRI generation, challenges remain in preserving anatomical fidelity and minimizing synthesis artifacts. In this work, we build upon the Hybrid Fusion GAN (HF-GAN) framework, introducing several enhancements aimed at improving synthesis quality and generalization across tumor types. Specifically, we incorporate z-score normalization, optimize network components for faster and more stable training, and extend the pipeline to support multi-view generation across various brain tumor categories, including gliomas, metastases, and meningiomas. Our approach focuses on refining 2D slice-based generation to ensure intra-slice coherence and reduce intensity inconsistencies, ultimately supporting more accurate and robust tumor segmentation in scenarios with missing imaging modalities. Our source code is available at https://github.com/AImageLab-zip/BraSyn25.

Keywords: Image Synthesis · MRI · Multimodal · BraTS · Brain Tumor Imaging · GANs · Medical Imaging

1 Introduction

In recent years, deep learning has significantly advanced medical image analysis, particularly for tasks such as segmentation and classification across various imaging modalities [8,10,20,23,39,41]. Moreover, generative models have also emerged as a powerful technique to produce fully synthetic datasets or expand existing ones, thereby increasing data variability, mitigating class imbalance, and supporting the development of more robust and generalizable deep learning models [11,17,24,33,38]. In this context, while certain applications involve

O. Carpentiero and K. Marchesini—Equal contribution. Authors are allowed to list their name first on their CVs.

S. Bakas et al. (Eds.): MICCAI 2025, LNCS 16377, pp. 15–28, 2026.
https://doi.org/10.1007/978-3-032-16370-7_2

distinct anatomical structures that can be accurately analyzed using a single image modality [7,29], many clinical scenarios require multi-modal imaging to effectively capture complex anatomical and pathological variations, lesion heterogeneity, and enhance tissue contrast [37]. Among the latter, the diagnosis and monitoring of brain tumors rely on multi-parametric Magnetic Resonance Imaging (MRI), considered the standard due to its superior capability in delineating tumor boundaries, quantifying tumor volumes, and guiding therapeutic decisions [4,7]. Specifically, clinical practice typically employs four complementary MRI sequences: T1-weighted images (T1), T1-weighted images with contrast enhancement (T1c), T2-weighted images (T2), and Fluid-Attenuated Inversion Recovery (FLAIR). Each modality highlights distinct tumor sub-regions, facilitating comprehensive analysis. However, acquiring all four MRI modalities is not always feasible in clinical practice due to constraints such as differing acquisition protocols, scanner limitations, or patient-specific issues like allergies to contrast agents (in the case of T1c modality). This absence of modalities, which can compromise the accuracy of diagnostic tasks, in particular tumor segmentation, has motivated extensive research into synthesizing missing MRI modalities from available ones. Recently, generative approaches spanning from Generative Adversarial Networks (GANs) to diffusion models, have been proposed to preserve the informative characteristics of each modality [22].

GAN-based Modality Synthesis. GANs have been widely used for cross-modality MRI translation, yielding promising results in producing realistic missing scans. Early works focused on paired image-to-image translation, adapting state-of-the-art general frameworks, such as Pix2Pix [6,14,40,45], to the MRI domain. Several other works demonstrated that GANs can produce anatomically plausible MRI sequences, if integrated with specific losses, such as a cycle-consistency loss [12,28], an edge-aware loss [45], a frequency loss [6], or masked versions of common losses to penalize more the errors in tumor regions [6]. Authors proved that synthetic modalities produced by GAN methods retain critical tumor information, leading to improved segmentation performance [34,42].

Diffusion Models. Diffusion models have recently emerged as a strong alternative to GANs for cross-modality MRI synthesis, offering higher fidelity via explicit likelihood modeling and gradual denoising [35]. Approaches include latent-space diffusion [21,46], which conditions on compressed representations to save memory, and modality-masked diffusion, like M2DN [30], which treats missing channels as noise for inpainting. The second and third place teams in the BraSyn 2024 challenge [16,18] used wavelet-domain diffusion, showing that denoising in wavelet space improves full-volume reconstruction and reduces 3D artifacts.

Hybrid and Multi-stage Methods. Recent work explored hybrid architectures and cascades to improve synthesis quality [19,22,35,36]. Hybrid Fusion GAN (HF-GAN) [22], the basis of our model, uses a hybrid generator with attention-based fusion to integrate modality-specific features, which are then mapped to the target sequence via a modality infuser. The BraSyn 2024 winner [22] extended HF-GAN with an intensity encoder for global context and a 3D Refiner to reduce artifacts and improve tumor segmentation.

In this work, we refine the HF-GAN framework by adding z-score normalization, optimizing network components, and adapting the training pipeline for multiview generation of tumors such as gliomas, metastases, and meningiomas. We focus on improving 2D generation to produce coherent slices and reduce intra-slice artifacts like intensity discrepancies.

2 Method

2.1 Preliminaries

We adopted HF-GAN [22] as our baseline model, using a lighter 2D pipeline to improve training and inference performance. The framework consists of a generator that synthesizes 2D brain slices from preprocessed 3D volumes and a discriminator for GAN-style adversarial learning. To enable the synthesis using a unified network independently from the missing modality scenario, the generator is composed of 4 modality-specific late-fusion encoders (one for each modality), an early fusion encoder that takes as input all the available modalities, a channel attention feature fusion module, a modality infuser, and a decoder. The encoder-decoder architecture is based on a U-Net structure.

The late fusion encoders, composed of residual convolutional blocks, with SiLU activation [15] and group normalization [44], are used for modality-specific feature extraction. The early-fusion encoder, architecturally identical to the specific encoders, accepts a stacked 4-channel image to extract complementary information from all the modalities, masking the missing ones.

Then, a feature fusion module integrates global and modality-specific information, with channel attention using global average pooling and softmax. A modality-infuser, made of Transformer blocks [43], infuses information about the missing modality into the hidden space. The decoder expands the feature maps using upsampling blocks characterized by a nearest neighbor interpolation layer followed by a 3×3 2D-convolution layer to smooth the image.

As for the standard U-Net architecture, the model incorporates skip connections between corresponding layers of the encoder and decoder to preserve spatial information and facilitate gradient flow.

2.2 Dataset and Preprocessing

Data. The Brain Tumor Segmentation (BraTS) challenge series has been organized annually since 2012, providing standardized multimodal MRI datasets and benchmarks that have driven progress in AI-based brain tumor analysis [3,27,31]. The BraSyn-2025 dataset is based on datasets containing different tumor cases, i.e., the BraTS-GLI 2023 (Glioma, GLI), BraTS-METS 2023 (Metastasis, MET) [32], and BraTS-MEN (Meningioma, MEN) [26]. The resulting dataset contains a retrospective collection of brain tumor mpMRI (multiparametric MRI) scans acquired from multiple institutions under standard clinical conditions but with different equipment and imaging protocols, resulting in a

Table 1. MRI intensity values of the training set before and after applying the 99.5th percentile clipping and normalization strategies.

Value	Clipp.	Norm.	T1c	T1n	T2f	T2w
Max.	✗	✗	2,120,538	155,724	612,368	4,563,634
Max.	✓	✗	8,664	7,315	8,842	8,233
Avg.	✓	✗	1,066.34	781.22	510.99	673.44
Std.	✓	✗	1,301.70	944.34	769.42	804.39
Min.	✓	✓	-0.8192	-0.8273	-0.6641	-0.8372
Max.	✓	✓	5.8367	6.9189	10.8277	9.3979

vastly heterogeneous image quality reflecting diverse clinical practice across different institutions. The training set is composed of 1,251 complete sequences from the BraTS-GLI dataset and 238 complete sequences from the BraTS-METS. All samples are annotated with a segmentation mask with 3 tumor structures: Enhancing Tumor (ET), Non-Enhancing Tumor Core (NETC), and peritumoral EDema (ED) [5]. The evaluation is always performed on an aggregation of these classes, namely Whole Tumor (WT) = ET + NETC + ED and Tumor Core (TC) = NETC + ET, as well as on the Enhancing Tumor (ET) region individually. The validation set is composed of 219 complete sequences from the BraTS-GLI dataset and 31 complete sequences from the BraTS-METS. Finally, the test set is composed of 219 complete sequences from the BraTS-GLI dataset, 59 complete sequences from the BraTS-METS, and 283 sequences from BraTS-MEN.

In contrast to previous editions, this year's challenge subtask introduces MET cases into both the training and validation sets and includes GLI, MET and MEN cases in the test set. This design aims to evaluate the models' ability to generalize across different tumor types. During the validation and test phases, ground-truth segmentation masks are not provided, and one of the four imaging modalities is randomly withheld ("modality dropout") for each subject.

Data Preprocessing. Our contribution begins by modifying the original HF-GAN data preprocessing pipeline. Since MRI intensities are unbounded and often contain extreme outliers, we first applied intensity clipping at the 99.5th percentile after setting all negative values to zero and excluding zero-valued background pixels from the calculation. This step helps mitigate the influence of outlier voxels while preserving the meaningful dynamic range of the brain tissue. The original maximum values across modalities in the training before and after the clipping are reported in Table 1.

Moreover, instead of linearly projecting the data into the $[-1, 1]$ range as done in the original work [22], we adopt *dataset-wise z-score normalization*, computing the global mean (Avg.) and standard deviation (Std.) across all training volumes from both the GLI and MET datasets. These statistics are computed after applying a 99.5th percentile intensity clipping and are reported in Table 1, along with the resulting voxel intensity ranges post-normalization.

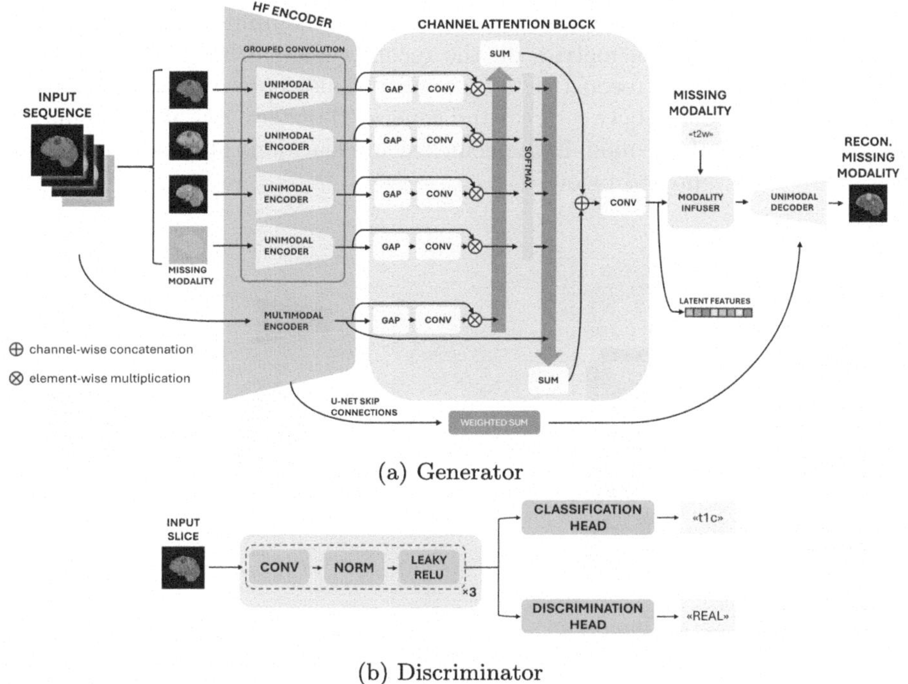

(a) Generator

(b) Discriminator

Fig. 1. Architecture of the proposed model.

To maintain compatibility with the original HF-GAN framework, we standardized background voxel values across all modalities. Specifically, all background voxels (i.e., those originally equal to zero) were reassigned a constant value of -1, which also serves as the placeholder for masked input slices.

To adapt our 2D framework to the dataset's 3D nature, we extracted axial, sagittal, and coronal slices, discarding those with fewer than 2,000 foreground pixels per modality ($< 3.47\%$ brain tissue). Sagittal and coronal slices were symmetrically padded to 240×240; padding was precomputed for training and applied on-the-fly at inference.

2.3 The Proposed Solution

As a GAN-based architecture, our framework consists of a Generator and a Discriminator, with the addition of a 2D Segmenter to guide the generation process. The generator receives three available modalities and a masked placeholder to reconstruct the missing one; this synthetic image is then combinedwith the originals to form a four-channel input for the tumor segmenter, which performs tumor segmentation. The resulting segmentation is used to compute a task-specific loss to enhance segmentation metrics on the reconstructed volumes. Following the typical GAN setup, the reconstructed modality is also passed to the Discriminator, which distinguishes between real and generated images, but also classifies the modality type to enforce modality-specific feature learning. The details regarding each module are reported below.

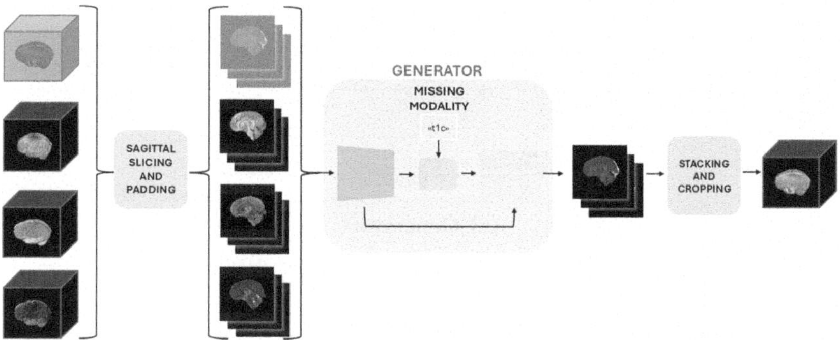

Fig. 2. Full inference pipeline. The input is split into slices, processed by the generator, then stacked to form the 3D volume. Padding and cropping are applied only to non-square sagittal slices.

Generator. Our model incorporates four modality-specific encoders and a shared fusion encoder. Each encoder consists of five downsampling stages with channel dimensions of $[64, 128, 256, 512, 640]$. Each stage includes a convolutional residual block, composed of normalization, SiLU activation, and a 3×3 convolution (stride 1, padding 1), followed by a downsampling block implemented as a 3×3 convolution with stride 2 and no padding. The fusion encoder is implemented using grouped convolutions to parallelize modality processing, replacing the previous sequential approach. Feature fusion, performed by the channel attention module is followed by a FlashAttention-compatible multi-head attention module, composed of four stages, replacing the previous custom implementation. This module is responsible for infusing modality information into the hidden space and can optionally incorporate view-specific information for multi-view generation tasks. Due to the use of z-score normalization, which preserves intensity structure while improving robustness to inter-slice variation, the intensity encoding modules were removed. The decoder mirrors the encoder with five upsampling stages, each comprising a convolutional residual block (as above) and an upsampling block using nearest-neighbor interpolation followed by a 3×3 convolution. Skip connections link each encoder stage to its corresponding decoder stage, merged by a weighted sum of the feature vectors: encoders corresponding to available modalities share the contribution equally, so that the total sum of coefficients is 1; encoders of missing modalities contribute 0, while the early-fusion encoder always contributes with full weight (1). The complete architecture of the generator is represented in Fig. 1a.

Segmenter. To guide the generation process and improve segmentation accuracy, we trained a lightweight 2D segmentation model to segment brain tumor subregions. Specifically, we adopted a nnU-Net-based architecture with four downsampling-upsampling stages and feature dimensions of [32, 64, 128, 256], employing SiLU as the activation function.

The model was trained on a subset of the training data consisting exclusively of slices containing at least 0.1% tumor tissue, thereby focusing the learning process on informative regions. To enhance generalizability, the segmenter was trained across all anatomical views (axial, coronal, and sagittal) and tumor types (GLI, MET), with the view and tumor type information incorporated into the input via one-hot encoding. This design enabled a compact yet effective model comprising only 1.79 million parameters. The resulting model achieved robust performance, with validation Dice scores of 0.74, 0.80, and 0.82 on the NETC, ED, and ET classes, respectively. The model was trained using the Focal Tversky loss [1], due to its ability to provide better performance in contexts where the different classes are highly imbalanced. The segmenter was independently trained, and then frozen during the training of the generation pipeline.

Discriminator. The discriminator, shown in Fig. 1b, is based on the PatchGAN architecture [13], which classifies local image patches rather than the whole image. It uses three downsampling layers and starts with 32 filters. Each block includes a 4×4 convolution with stride 2 (except the last, which uses stride 1), group normalization, and LeakyReLU activations. The final convolution outputs a single-channel map for real/fake classification. An auxiliary classifier branch predicts 4 class logits per image, one for each modality.

Final Generation. To correctly reconstruct a volume from 2D slices, the generator processes batches of slices, and then the outputs stacked (Fig. 2). After stacking, the image is de-normalized, and background pixels are set to zero. Padding is removed for 3D volumes generated from the sagittal view.

To enable a faster pipeline for training and evaluation, we rely on efficient GPU implementations of image processing algorithms [2,9] . The entire process, includ-ing data loading, preprocessing,and saving, requires, on average,13.4 seconds per sample on an RTX5000 16GB.

2.4 The Loss

Our model leverages a combination of different loss functions used to guide the architecture toward learning more robust and balanced representations. The overall loss function is:

Table 2. List of loss components.

Term	Role
$\mathcal{L}_{\text{recon}}$	Enforces pixel-level accuracy.
$\mathcal{L}_{\text{adv}}$	Encourages realistic outputs.
$\mathcal{L}_{\text{class}}$	Encourages modality specific features.
$\mathcal{L}_{\text{feat}}$	Promotes consistency in the latent space.
$\mathcal{L}_{\text{cycle}}$	Promotes cycle consistency.
$\mathcal{L}_{\text{SSIM}}$	Improves structural fidelity.
$\mathcal{L}_{\text{Tversky}}$	Promotes better downstream segmentation.

$$\mathcal{L}_{\text{total}} = 10\cdot\mathcal{L}_{\text{recon}} + 0.25\cdot\mathcal{L}_{\text{adv}} + 0.25\cdot\mathcal{L}_{\text{class}} + \mathcal{L}_{\text{feat}} + \mathcal{L}_{\text{cycle}} + 5\cdot\mathcal{L}_{\text{SSIM}} + 5\cdot\mathcal{L}_{\text{Tversky}}$$

Table 3. Characterization of settings employed in different experiments. Unmentioned losses are always present.

RunID	Losses					Train		View	
	$\mathcal{L}_{\text{cycle}}$	$\mathcal{L}_{\text{feat}}$	$\mathcal{L}_{\text{SSIM\_whole}}$	$\mathcal{L}_{\text{SSIM\_dual}}$	$\mathcal{L}_{\text{Tversky}}$	GLI	MET	Axial	Sagit.
R1	✓	✓	✗	✗	✗	✓	✗	✓	✗
R2	✓	✓	✗	✓	✗	✓	✗	✓	✗
R3	✓	✓	✗	✓	✗	✓	✗	✓	✗
R4	✓	✓	✓	✗	✗	✓	✗	✓	✗
R5	✗	✗	✗	✗	✗	✓	✗	✓	✗
R6	✓	✓	✗	✓	✓	✓	✗	✓	✗
R7	✓	✓	✗	✓	✓	✓	✗	✗	✓
R8A	✓	✓	✗	✓	✗	✓	✓	✓	✓
R8S	✓	✓	✗	✓	✗	✓	✓	✓	✓
R9	✓	✓	✗	✓	✓	✓	✗	✓	✓
R10	✓	✓	✗	✓	✗	✓	✓	✓	✓

Each loss targets a specific aspect of the task: a summary is reported in Table 2 and detailed in the following. The reconstruction loss $\mathcal{L}_{\text{recon}}$, based on the mean absolute error (MAE), serves as the dominant loss term, prioritizing pixel fidelity between the synthesized and ground-truth images. To enhance perceptual quality, we incorporate Structural Similarity Index (SSIM) losses $\mathcal{L}_{\text{SSIM}}$, computed as 1-SSIM on a per-pixel basis, and aggregated only over the regions of interest. We implement two variants of this loss: one that considers the entire volume, and another that produces two separate terms, one for healthy brain tissue and one for tumor tissue, which are equally weighted during training. The adversarial loss $\mathcal{L}_{\text{adv}}$ is used to encourage realism in the generated outputs and to suppress common synthesis artifacts. Cycle consistency is enforced through a two-step generation process. In the first step, the generator synthesizes a missing modality using ground truth modalities. In the second step, this previously generated output replaces the corresponding placeholder, one of the available modalities is randomly masked (selected from a uniform distribution, so each maskable modality has equal probability of being chosen), and the generator is applied again using the two remaining ground truth modalities along with the generated one. The cycle loss $\mathcal{L}_{\text{cycle}}$ is defined as the MAE between the output of the second generation and the ground truth of the corresponding modality. To further promote consistency at the representational level, a feature loss $\mathcal{L}_{\text{feat}}$ is included, defined as the cosine similarity between the hidden features of the bottleneck layer extracted during the first and second generation passes. Finally, the Tversky-focal loss [1] $\mathcal{L}_{\text{Tversky}}$ is introduced to guide the generator to produce outputs that are easier to segment, particularly in the presence of class imbalance. As in the default HF-GAN framework, forward propagation is performed twice, for cycle consistency, to generate each modality, resulting in a total of 8 forward passes on the same network (not along different paths). Gradients from these multiple forwards are aggregated by combining the corresponding losses into a single scalar and performing backpropagation once.

3 Experiments and Results

3.1 Assessment Metrics

Different algorithms are assessed using a combination of image quality and segmentation metrics. The evaluation relies on multiple quantitative metrics.

Structural Similarity Index Measure (SSIM), as an image quality metric, it is employed to measure the realism of the reconstructed volume. It is independently computed on the Whole Tumor (WT) area and on the Healthy Tissue (HT) part of the brain, resulting in two scores for each test subject.

Dice score and Normalized Surface Distance (NSD) are used to evaluate the effect of reconstructed volumes on segmentation masks and boundaries. Metrics are computed for three tumor structures: Enhancing Tumor (ET), Tumor Core (TC), and Whole Tumor (WT). Segmentation pseudo-labels for the validation set are generated using state-of-the-art algorithms from the BraTS python package [25], then compared to segmentations from sequences where one modality was masked and reconstructed.

3.2 Results

All experimental results from our analysis, on the validation set, are summarized in Table 4, where each run is identified by a unique identifier (e.g., R1, R2) and corresponds to a specific configuration of the generator's training process. The details of each configuration are provided in Table 3. All runs are trained for an equivalent number of steps, corresponding to 10 epochs on the GLI dataset, with the exception of R6 and R7. Notably, R1, R2, R4, and R6 differ from the others in how the input modalities are provided to the network, since the number of available modalities varies between 1, 2, or 3, whereas in the other runs it is fixed to 3. Runs R6 and R7 resume training from the checkpoint of R3 and are further optimized for 3 additional epochs, adding the Tversky loss. Runs R8A, R8S, and R10 share the same model, which is trained on multiple views and on the combined GLI+MET dataset, but are evaluated under three different settings: R8A generates axial views, R8S generates sagittal views, and R10 combines both views by averaging the outputs. Similarly, R9 aggregates the axial predictions from R6 and the sagittal predictions from R7. All models were evaluated on the combined GLI+MET validation set to assess their generalization capabilities across different tumor types. Table 5 reports the results on the hidden test set, provided by the challenge organizers. Additionally, Fig. 3 reports a comparison of the original and reconstructed slices sampled from all four modalities of random patients. The figure shows that although no 3D refinement was used, the slices show little to no striping artifacts, which are typical of 2D generation approaches.

Table 4. Experimental results obtained combining different losses, leveraging different training sets and 2D views. The Run IDs are explained in Table 3.

Metric	Val.Set	Class	Run ID										
			R1	**R2**	**R3**	**R4**	**R5**	**R6**	**R7**	**R8A**	**R8S**	**R9**	**R10**
SSIM	ALL	WT	99.73	**99.77**	99.76	99.74	99.71	99.76	99.75	99.76	**99.77**	99.75	99.76
		HT	93.31	94.07	94.05	93.82	93.15	**94.09**	93.91	93.79	93.89	94.07	93.79
	GLI	WT	99.72	**99.76**	**99.76**	99.74	99.70	99.75	99.74	99.75	99.75	99.74	99.75
		HT	93.69	94.47	94.44	94.22	93.52	**94.49**	94.28	94.10	94.20	94.47	94.11
	MET	WT	99.79	99.81	99.82	99.80	99.78	99.82	99.82	**99.84**	**99.84**	99.82	**99.84**
		HT	90.62	91.23	91.23	90.94	90.52	91.29	91.27	91.59	**91.73**	91.27	91.59
DICE	ALL	ET	53.62	57.13	54.16	54.16	52.43	57.02	57.70	55.98	**57.86**	57.00	56.42
		TC	73.86	76.49	75.48	75.48	73.89	76.88	75.11	75.28	**77.55**	76.88	75.28
		WT	71.74	73.63	71.89	71.89	70.41	74.07	74.97	73.57	**74.45**	74.07	73.58
	GLI	ET	52.94	56.67	53.82	53.82	51.87	56.58	57.40	55.90	**57.14**	56.58	55.90
		TC	72.28	75.27	74.24	74.24	72.55	75.59	73.55	73.88	**76.16**	75.58	73.85
		WT	69.75	71.91	70.01	70.01	68.47	72.25	**73.26**	71.79	72.50	72.25	71.79
	MET	ET	58.44	60.36	56.51	56.51	56.40	60.11	59.77	56.52	**62.92**	59.98	60.09
		TC	85.03	85.06	84.28	84.28	83.35	86.05	86.14	85.17	**87.38**	86.00	85.33
		WT	85.78	85.83	85.15	85.15	84.16	86.93	87.03	86.13	**88.26**	86.92	86.18
NSD	ALL	ET	54.06	56.48	57.66	54.38	52.55	56.96	**58.03**	56.81	57.92	56.96	56.81
		TC	63.27	66.80	68.55	65.83	63.06	67.46	65.73	65.79	**68.30**	67.48	65.79
		WT	52.80	55.54	56.51	53.02	51.32	56.11	**57.30**	55.41	56.64	56.11	55.41
	GLI	ET	52.68	55.41	56.86	53.43	51.34	55.84	**57.08**	55.51	56.40	55.85	55.51
		TC	61.11	65.04	**66.94**	64.22	61.26	65.32	63.42	63.65	66.25	65.35	63.65
		WT	49.19	52.17	53.20	49.60	47.90	52.35	**53.79**	51.78	52.88	52.36	51.78
	MET	ET	63.82	64.05	63.25	61.12	61.10	64.87	64.74	66.00	**68.64**	64.81	66.00
		TC	78.47	79.24	79.88	77.22	75.73	82.62	82.08	80.89	**82.82**	82.58	80.89
		WT	78.30	79.34	79.91	77.15	75.48	82.65	82.13	81.12	**83.23**	82.64	81.12

3.3 Discussion

All of our experiments demonstrate strong MRI synthesis performance and good generalization to unseen data. In particular, models trained exclusively on the GLI dataset still perform reasonably well when tasked with generating MET volumes, highlighting the robustness of the framework. R1, even without the SSIM loss term, achieves strong perceptual quality. Subsequent runs focus on incremental improvements. Introducing the SSIM loss on R2, split into two terms for healthy and tumor tissue, improves structural similarity metrics. In contrast, R3 applies the SSIM loss over the entire volume without differentiating between tissue types, which leads to worse performance, highlighting the importance of spatially targeted perceptual losses. The original framework supports cases with 1, 2, or 3 missing modalities. By always providing three known modalities as input, convergence is faster, but final scores showed minimal variation, as evidenced by the comparison between R2, which used variable input modalities, and R3, where three known modalities were always provided. We also experiment with removing the cycle consistency and feature losses on R5. This leads

Table 5. Quantitative results on the hidden test set for the submitted best-performing run (R8S), as provided by the challenge organizers.

Dataset		**DICE**			**NSD**			**SSIM**
		ET	TC	WT	ET	TC	WT	Whole
GLI	Mean	74.06	80.86	90.46	53.44	46.97	47.63	93.37
	Std.	31.13	27.79	12.04	29.52	29.36	20.16	5.43
MEN	Mean	72.26	73.95	78.42	56.65	56.87	53.54	93.41
	Std.	38.54	37.14	32.28	34.75	34.54	28.02	2.05
ALL	Mean	72.34	77.50	85.29	53.47	49.54	48.34	93.33
	Std.	33.97	31.87	22.83	31.17	31.28	23.43	4.49

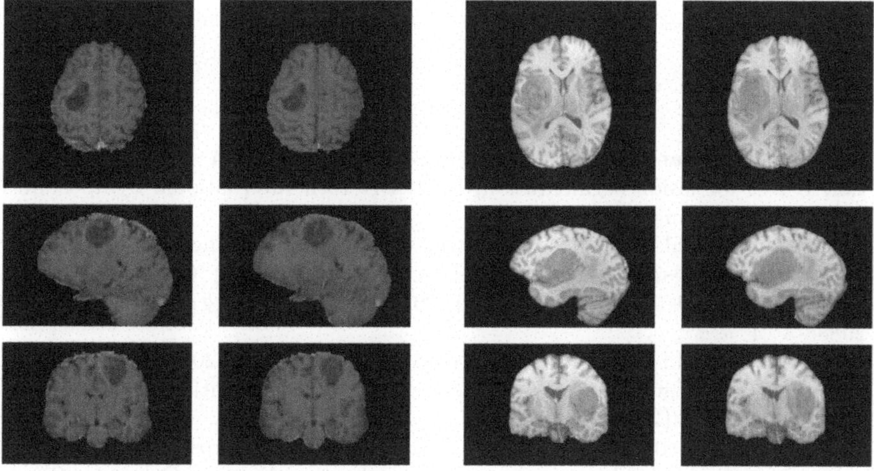

Fig. 3. Comparisons of real (left) and reconstructed (right) for two different patients sampled from the GLI validation dataset.

to performance degradation, confirming their contribution to training stability and reconstruction quality. However, the inclusion of cycle consistency roughly doubles training time and memory utilization. Incorporating the Tversky loss, intended to improve segmentation quality, did not yield significant gains. Similarly, using a simple mean of multiview predictions did not enhance performance. Our best-performing model, R8S, is trained using both axial and sagittal views and does not include the Tversky loss. It produces slices in the sagittal plane and benefits from the increased diversity of input representations.

4 Conclusion

We proposed an enhanced 2D MRI synthesis framework based on HF-GAN, introducing z-score normalization, architectural optimizations, and multi-view training to improve synthesis quality and generalization across tumor types. Our method achieves high structural fidelity and supports robust tumor segmentation, even with missing modalities. Results show strong cross-dataset performance, confirming the effectiveness of our design.

Acknowledgments. This work was supported by the University of Modena and Reggio Emilia and Fondazione di Modena through the "Fondo di Ateneo per la Ricerca - FAR 2024" (CUP E93C24002080007) and FARD-2024.

Disclosure of Interests. The authors have no conflicts of interest to declare.

References

1. Abraham, N., Khan, N.M.: A novel focal tversky loss function with improved attention U-Net for lesion segmentation. In: IEEE 16th International Symposium on Biomedical Imaging (2019)
2. Allegretti, S., et al.: How does connected components labeling with decision trees perform on GPUs? In: Vento, M., Percannella, G. (eds.) CAIP 2019. LNCS, vol. 11678, pp. 39–51. Springer, Cham (2019). https://doi.org/10.1007/978-3-030-29888-3_4
3. Baid, U., et al.: The RSNA-ASNR-MICCAI BraTS 2021 Benchmark on Brain Tumor Segmentation and Radiogenomic Classification. arXiv preprint arXiv:2107.02314 (2021)
4. Baid, U., et al. (eds.): Brain Tumor Segmentation, and Cross-Modality Domain Adaptation for Medical Image Segmentation, Lecture Notes in Computer Science, vol. 14669 (2023)
5. Bakas, S., et al.: Advancing the cancer genome atlas glioma MRI collections with expert segmentation labels and radiomic features. Scientific Data **4**(1) (2017)
6. Baltruschat, I.M., Janbakhshi, P., Lenga, M.: BraSyn 2023 challenge: missing MRI synthesis and the effect of different learning objectives. In: International Challenge on Cross-Modality Domain Adaptation for Medical Image Segmentation (2023)
7. Bolelli, F., et al.: Segmenting maxillofacial structures in CBCT volumes. In: IEEE/CVF Conference on Computer Vision and Pattern Recognition (2025)
8. Bontempo, G., Bolelli, F., Porrello, A., Calderara, S., Ficarra, E.: A graph-based multi-scale approach with knowledge distillation for WSI classification. IEEE Trans. Med. Imaging (2023)
9. Cardoso, M.J., et al.: Monai: an open-source framework for deep learning in healthcare. arXiv preprint arXiv:2211.02701 (2022)
10. Cipriano, M., et al.: Deep segmentation of the mandibular canal: a new 3D annotated dataset of CBCT volumes. IEEE Access **10** (2022)
11. Cipriano, M., Allegretti, S., Bolelli, F., Pollastri, F., Grana, C.: Improving segmentation of the inferior alveolar nerve through deep label propagation. In: IEEE/CVF Conference on Computer Vision and Pattern Recognition (2022)
12. Dar, S.U., et al.: Image synthesis in Multi-Contrast MRI with conditional generative adversarial networks. IEEE Trans. Med. Imaging **38**(10) (2019)

13. Demir, U., Unal, G.: Patch-Based Image Inpainting with Generative Adversarial Networks. arXiv preprint arXiv:1803.07422 (2018)
14. Eker, A.G., Pehlivanoğlu, M.K., Duru, N., Duendar, T.T.: BrainPixGAN: Generating intraoperative MRI images with mask-based generative networks. Eng. Sci. Technol. Int. J. **58** (2024)
15. Elfwing, S., Uchibe, E., Doya, K.: Sigmoid-weighted linear units for neural network function approximation in reinforcement learning. Neural Networks (2018)
16. Ferreira, A., et al.: Brain Tumour Removing and Missing Modality Generation Using 3D WDM. arXiv preprint arXiv:2411.04630 (2024)
17. Frid-Adar, M., et al.: GAN-based synthetic medical image augmentation for increased CNN performance in liver lesion classification. Neurocomputing (2018)
18. Friedrich, P., Durrer, A., Wolleb, J., Cattin, P.C.: cWDM: Conditional Wavelet Diffusion Models for Cross-Modality 3D Medical Image Synthesis. arXiv preprint arXiv:2411.17203 (2024)
19. Hamghalam, M., Lei, B., Wang, T.: High Tissue Contrast MRI Synthesis Using Multi-Stage Attention-GAN for Segmentation. In: Proceedings of the AAAI Conference on Artificial Intelligence, vol. 34 (2020)
20. Huang, S.C., et al.: Self-supervised learning for medical image classification: a systematic review and implementation guidelines. NPJ Digital Med. **6**(1) (2023)
21. Jiang, L., Mao, Y., Wang, X., Chen, X., Li, C.: CoLa-Diff: conditional latent diffusion model for multi-modal MRI synthesis. In: International Conference on Medical Image Computing and Computer-Assisted Intervention (2023)
22. Jihoon, C., Jonghye, W., Jinah, P.: A unified framework for synthesizing multisequence brain MRI via hybrid fusion. Med. Image Anal. (2024)
23. Karargyris, A., et al.: Federated benchmarking of medical artificial intelligence with MedPerf. Nat. Mach. Intell. **5**(7) (2023)
24. Kazeminia, S., et al.: GANs for medical image analysis. AIME **109** (2020)
25. Kofler, F., et al.: BraTS orchestrator : democratizing and disseminating state-of-the-art brain tumor image analysis. arXiv preprint arXiv:2506.13807 (2025)
26. LaBella, D., et al.: The ASNR-MICCAI Brain Tumor Segmentation (BraTS) Challenge 2023: Intracranial Meningioma. arXiv preprint arXiv:2305.07642 (2023)
27. Li, H.B., et al.: The Brain Tumor Segmentation (BraTS) Challenge 2023: Brain MR Image Synthesis for Tumor Segmentation (BraSyn). ArXiv (2024)
28. Li, H., et al.: DiamondGAN: unified multi-modal generative adversarial networks for MRI sequences synthesis. In: Shen, D., et al. (eds.) MICCAI 2019. LNCS, vol. 11767, pp. 795–803. Springer, Cham (2019). https://doi.org/10.1007/978-3-030-32251-9_87
29. Lumetti, L., et al.: U-Net Transplant: the role of pre-training for model merging in 3D medical segmentation. In: 28th International Conference on Medical Image Computing and Computer Assisted Intervention (2025)
30. Meng, X., Sun, K., Xu, J., He, X., Shen, D.: Multi-modal modality-masked diffusion network for brain MRI synthesis with random modality missing. IEEE Trans. Med. Imaging **43**(7) (2024)
31. Menze, B.H., Jakab, A., et al.: The multimodal brain tumor image segmentation benchmark (BRATS). IEEE Trans. Med. Imaging **34**(10) (2014)
32. Moawad, A.W., et al.: The Brain Tumor Segmentation - Metastases (BraTS-METS) Challenge 2023: Brain Metastasis Segmentation on Pre-treatment MRI. ArXiv (2024)
33. Morelli, N., et al.: Enhancing testicular ultrasound image classification through synthetic data and pretraining strategies. In: Image Analysis and Processing – ICIAP 2025 (2025)

34. Osuala, R., et al.: Pre- to post-contrast breast mri synthesis for enhanced tumour segmentation. In: Medical Imaging 2024: Image Processing, vol. 12926 (2024)
35. Özbey, M., et al.: Unsupervised medical image translation with adversarial diffusion models. IEEE Trans. Med. Imaging **42**(12) (2023)
36. Pan, S., Eidex, Z., Safari, M., Qiu, R., Yang, X.: Cycle-guided denoising diffusion probability model for 3D Cross-modality MRI synthesis. In: Medical Imaging 2025: Clinical and Biomedical Imaging, vol. 13410 (2025)
37. Pipoli, V., et al.: IM-Fuse: A mamba-based fusion block for brain tumor segmentation with incomplete modalities. In: 28th International Conference on Medical Image Computing and Computer Assisted Intervention (2025)
38. Pollastri, F., et al.: Improving skin lesion segmentation with generative adversarial networks. In: IEEE 31st International Symposium on Computer-Based Medical Systems (2018)
39. Pollastri, F., et al.: Confidence calibration for deep renal biopsy immunofluorescence image classification. In: 2020 25th International Conference on Pattern Recognition (2021)
40. Preetha, C.J., et al.: Deep-learning-based synthesis of post-contrast T1-weighted MRI for tumour response assessment in neuro-oncology: a multicentre, retrospective cohort study. Lancet Digital Health **3**(12) (2021)
41. Sistaninejhad, B., Rasi, H., Nayeri, P.: A review paper about deep learning for medical image analysis. Comput. Math. Methods Med. **2023**(1) (2023)
42. Thomas, M.F., et al.: Improving automated glioma segmentation in routine clinical use through artificial intelligence-based replacement of missing sequences with synthetic magnetic resonance imaging scans. Invest. Radiol. **57**(3) (2022)
43. Vaswani, A., et al.: Attention is all you need. Adv. Neural Inf. Process. Syst. **30** (2017)
44. Wu, Y., He, K.: Group Normalization. Int. J. Comput. Vis. (2020)
45. Yu, B., et al.: Ea-GANs: Edge-Aware generative adversarial networks for cross-modality MR image synthesis. IEEE Trans. Med. Imaging **38**(7) (2019)
46. Zhu, L., et al.: Make-a-volume: leveraging latent diffusion models for cross-modality 3D brain MRI synthesis. In: International Conference on Medical Image Computing and Computer-Assisted Intervention (2023)

Latent-Space Ensemble Synthesis of Missing Brain Tumor MRI Modalities for BraTS Challenge

Agustin Cartaya Lathulerie(✉), Valeriia Abramova, Micaela Rivas Díaz, Uma M. Lal-Trehan Estrada, Cansu Yalcin, Rachika E. Hamadache, Clara Lisazo, Adriá Casamitjana, Arnau Oliver, and Xavier Lladó

Computer Vision and Robotics Research Group, University of Girona, Girona, Spain
agustin.cartaya@udg.edu

Abstract. Missing MRI modalities is a frequent challenge in clinical brain tumor imaging, limiting the effectiveness of multimodal segmentation models. In this work, we propose an ensemble framework for synthesizing missing MRI modalities from the available ones. It combines a Modality Translation Encoder-Decoder and a Modality Translation Brownian Bridge Diffusion Model, both operating in a compact latent space generated by a pretrained Volumetric Compression Network. This design enables whole-volume 3D synthesis with moderate computational demands and improved anatomical coherence. Each model is trained and validated on the BraSyn 2025 dataset, and their outputs are fused to increase robustness against structural and contrast variability. Evaluation on the validation set shows that the synthetic images produced by our ensemble closely resemble the original missing modalities and, when combined with the available ones, support effective tumor segmentation, demonstrating the method's effectiveness for clinical data completion.

Keywords: Brain tumor · MRI · Synthesis · Ensemble · Autoencoder

1 Introduction

Central nervous system tumors, particularly those in the brain, pose a significant and growing global health challenge, with currently over 320,000 new cases worldwide each year and a projected increase of nearly 50% by 2045 due to population aging and growth [1–3]. These tumors are difficult to manage due to their high mortality and the complexity of diagnosis and treatment. Accurate brain tumor segmentation in magnetic resonance imaging (MRI) is essential for guiding diagnosis and therapy [4], however manual segmentation is labor-intensive, time-consuming, and prone to inter-expert variability.

Deep learning has recently enabled fast and accurate brain tumor segmentation [5]. However, these models typically rely on multiple MRI modalities such as T1-weighted (T1w), T1-weighted with contrast (T1ce), T2-weighted (T2w), and

S. Bakas et al. (Eds.): MICCAI 2025, LNCS 16377, pp. 29–41, 2026.
https://doi.org/10.1007/978-3-032-16370-7_3

FLAIR, for high precision, but one or more are often missing in clinical practice due to time and cost constraints or motion artifacts [6]. To address this, synthesizing missing modalities may become a key strategy for robust segmentation in incomplete datasets. In this context, the BraTS 2025 Challenge re-introduced Task 8, the Brain MR Image Synthesis (BraSyn) Challenge [12], which focuses on generating missing MRI volumes from available ones.

Common approaches to solve the missing modality problem include Generative Adversarial Networks (GANs), Variational Autoencoders (VAEs), and Diffusion Models (DMs) [6–10], which are designed to reconstruct anatomically plausible images. Although many have shown promising results, most operate on 2D slices or small 3D patches, limiting anatomical coherence and inter-slice consistency [6–8]. Additionally, adversarial training, used in GANs, is often unstable and highly sensitive to hyperparameter settings, making it difficult to generate consistent and realistic outputs [11].

To address these challenges, we propose an ensemble method that synthesizes missing MRI modalities by combining two generative models: a Modality Translation Encoder-Decoder (MT-ED) and a Modality Translation Brownian Bridge Diffusion Model (MT-BBDM). This ensemble seeks to enhance robustness against contrast variability and structural inconsistencies often seen in single-model synthesis. To enable volumetric training without excessive memory use, and to avoid slice- or patch-based artifacts, we compress 3D images into a compact latent space. This is done using a pretrained Volumetric Compression Network (VCN), based on a Variational Autoencoder, which reduces spatial resolution while preserving anatomical structure. Figure 1, provides an overview of the entire pipeline. We evaluate both individual models and the ensemble on the BraTS Syn Task 8 validation set, using the task's official metrics [12].

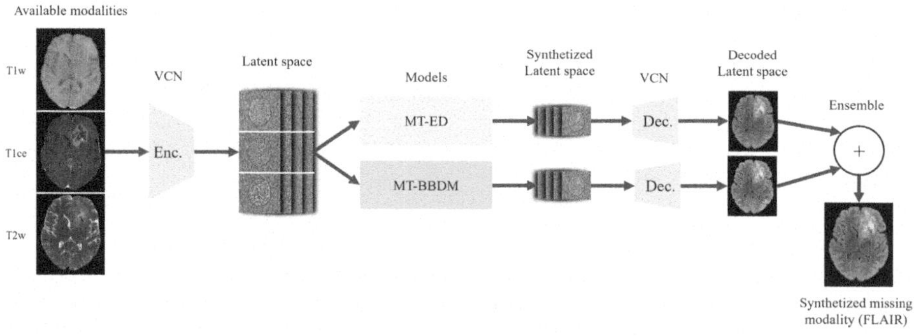

Fig. 1. Global overview of the complete pipeline when FLAIR modality is missing.

2 Materials and Methods

2.1 Dataset and Preprocessing

This work uses the BraSyn 2025 dataset [12–18], containing multimodal MRI scans of 2,300 subjects with glioma, metastases, and meningioma tumors. The training set includes 1,251 glioma and 238 metastasis cases; validation has 219 glioma and 31 metastasis; and the test set contains 219 glioma, 59 metastasis, and 283 meningioma cases. Each patient has four MRI sequences (T1w, T1ce, T2w, FLAIR). All modalities are available in training and validation, while one is randomly missing per subject in testing. Tumor segmentation masks are provided only for training.

The BraSyn 2025 dataset provided scans that were preprocessed as described in [12], including registration to a common space, resampling to 1 mm^3, and skull-stripping, yielding volumes of $240 \times 240 \times 155$ voxels. Subsequently, to enable whole-volume synthesis without using slice- or patch-based methods, we further preprocessed each volume by normalizing it to the range $[0, 1]$, zero-padded to $256 \times 256 \times 160$, and encoded into a compact latent space using a VCN. This latent space contains $K = 4$ latent channels with spatial dimensions of $64 \times 64 \times 40$ (i.e., $4 \times 64 \times 64 \times 40$).

2.2 Background

Brownian Bridge Diffusion Models. DMs have emerged as powerful tools for image generation, surpassing GANs in stability and output quality [19]. While they provide fine control over sample fidelity and diversity, their adaptation to image-to-image translation is nontrivial, as classical DMs are not explicitly conditioned on input images. In the standard setup, noise is gradually added to a clean image x_0 over T time steps, producing a sequence $x_1, x_2, \ldots, x_T$, where x_T is nearly pure Gaussian noise. Then a model is trained to help reverse this process step-by-step to recover x_0 from x_T. This generative process is detailed in [20].

To enable conditioning on known images, Brownian Bridge Diffusion Models (BBDM) reformulate the process as a Brownian bridge between two endpoints: input x_0 (e.g., missing modality) and target $x_T = y$ (e.g., available modality). As detailed in [21], the forward process is defined as:

$$q_{BB}(x_t \mid x_0, y) = \mathcal{N}\big(x_t; (1 - m_t)x_0 + m_t y, \delta_t I\big), \tag{1}$$

With $m_t = \frac{t}{T}$ and $\delta_t I$ controls noise variance. Then, during inference, the model reverses this process, conditioned on y:

$$p_\theta(x_{t-1} \mid x_t, y) = \mathcal{N}\big(x_{t-1}; \mu_\theta(x_t, t), \tilde{\delta}_t I\big), \tag{2}$$

Here, $\mu_\theta(x_t, t)$ is the mean of the noise predicted by a neural network, and $\tilde{\delta}_t$ denotes the reverse-step variance. During training, the model is also optimized to guide the reconstruction of x_0 from y, step-by-step, but unlike the standard setup, conditioning on y at each step.

Variational Autoencoders. The high dimensionality of medical imaging data, along with the large number of parameters in deep learning models, makes training computationally expensive. VAEs are often used to generate compressed full-volume latent representations that preserve anatomical coherence and support accurate reconstruction. These allow more efficient model training, reducing computational cost and enabling scalable 3D processing [22,23]. To address this, pretrained VAE foundation models trained on large multicenter cohorts [24] have emerged as more stable and generalizable solutions, significantly improving compression and reconstruction quality.

Proposal. Building on the BBDM and VAE frameworks, we implement an ensemble method for missing modality synthesis that integrates two generative models, an MT-ED and an MT-BBDM. Both models operate in the compressed latent space of the original 3D volumes and use the same U-Net architecture adapted to this space. They mainly differ in their output representations and training objectives, with the MT-ED producing direct reconstructions and the MT-BBDM learning denoising transitions. The latent space is obtained using the pretrained VCN proposed in [24], a 3D variational autoencoder trained with a combination of voxel-wise reconstruction loss, perceptual loss, adversarial loss, and KL regularization. This training was performed on a large dataset of CT and MRI volumes from different body regions, including skull-stripped brains, yielding a compact latent space and robust reconstructions. Due to computational constraints, we did not fine-tune the VCN on the BraSyn 2025 dataset and instead relied on the pretrained weights from the original work, which have been shown to generalize well to out-of-distribution datasets, including BraTS18. Further details about the VCN and U-Net architectures employed in our MT-ED and MT-BBDM can be found in [24].

2.3 Models

Given the latent representations of N different MRI modalities for a specific subject, denoted as $S = \{S_i\}_{i=1}^{N}$, where one modality S_m is missing and the remaining modalities $S_a = \{S_i\}_{i=1, i \neq m}^{N}$ are available, the proposed models aim to synthesize $\hat{S}_m$, an approximation of S_m given S_a.

Modality Translation Encoder-Decoder Model. This model employs an Encoder-Decoder architecture that encodes S_a, fuses them into a joint representation, and decodes it to generate $\hat{S}_m$ (see Fig. 2). The model is trained by minimizing a weighted L2 loss between $\hat{S}_m$ and S_m, computed separately for each of the four latent channels. The total loss $L_{\text{MT-ED}}$ is defined as:

$$L_{\text{MT-ED}} = \frac{1}{\sum_{k=1}^{4} w_k} \sum_{k=1}^{4} w_k \|\hat{S}_{mk} - S_{mk}\|_2^2$$

where $\hat{S}_{mk}$ and S_{mk} denote the kth latent channel of $\hat{S}_m$ and S_m, respectively. The weights w_k, set to $w_1 = 0.51$, $w_2 = 0.12$, $w_3 = 0.20$, and $w_4 = 0.16$, were determined in advance by encoding each modality with the VCN encoder, masking channel k of the latent space, decoding it with the VCN decoder, and computing the RMSE against the original image. This procedure was repeated across all modalities in the training set to obtain the mean error for channel k. The channel errors were then normalized by their sum so that the weights reflect each channel's contribution to reconstructing the original image.

Modality Translation Brownian Bridge Diffusion Model. This second model applies a Brownian diffusion process starting from S_a and iteratively denoises it to recover S_m. Since Eqs. 1 and 2 require the diffusion process's start and end to have the same dimension, the input includes S_a plus a null latent space S_0, while the output predicts $\hat{S}$, from which only $\hat{S}_m$ is extracted (see Fig. 2). The loss function is the weighted L2 norm between predicted and true noise ($\hat{n}$ and n), computed for S_m across each latent channel and for tumor and healthy regions individually. The total loss $L_{\text{MT-BBDM}}$ is defined as:

$$L_{\text{MT-BBDM},k} = \frac{\|\hat{n}_{\text{tumor},k} - n_{\text{tumor},k}\|_2 + \|\hat{n}_{\text{healthy},k} - n_{\text{healthy},k}\|_2}{2}$$

$$L_{\text{MT-BBDM}} = \sum_{k=1}^{4} w_k L_{\text{MT-BBDM},k}$$

Modality Conditioning. The original architecture of the models allows predicting any of the four modalities using a one-hot vector of dimension 4 to indicate the target modality. However, we also trained separate models specialized for each modality.

Implementation. All models were implemented in Python using PyTorch and MONAI, and trained on a single NVIDIA A30 GPU (24GB memory). Training was performed with a batch size of 4, the Adam optimizer with initial learning rate 1×10^{-4}, and a polynomial learning rate scheduler. The MT-ED model was trained for 540 epochs, while the MT-BBDM was trained for 1,080 epochs using 1,000 diffusion steps. The code of this work is available at: https://github.com/AgustinCartaya/brats2025-latent-ensemble-synthesis

2.4 Postprocessing and Ensemble Method

After synthesizing the latent space of the missing modality with each model, the results are reconstructed using the VCN. The reconstructed volumes are combined by computing the voxel-wise average, cropped to the original volume dimensions, and normalized to the [0, 1] range to obtain the final synthesized modality.

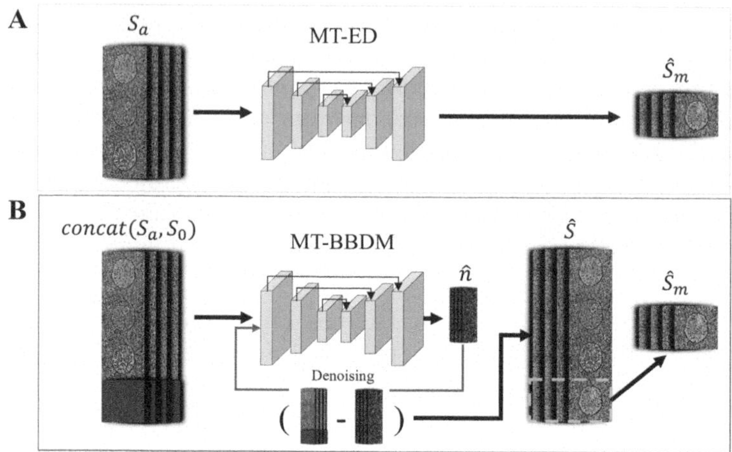

Fig. 2. Input-output schemes of the proposed models. **A:** MT-ED, fuses the preprocessed available modalities to reconstruct the missing one. **B:** MT-BBDM, denoises a concatenation of the preprocessed available modalities and a null latent space (S_0) to recover all modalities, from which the missing one is extracted.

3 Results

To evaluate our models, for each patient in the validation set, we synthesized each modality from the other three. For MT-BBDM synthesis we employed the accelerated sampling method from [21], reducing time steps from 1,000 to 50 to lower computation time while preserving quality. In contrast, MT-ED synthesis was performed directly. After generating the two synthetic latent spaces, we postprocessed and combined them as specified in Sect. 2.4. Following BraSyn 2025 [12], we conducted an evaluation including direct and indirect metrics, structured into three parts: (1) synthesis quality of specialized models versus original modalities, (2) versus reconstructed modalities, and (3) comparison between multimodal and specialized synthesis models. Finally, we present the official test set results reported in the BraSyn challenge during MICCAI 2025.

3.1 Evaluation Against Original Modalities

We evaluate synthesized modalities using original MR volumes as ground truth. For direct assessment, we computed the Structural Similarity Index Measure (SSIM) between synthesized and original volumes. Scores were calculated globally across the brain and separately within healthy and tumor regions. Table 1 reports global SSIM values, while Table 2 shows region-wise results.

We also assessed the utility of synthesized modalities in tumor segmentation using the FeTS framework [25–27]. Specifically, three original modalities combined with one synthesized modality were input to FeTS to generate segmentations of three subregions: Enhancing Tumor (ET), Peritumoral Edema (ED), and Necrotic Core (NCR). Segmentation performance was evaluated with Dice scores and Hausdorff Distances against ground-truth annotations. Results appear in Table 3. As the validation set lacks manual annotations, pseudo-ground-truth segmentations were generated using all four original modalities with FeTS.

To contextualize these results, we also report the performance of latent-space reconstructions of the original modalities, denoted as"Rec (GT)". For the direct assessment, we evaluated the reconstructed modality against the original one. For the indirect assessment, we used one reconstructed modality along with three original ones to compute the segmentation. These reconstructions represent an upper performance bound, limited only by the VCN reconstruction error. Figure 3, shows an example of original, reconstructed, and synthetic images for a patient in the validation set, along with their corresponding segmentations.

Table 1. SSIM between synthesized and original modalities over the whole brain. ↑ indicates higher is better. Best synthetic results are highlighted in bold.

Method	SSIM↑				
	T1w	T1ce	T2w	FLAIR	Average
MT-ED	0.9407	0.9133	0.9299	0.9191	0.9257
MT-BBDM	0.9395	0.9128	0.9295	0.9118	0.9234
Ensemble	**0.9467**	**0.9203**	**0.9372**	**0.9245**	**0.9322**
Rec (GT)	0.9768	0.9641	0.9780	0.9637	0.9706

Table 2. SSIM in healthy and tumor regions.

Healthy Region SSIM↑					
Method	T1w	T1ce	T2w	FLAIR	Average
MT-ED	0.9477	0.9223	0.9346	0.9241	0.9322
MT-BBDM	0.9465	0.9219	0.9343	0.9174	0.9300
Ensemble	**0.9530**	**0.9287**	**0.9415**	**0.9293**	**0.9381**
Rec (GT)	0.9793	0.9671	0.9792	0.9652	0.9727
Tumor Region SSIM↑					
Method	T1w	T1ce	T2w	FLAIR	Average
MT-ED	0.9973	0.9958	0.9972	0.9975	0.9969
MT-BBDM	0.9972	0.9958	0.9971	0.9971	0.9968
Ensemble	**0.9975**	**0.9960**	**0.9974**	**0.9976**	**0.9971**
Rec (GT)	0.9990	0.9989	0.9994	0.9992	0.9991

Table 3. Segmentation results using three original modalities plus one synthetic modality, with scores computed for the whole tumor (WT) and its three subregions. For the Hausdorff distance, lower values indicate better performance (↓).

Method	Dice score↑					Hausdorff distance↓			
	WT	NCR	ED	ET	Avg.	NCR	ED	ET	Avg.
MT-ED	0.9119	0.6563	0.8627	0.7779	0.8022	13.0892	**16.5477**	10.6731	13.4367
MT-BBDM	0.9054	0.6516	0.8530	0.7739	0.7960	**12.1101**	17.3885	9.7988	13.0991
Ensemble	**0.9185**	**0.6628**	**0.8702**	**0.7852**	**0.8092**	12.2401	16.6302	**9.7429**	**12.8711**
Rec (GT)	0.9697	0.8408	0.9553	0.9364	0.9256	7.3590	8.9666	5.4176	7.2478

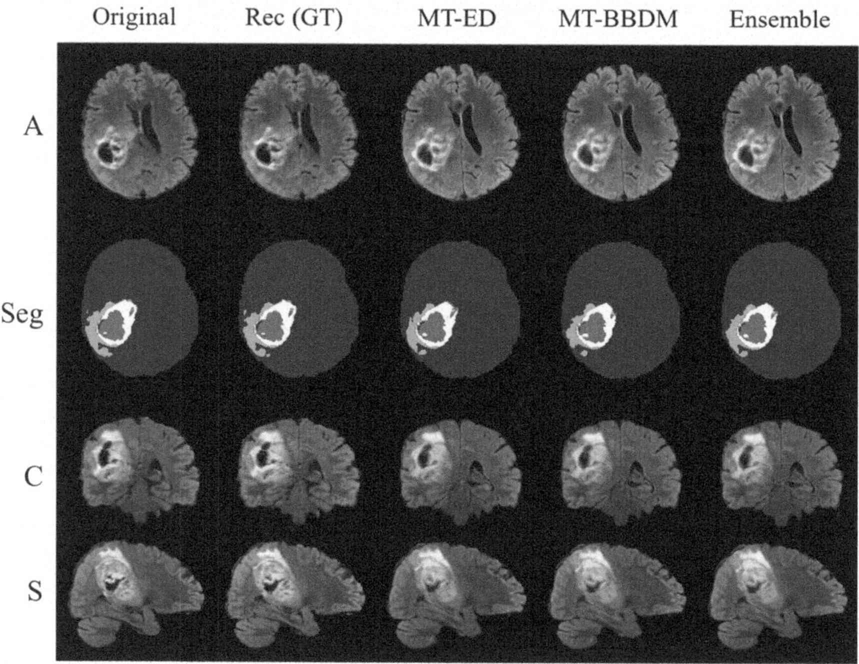

Fig. 3. Synthesis results from the different models when FLAIR MRI is missing, including Axial (A), Coronal (C), and Sagittal (S) planes, along with the corresponding segmentations.

3.2 Evaluation Against Reconstructed Modalities

To isolate the synthesis quality from the inherent reconstruction error introduced by the VCN, we repeated the evaluation using original reconstructed modalities as references. Table 4 reports the SSIM between synthesized and reconstructed modalities. For the indirect evaluation, shown in Table 5, segmentations were generated using one synthetic modality combined with three reconstructed modalities, and compared against segmentations obtained from all four reconstructed modalities.

Table 4. SSIM between synthesized and reconstructed modalities.

Method	SSIM↑				
	T1w	T1ce	T2w	FLAIR	Average
MT-ED	0.9468	0.9230	0.9363	0.9239	0.9325
MT-BBDM	0.9461	0.9228	0.9350	0.9168	0.9302
Ensemble	**0.9530**	**0.9308**	**0.9436**	**0.9296**	**0.9393**

Table 5. Segmentation results using three reconstructed and one synthetic modality.

Method	Dice score↑					Hausdorff distance↓			
	WT	NCR	ED	ET	Avg.	NCR	ED	ET	Avg.
MT-ED	0.9189	0.6633	0.8679	0.7791	0.8073	13.0634	**14.0625**	11.7730	12.9663
MT-BBDM	0.9109	0.6562	0.8587	0.7793	0.8013	**12.4031**	15.6647	**10.6763**	12.9147
Ensemble	**0.9221**	**0.6651**	**0.8731**	**0.7893**	**0.8124**	12.5115	14.0640	10.7912	**12.4556**

3.3 Multimodal Vs. Specialized Models

Finally, we compared the performance of a single multimodal synthesis MT-BBDM, trained to generate all target modalities simultaneously, with four specialized MT-BBDM models, each trained for a specific target modality. This comparison aimed to assess whether joint learning compromises quality in favor of generality. The multimodal model used for the comparison was trained for 540 epochs, while each specialized model was trained for 270 epochs. Figure 4, illustrates qualitative differences in the synthesized images.

3.4 Test Results

This section presents the results computed by the BraSyn challenge organizers on the test set using our ensemble method. The metrics reported in Table 6 correspond to those used for the final ranking, in which our approach achieved second place. Results are provided separately for two tumor types, Glioma and Meningioma, and the overall mean including Metastasis.

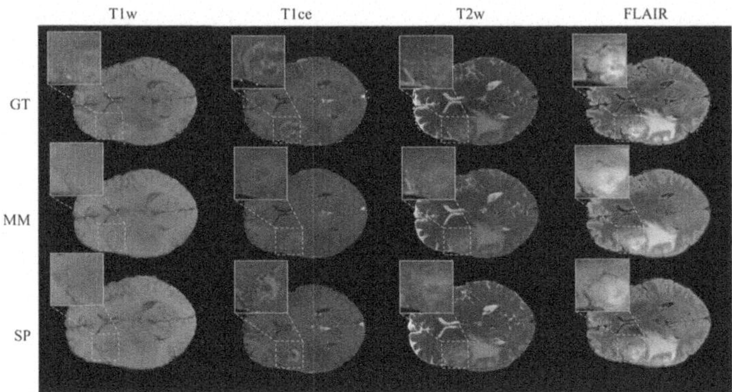

Fig. 4. Performance differences between multimodal (MM) and specialized (SP) models across different modalities compared with the ground truth (GT).

Table 6. Test set results. $NSD_{0.5}$ corresponds to the Normalized Surface Distance.

Tumor	Dice score↑			$NSD_{0.5}$↑			SSIM↑
	WT	NCR	ET	WT	NCR	ET	
Glioma	0.9137	0.8189	0.7597	0.4824	0.4697	0.5297	0.9369
Meningioma	0.7978	0.7487	0.7346	0.5440	0.5720	0.5724	0.9382
All	0.8619	0.7847	0.7393	0.4897	0.4963	0.5338	0.9371

4 Discussion

This work presents an ensemble approach for synthesizing missing brain MRI modalities using two generative models, MT-ED and MT-BBDM, both operating in a latent space. Our results show that combining these models improves both image similarity and segmentation accuracy compared to using each model alone.

Both models contributed positively to the synthesis task and produced visually similar outputs (Fig. 3). However, MT-ED achieved slightly better results on quantitative metrics, benefiting from its simplicity and efficiency. These characteristics make it a suitable choice when computational efficiency is a priority.

Using the pretrained VCN to compress full 3D volumes into a latent space reduced computational cost and preserved spatial continuity. This allowed the models to process entire volumes without relying on patching or slicing, which is particularly important for clinical tasks like tumor segmentation where anatomical consistency is critical. Despite this, the results showed that compression introduced some loss of fine detail, especially in lesion regions, which affected segmentation accuracy. Fine-tuning the VAE on the target dataset may help recover this detail and improve alignment with the original images.

The ensemble method was able to merge complementary information from the two models despite using a simple averaging strategy. Future work could investigate more advanced fusion methods, including uncertainty-aware weighting or attention-based blending [28], to further enhance synthesis results. This may be especially beneficial in complex regions like tumor boundaries or for modalities with lower synthesis quality, such as FLAIR and T1ce.

Training specialized models for each target modality seems to improve performance, as shown in Fig. 4, where early specialized models captured more detail than the multimodal ones. However, this came with higher training time and deployment complexity. Future work could explore multimodal learning techniques that use shared latent representations [8] to build more scalable models without compromising performance.

The ensemble strategy combines the strengths of both models. MT-ED provides speed and anatomical precision, while MT-BBDM contributes robustness and diversity. Together with latent-space processing, this method offers a promising approach for synthesizing missing modalities in multi-modal MRI workflows.

Acknowledgments. Agustin Cartaya Lathulerie and Valeriia Abramova hold FPI grants from the Ministerio de Ciencia, Innovación y Universidades, with reference numbers PREP2023-001473 and PRE2021-099121, respectively. Micaela Rivas Díaz is supported by the DEXCOM Chair grant TSI-100932-2023-1. Uma M. Lal-Trehan Estrada and Rachika E. Hamadache hold IFUdG2022 and IFUdG2024 grants from Universitat de Girona. Cansu Yalcin and Clara Lisazo hold FI grants from the Catalan Government, with reference numbers 2023 FI-1 00096 and 2024 FI-1 00103. Adrià Casamitjana holds a POSTDOC-UdG2023 grant. This work was also supported by PID2023-146187OB-I00 from the Ministerio de Ciencia, Innovación y Universidades and by the ICREA Academia program.

References

1. Zhou, J., Gu, L., Du, F., et al.: The global, regional, and national brain and CNS cancers burden and trends from 1990 to 2021. Sci. Rep. **15**, 19228 (2025). https://doi.org/10.1038/s41598-025-04636-7
2. Ilic, I., Ilic, M.: International patterns and trends in the brain cancer incidence and mortality: an observational study based on the global burden of disease. Heliyon **9**(7), e18222 (2023). https://doi.org/10.1016/j.heliyon.2023.e18222
3. Filho, A.M., Znaor, A., Sunguc, C., Zahwe, M., Marcos-Gragera, R., Figueroa, J.D., Bray, F.: Cancers of the brain and central nervous system: global patterns and trends in incidence. J. Neurooncol. **172**(3), 567–578 (2025). https://doi.org/10.1007/s11060-025-04944-y
4. Wen, P.Y., Macdonald, D.R., Reardon, D.A., et al.: Updated response assessment criteria for high-grade gliomas: response assessment in neuro-oncology working group. J. Clin. Oncol. **28**(11), 1963–1972 (2010). https://doi.org/10.1200/JCO.2009.26.3541
5. Vollmuth, P., Foltyn, M., Huang, R.Y., et al.: Artificial intelligence (AI)-based decision support improves reproducibility of tumor response assessment in neuro-oncology: an international multi-reader study. Neuro Oncol. **25**(3), 533–543 (2023). https://doi.org/10.1093/neuonc/noac189

6. Conte, G.M., Weston, A.D., Vogelsang, D.C., et al.: Generative adversarial networks to synthesize missing T1 and FLAIR MRI sequences for use in a multisequence brain tumor segmentation model. Radiology **299**(2), 313–323 (2021). https://doi.org/10.1148/radiol.2021203786
7. Li, H., et al.: DiamondGAN: unified multi-modal generative adversarial networks for MRI sequences synthesis. In: Shen, D., et al., (eds.) MICCAI 2019. LNCS, vol. 11767, pp. 795–803. Springer, Cham (2019). https://doi.org/10.1007/978-3-030-32251-9_87
8. Cho, J., Woo, J., Park, J.: A Unified Framework for Synthesizing Multisequence Brain MRI via Hybrid Fusion (2024). https://doi.org/10.48550/arXiv.2406.14954
9. Xiong, H., Wang, Y., Shen, Z., et al.: Learning contrast and content representations for synthesizing magnetic resonance image of arbitrary contrast. Med. Image Anal. **104**, 103635 (2025). https://doi.org/10.1016/j.media.2025.103635
10. Friedrich, P., Wolleb, J., Bieder, F., Durrer, A., Cattin, P.C.: WDM: 3D wavelet diffusion models for high-resolution medical image synthesis. In: Deep Generative Models, pp. 11–21. Springer Nature Switzerland (2024). https://doi.org/10.1007/978-3-031-72744-3_2
11. Ni, Y.: Enhancing the stability of generative adversarial networks: a survey of progress and techniques. Appl. Comput. Eng. **74**, 21–26 (2024).https://doi.org/10.54254/2755-2721/74/20240427
12. Li, H.B., Conte, G.M., Hu, Q., et al.: The brain tumor segmentation (BraTS) challenge 2023: brain MR image synthesis for tumor segmentation (BraSyn). arXiv preprint arXiv:2305.09011v6 (2024). PMID: 37608932; PMCID: PMC10441440
13. Karargyris, A., Umeton, R., Sheller, M.J., et al.: Federated benchmarking of medical artificial intelligence with MedPerf. Nat. Mach. Intell. **5**, 799–810 (2023)
14. Baid, U., et al.: The RSNA-ASNR-MICCAI BraTS 2021 Benchmark on Brain Tumor Segmentation and Radiogenomic Classification. arXiv preprint arXiv:2107.02314 (2021)
15. Menze, B.H., Jakab, A., Bauer, S., et al.: The multimodal brain tumor image segmentation benchmark (BRATS). IEEE Trans. Med. Imaging **34**(10), 1993–2024 (2015). https://doi.org/10.1109/TMI.2014.2377694
16. Bakas, S., Akbari, H., Sotiras, A., et al.: Advancing the cancer genome atlas glioma mri collections with expert segmentation labels and radiomic features. Sci. Data **4**, 170117 (2017). https://doi.org/10.1038/sdata.2017.117
17. Bakas, S., Akbari, H., Sotiras, A., et al.: Segmentation labels and radiomic features for the pre-operative scans of the TCGA-GBM collection. Cancer Imaging Archive (2017). https://doi.org/10.7937/K9/TCIA.2017.KLXWJJ1Q
18. Bakas, S., Akbari, H., Sotiras, A., et al.: Segmentation labels and radiomic features for the pre-operative scans of the TCGA-LGG collection. Cancer Imaging Archive (2017). https://doi.org/10.7937/K9/TCIA.2017.GJQ7R0EF
19. Ho, J., Jain, A., Abbeel, P.: Denoising diffusion probabilistic models. In: Advances in Neural Information Processing Systems (NeurIPS), vol. 33, pp. 6840–6851. Curran Associates Inc. (2020)
20. Sohl-Dickstein, J., Weiss, E.A., Maheswaranathan, N., Ganguli, S.: Deep unsupervised learning using nonequilibrium thermodynamics. In: Proc. of the 32nd Int. Conf. on Machine Learning (ICML), vol. 37, pp. 2256–2265 (2015)
21. Li, B., Xue, K., Liu, B., Lai, Y.-K.: BBDM: image-to-image translation with brownian bridge diffusion models. In: Proc. CVPR 2023, pp. 1952–1961. IEEE (2023). https://doi.org/10.1109/CVPR52729.2023.00194
22. Kingma, D.P., Welling, M.: An introduction to variational autoencoders. Found. Trends Mach. Learn. **12**(4), 307–392 (2019)

23. Cheng, L., Guan, P., Taherkordi, A., Liu, L., Lan, D.: Variational autoencoder-based neural network model compression (2024). https://doi.org/10.48550/arXiv.2408.14513
24. Guo, P., Zhao, C., Yang, D., et al.: MAISI: Medical AI for Synthetic Imaging (2024). https://doi.org/10.48550/arXiv.2409.11169
25. Pati, S., Baid, U., Edwards, B., et al.: Federated learning enables big data for rare cancer boundary detection. Nat. Commun. **13**, 7346 (2022). https://doi.org/10.1038/s41467-022-33407-5. Erratum. In: Nat. Commun. **14**(436), 10 (2023). 10.1038/s41467-023-36188-7
26. Pati, S., Baid, U., Edwards, B., et al.: The federated tumor segmentation (FeTS) tool: an open-source solution to further solid tumor research. Phys. Med. Biol. **67**(20), (2022). https://doi.org/10.1088/1361-6560/ac9449
27. Pati, S., Bakas, S.: FETS-AI/Front-End: Release for Zenodo. Version 0.0.8. Zenodo (2022). https://doi.org/10.5281/zenodo.7036038
28. Baumgartner, C.F., et al.: PHiSeg: capturing uncertainty in medical image segmentation. In: Shen, D., et al., (eds.) MICCAI 2019. LNCS, vol. 11765, pp. 119–127. Springer, Cham (2019). https://doi.org/10.1007/978-3-030-32245-8_14

MISFIT: Modality Inference via Style Fusion and Invertible Translation for Cross-Modality Synthesis of 3D MRI Volumes

Mohor Banerjee, Qiankun Ji, Sarim Hashmi, Abdelrahman Elsayed(✉), Daniil Tikhonov, Matheus Ferracciu Scatolin, Ahmed Jaheen, Damir Kim, Hu Wang, Mostafa Salem, and Mohammad Yaqub

Mohamed bin Zayed University of Artificial Intelligence (MBZUAI), Abu Dhabi, United Arab Emirates
{mohorbanerjee,qiankunji,sarimhashmi,abdelrahmanelsayed,daniiltikhonov, matheusferracciuScatolin,ahmedjaheen,damirkim,huwang,mostafasalem, mohammadyaqub}@mbzuai.ac.ae

Abstract. Robust synthesis of missing MRI modalities is essential for enabling the deployment of brain tumor segmentation pipelines in real-world clinical settings, where complete multi-modal scans are possibly unavailable due to acquisition constraints, scanner limitations, or patient-specific factors. This critical limitation is the focus of the Brain MR Image Synthesis Challenge (BraSyn), Task 8 of the BraTS-Lighthouse 2025 Challenge, which aims to foster generalizable and clinically deployable methods for synthesizing missing MRI modalities from available ones. To tackle this, we propose MISFIT – Modality Inference via Style Fusion and Invertible Translation – a novel two-stage generative framework for 3D brain MRI synthesis that operates entirely in the wavelet domain. MISFIT enhances the conditional wavelet diffusion paradigm by incorporating a Channel Attention Feature Fusion (CAFF) module for modality-aware representation learning and a Multi-Switchable SPADE block for style-conditioned generation. In Stage I, fused wavelet representations of the input modalities are used to generate a coarse approximation of the target modality. In Stage II, a denoising diffusion model - conditioned on both Stage I outputs and the original wavelet subbands - progressively reconstructs the final high-fidelity target volume. Evaluated on the BraSyn 2025 validation set, MISFIT achieves a PSNR of 18.65 dB and SSIM of 0.8041 in the randomized setting, demonstrating the viability of wavelet-based diffusion with adaptive fusion for medical image reconstruction. https://github.com/mohrsalt/MISFIT

Keywords: BraSyn · Brain MRI · 3D MRI synthesis · Wavelet diffusion · MISFIT · CAFF · SPADE

S. Bakas et al. (Eds.): MICCAI 2025, LNCS 16377, pp. 42–53, 2026.
https://doi.org/10.1007/978-3-032-16370-7_4

1 Introduction

Deep learning has become a cornerstone of brain tumor segmentation in magnetic resonance imaging (MRI), offering accurate, reproducible alternatives to manual delineation and demonstrating strong clinical potential [1–3]. Recent state-of-the-art methods typically rely on a complete set of four MRI modalities: T1-weighted (T1), contrast-enhanced T1 (T1ce), T2-weighted (T2), and fluid-attenuated inversion recovery (FLAIR), each capturing distinct anatomical and pathological characteristics. Despite these advancements, in practice, one or more sequences are often missing due to time constraints, patient movement, or protocol variability, limiting the reliability of such models in real-world clinical settings [4,5].

The BraTS 2025 Brain MR Image Synthesis Challenge addresses this issue directly by encouraging the development of generative methods that can reconstruct missing modalities from the remaining ones [6]. By enabling the recovery of a complete input set, these approaches support the robust deployment of segmentation pipelines given incomplete data scenarios. However, the task presents notable challenges: MR volumes are inherently three-dimensional and high-resolution, making full-volume modeling computationally demanding. As a result, many existing solutions decompose the task into smaller slices or patches, which are later reassembled, often at the cost of spatial coherence and inter-slice consistency.

Recent work has demonstrated that modeling in the wavelet domain [7,8] offers a promising direction for high-fidelity medical image synthesis. The conditional Wavelet Diffusion Model (cWDM) [9], for instance, achieves strong results by operating on wavelet-transformed 3D MR volumes and conditioning the generation process through direct concatenation of the available modalities at each denoising step. Although effective, this approach treats each input modality independently and does not explicitly model their interactions or adapt to the specific characteristics of the missing modality.

In this paper, we propose **MISFIT** - **M**odality **I**nference via **S**tyle **F**usion and **I**nvertible **T**ranslation - a generative framework for missing MR modality synthesis. MISFIT retains the concatenation-based conditioning strategy of cWDM but enhances it with two key additions: a Channel Attention Feature Fusion (CAFF) module [10] that learns to combine information from the wavelet-transformed inputs, and a Multi-Switchable Spatially-Adaptive Denormalization (MS-SPADE) block [11,12] that transforms the fused features to match the style of the target modality. The outputs of both CAFF and MS-SPADE, along with the original wavelet-transformed inputs, are concatenated with the noise sample at each denoising step to guide generation. This design enables MISFIT to produce anatomically consistent, modality-specific 3D outputs. This paper makes the following contributions:

- A modality-aware wavelet-domain pipeline for cross-modality 3D brain MRI synthesis in the BraTS 2025 Challenge.
- A two-phase strategy that separates modality fusion from diffusion-based synthesis to better disentangle structural priors and generative detail.

– Integration of CAFF and Multi-Switchable SPADE for adaptive conditioning to fuse inter-modality features while preserving contrast and spatial fidelity.

2 Related Work

Generative Adversarial Networks (GANs) [13–17] have been widely used for image-to-image translation, especially in settings where paired data is available. Early methods like pix2pix [18] model the conditional distribution between source and target modalities, while later extensions support unpaired translation using techniques such as cycle consistency or representation disentanglement. In medical imaging, GAN-based methods have been applied to 3D modality synthesis and offer fast inference, but they are often unstable to train, particularly on volumetric data, and are prone to issues such as mode collapse.

Denoising Diffusion Models (DDMs) [19] have recently outperformed GANs in synthesis quality and training stability, and have been adapted for translation tasks, including 3D medical imaging [20–22]. However, due to their high computational costs, they can be difficult to scale to high-resolution 3D volumes and thus, many implementations rely on 2D slices and pseudo-3D setups instead.

To reduce this overhead, Latent Diffusion Models (LDMs) perform the diffusion process in a learned compressed space, enabling efficient training and high-resolution outputs [23–25]. Building on this, the Adaptive Latent Diffusion Model (ALDM) introduces Multi-Switchable SPADE blocks to condition on different target modalities, allowing one-to-many translation in full 3D volumes without patch-based training [12]. These approaches highlight the potential of combining latent-space modeling with structured conditioning to support flexible and accurate modality synthesis.

While effective, latent diffusion models often require complex encoders and decoders to be trained and can lose spatial details during compression. Recently, Wavelet Diffusion Models (WDMs) have addressed this by operating directly in the wavelet-transformed image domain, preserving fine spatial information while still offering computational efficiency [8]. In the BraTS 2024 Modality Synthesis Challenge, WDM's conditional extension cWDM (Conditional Wavelet Diffusion Model) enabled paired 3D image-to-image translation by conditioning wavelet-domain diffusion on multiple source modality inputs [9].

Also featured in the same challenge, the Hybrid Fusion GAN (HF-GAN) proposed a strategy where modality-specific features are first fused in 2D using a Channel Attention Feature Fusion (CAFF) module and subsequently refined in 3D to enhance structural consistency and tumor visibility [26]. Notably, HF-GAN was the top-ranked submission in the competition.

However, prior methods remain limited in several ways: GAN-based models are challenging to train stably on 3D data and often produce anatomically inconsistent results; ALDM requires training a separate encoder-decoder and performs one-to-many translation without leveraging cross-modal interactions; and cWDM simply concatenates inputs without any explicit fusion mechanism to model relationships between modalities. Our proposed method, MISFIT, addresses these limitations by operating entirely in the wavelet domain and combining conditional diffusion with channel-aware fusion and SPADE-style modulation. This enables more informed conditioning on available modalities to capture inter-modal relationships, while sidestepping the complexity of training a separate encoder-decoder model by generating directly in the wavelet-transformed space.

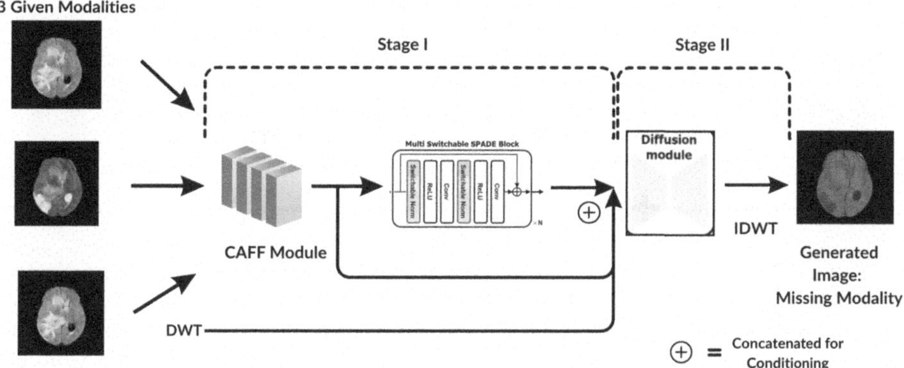

Fig. 1. Overall MISFIT pipeline for missing modality synthesis using CAFF, Multi-Switchable SPADE, and conditional wavelet-domain diffusion.

3 Method

We propose a two-stage training pipeline for 3D MRI modality synthesis that integrates frequency-aware representation with structured conditioning and invertible translation. The model operates entirely in the wavelet-transformed domain, preserving spatial fidelity while enabling efficient learning. The first phase of training performs wavelet-domain feature fusion and class-conditioned generation of an initial target estimate. The second phase uses a denoising diffusion model - conditioned on the Stage I outputs and the wavelet-transformed source modalities - to produce the final target in the wavelet domain. The complete MISFIT pipeline is depicted in Fig. 1.

3.1 Stage I: Wavelet Fusion and SPADE-Modulated Style Transfer

Given three source modalities (X_1, X_2, X_3) and a target class label y, the overall Stage 1 pipeline (outlined in Algorithm 1) begins by applying a 3D Haar Discrete Wavelet Transform (DWT) to each modality, producing 8 frequency subbands per modality. These subbands are concatenated along the channel axis to form a compact wavelet-domain representation for each modality.

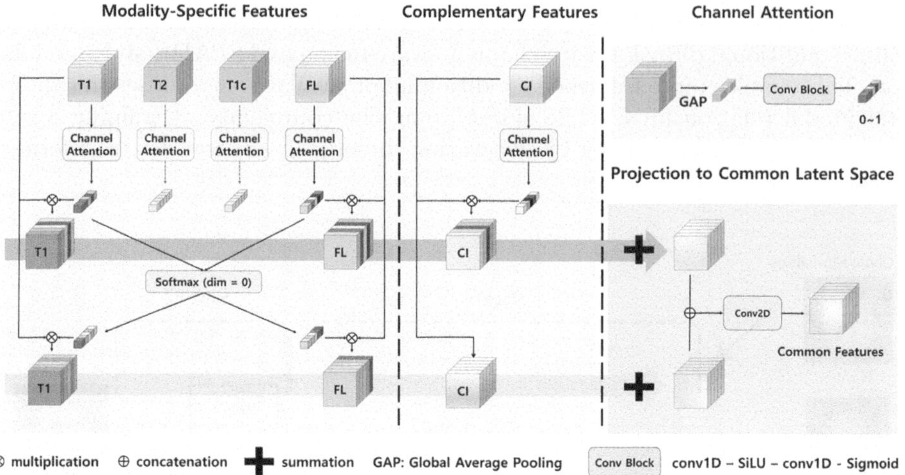

Fig. 2. The Channel Attention Feature Fusion (CAFF) module applies channel attention (GAP → Conv1D–SiLU–Conv1D–Sigmoid) to compute importance weights, which modulate each modality via element-wise multiplication. Weighted features are fused using softmax-based aggregation and projected to a shared latent space via Conv2D, enhancing cross-modality integration. Adapted from [10].

To combine these modality-specific representations, we implement a Channel Attention Feature Fusion (CAFF) module, illustrated in Fig. 2. For each sample, two complementary fusion strategies are applied: (i) a spatial fusion using learned channel-wise attention weights from modality-specific attention blocks, and (ii) a softmax-normalized fusion that enforces inter-modality competition. The resulting spatial and soft attention-weighted representations are concatenated and projected using a 1×1 convolution to obtain the fused latent representation.

This fused representation is passed to a conditional generator based on the Spatially-Adaptive Denormalization (SPADE) framework, where the target label y modulates the decoding process through feature-wise affine transformations. The output comprises 8 predicted wavelet subbands that reconstruct the target modality

The model is trained using a weighted combination of wavelet-domain reconstruction loss and a conditional adversarial classification loss. The reconstruction objective minimizes the mean squared error (MSE) between the predicted and ground-truth wavelet subbands:

$$\mathcal{L}_{\text{rec}} = \frac{1}{B} \sum_{i=1}^{B} \|x_i - \hat{x}_i\|_2^2 ,$$

where x_i and $\hat{x}_i$ denote the ground-truth and predicted wavelet subbands for the i-th sample in a batch of size B. In parallel, the generator is optimized to produce outputs that a multi-class discriminator classifies as belonging to the correct modality class, using a cross-entropy loss:

$$\mathcal{L}_{\mathrm{G}} = \frac{1}{B}\sum_{i=1}^{B} \mathrm{CE}\left(D(\hat{x}_i), y_i\right),$$

where $D(\cdot)$ denotes the discriminator, and y_i is the target class label. The discriminator is trained to assign real samples to their true class and generated (fake) samples to a designated auxiliary class y_{fake}, with its loss defined as:

$$\mathcal{L}_{\mathrm{D}} = \frac{1}{2B}\sum_{i=1}^{B} \left[\mathrm{CE}(D(x_i), y_i) + \mathrm{CE}(D(\hat{x}_i), y_{\text{fake}})\right].$$

The total generator loss is computed as:

$$\mathcal{L}_{\text{total}} = \mathcal{L}_{\text{rec}} + \lambda_{\text{adv}} \cdot \mathcal{L}_{\mathrm{G}},$$

where λ_{adv} is a weighting factor progressively increased after a warm-up period. Generator and discriminator are updated alternately using separate Adam optimizers, with gradient clipping applied for stability.

Algorithm 1: Wavelet Fusion and SPADE-Modulated Style Transfer

Input: Source modalities (X_1, X_2, X_3); target class label y
Output: Predicted wavelet-domain subbands $\hat{Y}_0$
Step 1: Compute wavelet representations;
$h_1 \leftarrow \mathrm{DWT}(X_1)$;
$h_2 \leftarrow \mathrm{DWT}(X_2)$;
$h_3 \leftarrow \mathrm{DWT}(X_3)$;
Step 2: Fuse modality features via CAFF;
$z_{\text{fused}} \leftarrow \mathrm{CAFF}(h_1, h_2, h_3)$;
Step 3: Generate target subbands via MS-SPADE;
$\hat{Y}_0 \leftarrow \mathrm{MS} - \mathrm{SPADE}(z_{\text{fused}}, y)$;
Step 4: Return synthesized wavelet output;
return $\hat{Y}_0$;

3.2 Stage II: Conditional Wavelet Diffusion

In the second phase, we train a conditional denoising diffusion model that operates directly in the wavelet domain, as shown in Fig. 3. The goal is to reverse a predefined noise process in the wavelet domain, using output features from Stage I as conditioning, to recover the clean target. The overall procedure is outlined in Algorithm 2.

During training, the ground-truth target modality is transformed via DWT to obtain clean wavelet subbands, which are then perturbed by Gaussian noise using a cosine diffusion schedule. The conditioning input is constructed by running the Stage I model in evaluation mode to extract its CAFF and MS-SPADE

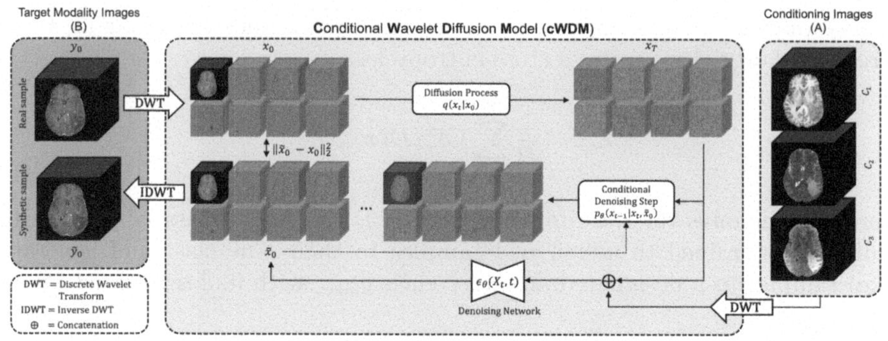

Fig. 3. The Conditional Wavelet Diffusion Model (cWDM) synthesizes missing MR modalities by learning to denoise wavelet-transformed target images under external conditioning. Noise is added to the DWT of the target y_0 to obtain x_T, which is iteratively denoised to produce $\tilde{x}_0$, then reconstructed via Inverse DWT to yield $\tilde{y}_0$. Adapted from [9].

outputs, which are then concatenated with the individual DWT representations of the three input modalities. The resulting 5-channel tensor serves as a fixed conditioning vector and remains constant across all timesteps.

At each step of the reverse process, the model receives the noisy wavelet input concatenated with the conditioning vector, following a Palette-style conditioning strategy [27], and predicts the denoised wavelet subbands. The model is trained using an MSE loss applied across all subbands, with equal weighting per channel. After the final timestep, the denoised wavelet representation is reconstructed to the spatial domain using the inverse DWT, yielding the synthesized target volume.

Algorithm 2: Conditional Wavelet Diffusion

Input: Conditioning modalities C_1, C_2, C_3; Stage I CAFF output z_{fused}; Stage I MS-SPADE output $\hat{Y}_0$

Output: Synthesized target image $\tilde{y}_0$

Step 1: Initialize latent noise and conditioning input;

$x_T \sim \mathcal{N}(0, I)$;

$c \leftarrow \text{DWT}(C_1) \oplus \text{DWT}(C_2) \oplus \text{DWT}(C_3) \oplus z_{\text{fused}} \oplus \hat{Y}_0$;

Step 2: Perform conditional denoising over T steps;

for $t = T$ **to** 1 **do**

- $X_t \leftarrow x_t \oplus c$;
- $\tilde{x}_0 \leftarrow \epsilon_\theta(X_t, t)$;
- $x_{t-1} \sim p_\theta(x_{t-1} \mid x_t, \tilde{x}_0)$;

Step 3: Invert wavelet transform to obtain output;

$\tilde{y}_0 \leftarrow \text{IDWT}(x_0)$;

return $\tilde{y}_0$;

4 Experimental Settings

4.1 Dataset

We evaluate MISFIT on the BraTS 2025 Modality Synthesis Challenge dataset, based on the RSNA-ASNR-MICCAI BraTS 2021 collection [28,34,35]. It includes multi-parametric 3D brain tumor MRI scans from multiple institutions, with four modalities per case: T1, T1ce, T2, and FLAIR. A total of 1489 training and 250 validation cases are provided, each with spatial dimensions of 155 × 240 × 240. All training samples include tumor segmentation masks, although our model is trained using only the raw image volumes.

4.2 Preprocessing Pipeline

All volumes are first spatially padded to 240Âă×Âă240Âă×Âă160, and then center-cropped to 224Âă×Âă224Âă×Âă160. Intensity values are clipped at the 0.1 and 99.9 percentiles and rescaled to the range $[-1, 1]$. For training, we apply random flipping along all three spatial axes. To accommodate the four different missing-modality scenarios, training is performed separately for each configuration. Accordingly, each sample is configured by selecting a fixed target modality specific to the training setup, with the remaining three modalities used as input. The target modality is also mapped to a class index, which is used for conditioning during training.

4.3 Training Strategy

We train separate models for each of the four missing-modality scenarios, with each model learning to synthesize a specific target modality conditioned on the other three. This aligns with the strategy adopted by cWDM [9]. Each model is trained in two phases: Stage I (Wavelet Fusion and MS-SPADE-based generation) is trained for 1000 epochs with a batch size of 1, using an adversarial loss and subband-wise MSE. Stage II (Conditional Wavelet Diffusion) is trained for 150,000 steps using cosine noise scheduling and DDPM-style denoising. All experiments are run on 4 NVIDIA A100 GPUs (40 GB each) using PyTorch Lightning's DDP strategy, with mixed precision enabled for memory efficiency.

4.4 Implementation Details

Wavelet transforms (DWT/IDWT) are applied using an 8-channel decomposition. In Stage I, the fused features from three source modalities are passed through a MS-SPADE-modulated generator conditioned on the target modality class. In Stage II, the CAFF output and MS-SPADE output from Stage I are concatenated with the DWT representations of the source inputs to form the conditioning for the denoising process. The denoising network ϵ_θ is a 3D U-Net with 64 base channels, operating entirely in the wavelet domain. Sampling uses 1000 steps with a cosine noise scheduler, and the final output is reconstructed via inverse DWT.

4.5 Evaluation Metrics

We evaluate modality synthesis quality using Structural Similarity Index Measure (SSIM) [31] and Peak Signal-to-Noise Ratio (PSNR) [32]. SSIM measures perceptual quality using local statistics on luminance, contrast, and structure, while PSNR quantifies pixel-wise accuracy via the MSE-based signal-to-error ratio in decibels.

5 Results

Table 1 shows the evaluation results for each of the four missing-modality configurations. In the first four rows, one modality is excluded from the input, and the respective model, which is trained to reconstruct that specific modality, is evaluated using the remaining three modalities as input.

The final row reports performance on a randomized pseudo-validation set, where a different modality is randomly omitted for each subject. This set was generated using the official script provided by the challenge organizers, with a fixed random seed to ensure reproducibility. All validation samples - both fixed and randomized - are drawn from the challenge-provided validation dataset.

To complement the quantitative evaluation, Fig. 4 presents representative real and synthetic MR slices, highlighting visual characteristics and limitations across modalities.

Table 1. Quantitative performance for reconstructing each held-out modality, including results on a randomized pseudo-validation set. Metrics are reported as mean $\pm$ standard deviation.

Missing Modality	PSNR ↑	SSIM ↑
T1	17.45 $\pm$ 0.99	0.7977 $\pm$ 0.0187
T1ce	20.15 $\pm$ 1.59	0.8064 $\pm$ 0.0171
T2	17.54 $\pm$ 1.43	0.8070 $\pm$ 0.0180
FLAIR	18.54 $\pm$ 1.87	0.8047 $\pm$ 0.0179
Random	18.65 $\pm$ 1.79	0.8041 $\pm$ 0.0179

6 Discussion

MISFIT exhibits consistent quantitative performance across all missing-modality settings, with SSIM values clustering around 0.80 and PSNR scores in the 17–20 dB range (Table 1). The similarity of results across both fixed and randomized validation splits suggests that the model reliably reconstructs diverse targets using the remaining three modalities. This indicates that the structured conditioning pathway - combining wavelet-domain decomposition with CAFF and

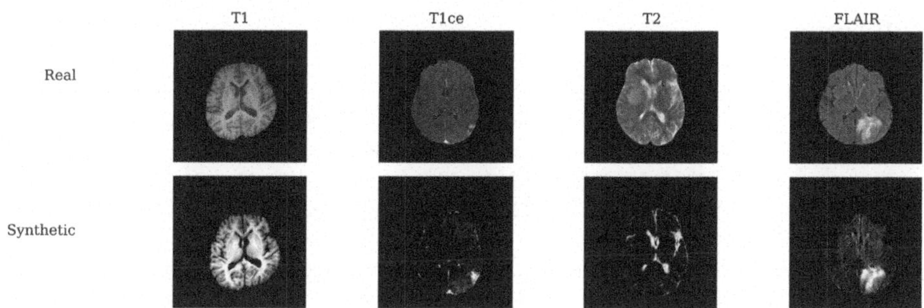

Fig. 4. Comparison of real and synthetic axial MR slices for T1, T1ce, T2, and FLAIR: the top row shows ground truth, the bottom row shows MISFIT-generated outputs conditioned on the remaining three modalities, serving as a qualitative reference.

MS-SPADE - effectively guides the synthesis process without requiring modality-specific encoders or shared decoder heads.

The qualitative results in Fig. 4 provide additional context, revealing that while basic structure is preserved, contrast loss and blurring are evident in several modalities. However, these limitations are less indicative of architectural shortcomings and more a consequence of the restricted training schedule. Due to computational budget constraints, Stage II was trained for only 150,000 steps - far fewer than the 1.2 million steps used in cWDM [9]. As contrast-sensitive and high-frequency features tend to emerge in later phases of training, the current results likely represent an intermediate convergence point rather than the model's full potential.

Thus, while the model performs well in capturing gross anatomical layout, the fidelity of subtle, modality-specific features may improve significantly with longer training. The current results, both quantitative and qualitative, should therefore be interpreted as a lower-bound estimate of MISFIT's representational capacity under limited optimization.

7 Conclusion

This work presents our submission to BraSyn (BraTS-Lighthouse 2025, Task 8), proposing a two-phase wavelet-domain framework that separates modality fusion (via CAFF and MS-SPADE) from generation (via diffusion). Despite limited training budgets, the model produces structurally consistent outputs across missing-modality settings. Future directions include unified modeling and improved conditioning.

Acknowledgments. We thank Salma Wael Fekry Hassan for her contributions; Padma Pavani, Walid Omari, and the MBZUAI Research IT team for computational support; and Teresa Lynn, Jingjing Huang, Aidar Alimbayev, and Ali Mekky for coordinating the UGRIP programme under which this project was conducted.

References

1. Dorfner, F.J., et al. A review of deep learning for brain tumor analysis in MRI. NPJ Precis. Onc. 9, 2 (2025). https://doi.org/10.1038/s41698-024-00789-2
2. Khan, MKH., et al.: Machine learning and deep learning for brain tumor MRI image segmentation. Exp Biol Med (Maywood). 2023 Nov;248(21):1974-1992. https://doi.org/10.1177/15353702231214259.Epub 2023 Dec 16. PMID: 38102956; PMCID: PMC10798183
3. Içn, A., Direkoğlu, C., çah, M.: Review of MRI-based brain tumor image segmentation using deep learning methods. Proc. Comput. Sci. 102:317-324, ISSN 1877-0509 (2016). https://doi.org/10.1016/j.procs.2016.09.407, https://www.sciencedirect.com/science/article/pii/S187705091632587X
4. Zaitsev, M., Maclaren, J., Herbst, M.: Motion artifacts in MRI: a complex problem with many partial solutions. J Magn Reson Imaging. 42(4):887-901 (2015). https://doi.org/10.1002/jmri.24850.Epub 2015 Jan 28. PMID: 25630632; PMCID: PMC4517972
5. Havsteen, I., et al.: Are movement artifacts in magnetic resonance imaging a real problem? - a narrative review. Front. Neurol. **8–2017**,(2017). https://doi.org/10.3389/fneur.2017.00232
6. Li, H. B., etal.: The brain tumor segmentation (BraTS) challenge 2023: brain MR image synthesis for tumor segmentation (BraSyn). arXiv [Eess.IV]. Retrieved from (2024). http://arxiv.org/abs/2305.09011
7. Phung, H., Dao, Q., Tran, A.: Wavelet diffusion models are fast and scalable image generators. Retrieved from (2023). http://arxiv.org/abs/2211.16152
8. Friedrich, P., Wolleb, J., Bieder, F., Durrer, A., Cattin, P. C.: WDM: 3D wavelet diffusion models for high-resolution medical image synthesis. In Deep Generative Models, pp. 11–21 (2024). https://doi.org/10.1007/978-3-031-72744-3_2
9. Friedrich, P., Durrer, A., Wolleb, J., Cattin, P. C.: cWDM: conditional wavelet diffusion models for cross-modality 3D medical image synthesis. Retrieved from (2024). http://arxiv.org/abs/2411.17203
10. Cho, J., Woo, J., Park, J.: A unified framework for synthesizing multisequence brain MRI via hybrid fusion. Retrieved from (2024). http://arxiv.org/abs/2406.14954
11. Park, T., Liu, M.-Y., Wang, T.-C., Zhu, J.-Y.: Semantic image synthesis with spatially-adaptive normalization. http://arxiv.org/abs/1903.07291
12. Kim, J., Park, H.: Adaptive latent diffusion model for 3d medical image to image translation: multi-modal magnetic resonance imaging study. In: 2024 IEEE/CVF Winter Conference on Applications of Computer Vision (WACV),pp. 7589–7598 (2024). https://doi.org/10.1109/wacv57701.2024.00743
13. Welander, P., Karlsson, S., Eklund, A.: Generative adversarial networks for image-to-image translation on multi-contrast MR images - a comparison of CycleGAN and UNIT (2018).http://arxiv.org/abs/1806.07777
14. Chen, G., Sun, M., Mao, Z.-H., Liu, K., Jia, W.: Mechanisms of generative image-to-image translation networks (2024). http://arxiv.org/abs/2411.10368
15. Ko, K., Yeom, T., Lee, M.: SuperstarGAN: generative adversarial networks for image-to-image translation in large-scale domains. Neural Netw. **162**, 330–339 (2023). https://doi.org/10.1016/j.neunet.2023.02.042
16. Gong, Y., et al.: E2GAN: efficient training of efficient gans for image-to-image translation (2024). http://arxiv.org/abs/2401.06127

17. Armanious, K., et al.: MedGAN: medical image translation using GANs. Comput. Med. Imaging Graph. **79**, 101684 (2020). https://doi.org/10.1016/j.compmedimag.2019.101684
18. Isola, P., Zhu, J.-Y., Zhou, T., Efros, A. A.: Image-to-image translation with conditional adversarial networks (2018). http://arxiv.org/abs/1611.07004
19. Ho, J., Jain, A., Abbeel, P.: Denoising diffusion probabilistic models (2020). http://arxiv.org/abs/2006.11239
20. Xia, B., et al.:DiffI2I: efficient diffusion model for image-to-image translation (2023). http://arxiv.org/abs/2308.13767
21. Kwon, G., Ye, J. C.: Diffusion-based image translation using disentangled style and content representation (2023). http://arxiv.org/abs/2209.15264
22. Özbey, M., et al.: Unsupervised medical image translation with adversarial diffusion models(2023). http://arxiv.org/abs/2207.08208
23. Rombach, R., Blattmann, A., Lorenz, D., Esser, P., Ommer, B.: High-resolution image synthesis with latent diffusion models. In: Proceedings of the IEEE/CVF conference on computer vision and pattern recognition, pp. 10684–10695 (2022)
24. Zhu, L., et al.: Make-a-volume: leveraging latent diffusion models for crossmodality 3d brain MRI synthesis. In: International Conference on Medical Image Computing and Computer-Assisted Intervention, pp. 592–601. Springer (2023)
25. Kebaili, A., Lapuyade-Lahorgue, J., Vera, P., Ruan, S.: 3D MRI synthesis with slice-based latent diffusion models: improving tumor segmentation tasks in data-scarce regimes (2024). http://arxiv.org/abs/2406.05421
26. Cho, J., Park, S., Park, J.: Two-stage approach for brain MR image synthesis: 2D image synthesis and 3D refinement (2024). http://arxiv.org/abs/2410.10269
27. Saharia, C., et al.: Palette: image-to-image diffusion models (2022). http://arxiv.org/abs/2111.05826
28. U.Baid, et al., The RSNA-ASNR-MICCAI BraTS 2021 benchmark on brain tumor segmentation and radiogenomic classification, arXiv:2107.02314 (2021)
29. Menze, B.H., et al.: The multimodal brain tumor image segmentation benchmark (BRATS). IEEE Trans. Med. Imaging **34**(10), 1993–2024 (2015). https://doi.org/10.1109/TMI.2014.2377694
30. Bakas, S., et al.: Advancing the cancer genome atlas glioma MRI collections with expert segmentation labels and radiomic features. Nature Scientific Data **4**, 170117 (2017). https://doi.org/10.1038/sdata.2017.117
31. Nilsson, J., Akenine-Möller, T.: Understanding SSIM (2020). http://arxiv.org/abs/2006.13846
32. Horé, A., D. Ziou.: Image quality metrics: PSNR vs. SSIM. In: 2010 20th International Conference on Pattern Recognition, Istanbul, Turkey, 2010, pp. 2366-2369. https://doi.org/10.1109/ICPR.2010.579.keywords: PSNR;Degradation;Image quality;Additives;Transform coding;Sensitivity;Image coding;PSNR;SSIM;image quality metrics,
33. Karargyris, A., et al.: Federated benchmarking of medical artificial intelligence with MedPerf. Nat Mach Intell 5, 799–810 (2023). https://doi.org/10.1038/s42256-023-00652-2
34. Bakas, S., et al.: Segmentation labels and radiomic features for the pre-operative scans of the TCGA-GBM collection. Cancer Img. Archive (2017). https://doi.org/10.7937/K9/TCIA.2017.KLXWJJ1Q
35. Bakas, S., et al.: Segmentation labels and radiomic features for the pre-operative scans of the TCGA-LGG collection. Cancer Imaging Archive (2017). https://doi.org/10.7937/K9/TCIA.2017.GJQ7R0EF

Fast-cWDM Brain MRI: Fast Conditional Wavelet Diffusion Model for Synthesis Brain MRI Modality

Timothy Sereda and Lina Chato(✉)

Department of Computer Science, University of South Dakota, Vermillion, USA
timothy.sereda@coyotes.usd.edu, lina.chato@usd.edu

Abstract. In this paper, we present a novel and efficient framework for cross-modality medical image synthesis, developed for BraSyn–Task 8. Our method combines the fast-sampling capabilities of the Fast-Denoising Diffusion Probabilistic Model (Fast-DDPM) with Discrete Wavelet-Transformed components, as used in Conditional Wavelet Diffusion Models. By reducing the number of denoising steps to 100 and using wavelet-transformed inputs, we accelerate both training and inference and reduce memory usage while preserving high image quality. The framework was trained on the BraTS 2025 dataset, which includes four magnetic resonance imaging (MRI) modalities: T1-weighted, contrast-enhanced T1-weighted (T1c), T2-weighted, and FLAIR. We developed four independent models, each synthesizing one missing modality from the remaining three. Evaluation on the BraSyn 2025 Task 8 public validation set demonstrated competitive performance using standard image metrics: mean squared error, signal-to-noise ratio, and structural similarity index. Our method achieved Third place in the challenge in the final test data, with fast inference times (average 41–67 s per case). To assess clinical relevance, we applied a pretrained nnU-Net segmentation model on the synthesized modalities. Segmentation results yielded high Dice coefficients: 0.877 for the whole tumor, 0.769 for the tumor core, and 0.667 for the enhancing tumor. These results confirm the effectiveness and reliability of our approach for missing-modality synthesis, enabling accurate downstream analysis in high-dimensional medical imaging tasks. Our team in **the challenge is USD-2025-Chato-Sereda (Team ID: 3551654)**. Github link: **https://github.com/tsereda/brats-synthesis**

Keywords: Discrete Wavelet Transform · Diffusion Denoising Probabilistic Model · U-Net · Synthesis MRI images · Fast Sampling · BraSyn

1 Introduction

Medical imaging systems, such as Magnetic Resonance Imaging (MRI), Computed Tomography (CT), mammography, ultrasound, and fundus photography are essential tools for non-invasive medical evaluations. These medical imaging plays a crucial role in diagnosing a wide range of diseases, including brain tumors, stroke, retinal disorders, breast cancer, and others [1, 2].

S. Bakas et al. (Eds.): MICCAI 2025, LNCS 16377, pp. 54–65, 2026.
https://doi.org/10.1007/978-3-032-16370-7_5

In recent years, numerous research efforts have explored the use of Artificial Intelligence (AI) to improve diagnostic processes and clinical outcomes in healthcare, particularly in the field of medical imaging [3–7].

AI, especially Deep Learning (DL), including generative models, has shown significant potential in enhancing both the quality and quantity of medical imaging data. Applications include image synthesis, denoising, automatic classification, segmentation, and disease detection. These advancements not only assist clinicians in achieving faster and more accurate diagnoses but also enable the development of robust computer-aided diagnostic systems.

One important case use is the identification and segmentation of brain tumors, including primary and secondary tumors. Accurate segmentation of tumor subregions of gliomas typically requires access to multiple MRI modalities, including T1-weighted (T1), T1 post-contrast (T1c), T2-weighted (T2), and Fluid-Attenuated Inversion Recovery (FLAIR) images. The Brain Tumor Segmentation (BraTS) Challenge has become a benchmark for evaluating the performance of automated algorithms in this domain [8]. However, in real-world clinical settings, it is common for one or more of these modalities to be missing due to cost constraints, time limitations, or acquisition errors.

Missing modalities can prevent benefits from the state-of-the-art segmentation models when these models mostly were developed based on multimodal input of either all four MRI modalities, (Tw1, T1wc, Tw2, and FLAIR), or three of them, excluding the T1 modality. To address this challenge, recent research has focused on generating missing modalities using generative models such as Generative Adversarial Networks (GANs) and Diffusion Models [9–11]. These methods aim to synthesize high-quality, clinically realistic images that can substitute missing inputs, thus preserving or even enhancing model performance.

Contributing to the BraTS 2025 Brain MRI Image Synthesis Challenge (BraSyn)-Global Missing Modality Task 8 [13], we propose a **Fast Conditional Wavelet Diffusion Model (Fast-cWDM)** for efficient cross-modality generation of 3D MRI medical images. Our work focuses on developing a generative model that can accurately synthesize missing MRI modalities to support downstream segmentation tasks and improve diagnostic reliability in incomplete imaging scenarios. By integrating the reduced-step sampling of Fast-DDPM [10] with wavelet-based spatial decomposition in cWDM [12], our approach achieves high-quality synthesis with significantly lower memory usage and faster inference, making it well-suited for practical clinical applications.

The remains of this paper are organized as follows: Sect. 2 describes the data and explains the proposed synthesis image generated models; Sect. 3 presents experiments conducted to develop and evaluate the best model and displays the results; Sect. 4 discusses the contributions and sets future directions to enhance the performance.

2 Methodology

2.1 Multimodal BraSyn 2025 Data for Missing MRI Modality

BraSyn-missing MRI modality task released multimodal MRI training data [13]: BraTS-GLI 2023 dataset [14], and BraTS-METS 2023 [15]. This data consists of 1251 glioma samples, and 238 Metastasis samples. Gliomas are primary brain tumors that arise from glial cells. Gliomas can be both low-grade and high-grade, depending on how aggressive they are. While **brain metastasis** tumors are a **secondary brain tumor** that originate **outside the brain** (in another organ) and spread (**metastasize**) to the brain through the bloodstream or lymphatic system. Each sample in the training data has four MRI modalities, (T1, T1c, T2, and Flair), in addition to a segmentation file. The segmentation file consists of a segmentation mask of the three brain tumor subregions (Peritumoral edema (ED), Enhancing tumor (ET), Necrotic and/or non-enhancing core (NCR/NETC), as well as healthy brain tissues and background), as shown in Fig. 1. The size of each MRI modality is (240 × 240 × 155) voxels. To test the developed models, two stages of test are released by BraSyn. In the first test stage, the challenge released validation data that consists of 219 samples of glioma tumors, and 31 samples of Metastasis tumors. The validation data contains all the four MRI modalities, excluding the segmentation file. While the final test stage contains 219 samples of Glioma, 59 samples of Metastasis, and 283 samples of Meningioma [16], excluding the segmentation file and randomly one of the MRI modalities in each sample. Meningioma is a type of primary brain tumor that arises from the meninges. This tumor is a usually benign, slow-growing brain tumor that forms outside the brain tissue but can compress adjacent brain structures.

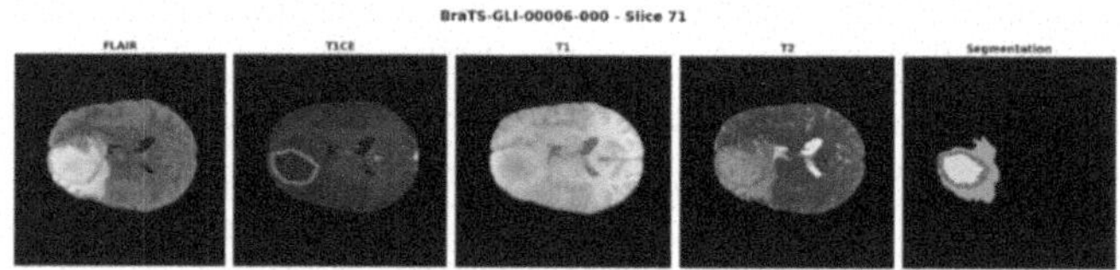

Fig. 1. A sample from BraSyn 2025 training data for missing MRI modality task [13]. The colors of the segmentation labels are as follows: Green: ED, Red: ET, Yellow: NCR/NETC.

2.2 3D Fast Conditional Wavelet Diffusion Model (3D Fast-cWDM)

Background

Denoising Diffusion Probabilistic Model (DDPM) is a type of generative model developed to produce high-quality, realistic images by gradually reversing a noise-adding process [11]. It operates in two main stages:

1. Forward Process: Noise is incrementally added to an image over many steps until it becomes pure noise.
2. Reverse Process: A neural network, such as a U-Net backbone, is trained to denoise the image step by step, reconstructing a clean image from the noisy input.

By learning to reverse this noise process, DDPMs can generate entirely new, realistic images from noise. However, this process usually requires thousands of denoising steps (often 1,000+), resulting in long sampling times. Generating a single image can take several minutes, and the time can increase significantly when generating full 3D/4D medical volumes, depending on computational resources and memory. To address this issue, Fast-DDPM [10] was introduced. The authors proposed a significantly more efficient diffusion process that reduces the number of denoising steps to just 10–25, while preserving image quality. This was achieved through: a) Novel noise schedulers (both uniform and non-uniform), which optimize the diffusion trajectory; b) Aligned training-time sampling, which ensures the model effectively learns denoising within the reduced number of steps. This approach reduced sampling time (by ~100×) and training costs (by ~5×), making Fast-DDPM practical for high-dimensional tasks like 3D MRI modality synthesis, without substantial degradation in image quality. Compared to the original DDPM, Fast-DDPM showed only a minor decrease in pixel-wise accuracy (e.g., PSNR, MSE), while maintaining or even improving structural similarity image quality (SSIM), making it well-suited for clinical and research applications. To further accelerate high-resolution medical image generation, the authors of [17] proposed training a diffusion probabilistic model using discrete wavelet components instead of raw images. This strategy offered multiple advantages: 1) Each wavelet component volume is 1/8 the size of the raw image, due to wavelet subsampling reducing spatial dimensions by a factor of 2 in each axis of a 3D image; the reduced input feature map size (1/8 of the original) results in a smaller U-Net, which significantly lowers memory and computational requirements. 2) The U-Net backbone processes these wavelet-based features instead of raw image data, allowing the network to learn from more informative and compact representations. In [17], the authors proposed a **Conditional Wavelet Diffusion Model (cWDM)** for cross-modality synthesis, contributing to the BraTS 2024 missing modality challenge. Their model achieved competitive results compared to standard DDPM. However, the method still involved high computational costs due to the use of 24 wavelet components for the conditional modalities (3 modalities × 8 components for each), in addition to 8 wavelet components for the target (missing) modality. Moreover, since the model was based on standard DDPM, it still required a large number of denoising steps to achieve high-quality outputs. Inspired by Fast-DDPM's reduced time steps and the efficiency of the cWDM approach, we propose a new framework that combines these techniques for cross-modality generation. Our approach aims to leverage the strengths of both methods: significantly faster inference and lower memory usage without compromising image fidelity, thereby enabling practical and scalable solutions for high-dimensional medical imaging tasks.

Modeling

Our proposed model, Fast Conditional Wavelet Diffusion Model (Fast-cWDM), operates in wavelet space, as shown in Fig. 2, to reduce computational complexity and leverages a reduced denoising step strategy to accelerate sampling.

We removed 8 pixels from each side of every slice in each MRI modality, and appended 5 additional slices using zero-padding to the final slice of each modality. This preprocessing step ensures a compatible input size of 224 × 224 × 160 for wavelet composition. Let the three available MRI modalities $x^1, x^2, x^3 \in \mathbb{R}^{224 \times 224 \times 160}$, and the target (missing) modality be x^m . Applying the 3D DWT $W(.)$, we obtain

$$w^i = W\left(x^i\right), \quad for\ i \in \left\{x^1, x^2, x^3, x^m\right\}$$

Each $w^i \in \mathbb{R}^{112 \times 112 \times 80 \times C}$, where C refers to the number of the wavelet subbands per modality. As we applied one level of 3D DWT for the volumetric image data, $C = 8$. The model takes $\{w^1, w^2, w^3\}$ as conditional inputs, and learns to generate w^m

i. **Forward Diffusion Process**

We define the forward noising process over the wavelet components of the missing modality. Let $w_0 = \omega^m$, the wavelet representation of the original missing modality. For time step $t \in \{1, \ldots, T\}$, the forward process is defined as:

$$q(w_t|w_{t-1}) = N\left(w_t; \sqrt{\overline{\alpha_t}}\, w_{t-1},\ (1 - \alpha_t\ )\, I\right)$$

$$\overline{\alpha_t} = \prod_{s=1}^{t} \alpha_s$$

Where N is a Normal Gaussian Noise, $\alpha_t = 1 - \beta_t$, and β_t is a small noise schedule for our Fast-cWDM (for this task, we used T = 100)

ii. **Reverse Process**

The denoising network is a U-Net variant ϵ_θ, trained to predict the added noise ϵ to the wavelet component of the missing MRI modality, w_t, at timestep t, and the condition set (the available three modalities) $\{w^1, w^2, w^3\}$:

$$\hat{\epsilon}_t = \epsilon_\theta\left(w_t, t, w^1, w^2, w^3\right)$$

The reverse process uses the predicted noise to reconstruct w_{t-1} from w_t

$$w_{t-1} = \frac{1}{\sqrt{\alpha_t}}\left(w_t - \frac{1 - \alpha_t}{\sqrt{1 - \overline{\alpha_t}}}\hat{\epsilon}_t\right) + \sigma_t z$$

When σ_t is the standard deviation of added noise, and $z \sim N(0, 1)$

The conditional U-Net backbone processes the noisy wavelet component of the missing modality and conditional wavelet inputs. Due to one level of the wavelet subsampling using Haar mother wavelet function, all input volumes are at 1/8 spatial scale, allowing for a lightweight architecture.

2.3 Evaluation Measures

To evaluate the performance of our image synthesis model, we adopt a combination of image quality metrics and segmentation-based metrics, reflecting both the visual realism and clinical utility of the generated images.

Image Quality Metrics: We assess how closely the synthesized modality resembles the real (acquired) image using the following pixel-level and perceptual metrics:

Mean Squared Error (MSE) quantifies the average squared difference between the synthesized image $\hat{x}$ and the ground truth image x:

$$MSE\ (x, \hat{x}) = \frac{1}{No}\sum_{i=1}^{No} (x_i - \hat{x}_i)^2$$

Where No is the number of the image in the test sets. Lower MSE values indicate better pixel-wise accuracy.

Peak Signal-to-Noise Ratio (PSNR) measures the ratio between the maximum possible pixel intensity and the distortion (noise) in the image. It is derived from MSE:

$$PSNR(x, \hat{x}) = 10\log_{10}\left(\frac{\text{MAX}^2}{MSE\ (x, \hat{x})}\right)$$

Higher PSNR values indicate better image fidelity.

Structural Similarity Index Measure (SSIM) evaluates perceptual similarity by comparing luminance, contrast, and structure between the synthesized image $\hat{x}$ and the ground truth image x:

$$SSIM\,(x, \hat{x}) = \frac{(2\mu_x\mu_{\hat{x}} + C_1)(2\sigma_{x\,\hat{x}} + C_2)}{\left(\mu_{\hat{x}}^2 + \mu_{\hat{x}}^2 + C_1\right)\left(\sigma_{\hat{x}}^2 + \sigma_{\hat{x}}^2 + C_2\right)}$$

Segmentation-Based Metrics: To assess clinical utility, we evaluate whether the synthesized modality enables accurate brain tumor segmentation using a pre-trained BraTS segmentation model. The following metrics are computed between the predicted and ground-truth labels for three tumor subregions:

Dice Similarity Coefficient (DSC)

$$Dice(P, G) = \frac{2|P \cap G|}{|P| + |G|}$$

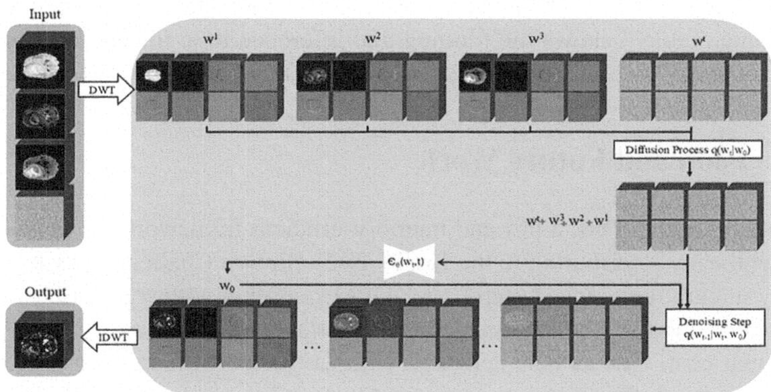

Fig. 2. Infrastructure of our Fast-cWDM. The noise image in the input column (left) is the missing modality, and the other available modalities are conditional inputs. The output image is the generated missing image (i.e., noisy image)

3 Experiment Setup and Results

We trained a Fast-DDPM model with a 3D U-Net backbone to predict the noise over a reduced number of diffusion steps. We conducted four experiments. For each experiment, we trained a separate model to synthesize one of the four modalities (T1, T1c,

T2, or FLAIR) from the remaining three as conditional inputs. Each MRI modality was preprocessed using Haar wavelet decomposition, producing eight subband components per modality, each size $112 \times 112 \times 80$. We used T = 100 diffusion steps with a uniform linear noise schedule, trained with the AdamW optimizer (learning rate = 1e-5, batch size = 1) for three stages: 47,500 iterations, 200,000 iterations, and 600,000 iterations using MSE loss. Inference was performed using the Denoising Diffusion Implicit Models (DDIM) solver, exploring uniform timestep sampling strategies. DDIM treats the reverse diffusion process as a deterministic Ordinary Differential Equation (ODE), enabling fast, non-Markovian sampling. All training and evaluation were conducted on four GPUs Nvidia A100 (each 40 GB), that were supported by Nautilus [18]. The U-Net architecture used in all models followed a standard 3D encoder–decoder design with skip connections and group normalization, tailored to handle 8-channel wavelet inputs for each modality. The model output predicted the denoised wavelet coefficients, which were subsequently reconstructed into the full MRI volume using Inverse Discrete Wavelet Transform (IDWT). Fig. 3 displays the training and validation loss for the four missing MRI models. Table 1 displays the results of image quantitative measures comparing the generated modality against the ground truth (real). All metrics were computed on the reconstructed image volumes in the original spatial domain. nnUnet segmentation model was also used to test the random missing synthesis modality in BraSyn validation dataset, and dice scores of the segmented brain tumor regions are presented in Table 2. The qualitative visualization evaluation is presented in Fig. 4. Some results from the validation data are presented in Fig. 5.

We submitted the four models (one for each missing MRI modality) that were trained with 600,000 iterations to the BraSyn team 2025 to be tested on the final test phase unlabeled data. Table 3 shows the training and inference time for the models. Table 4 presents the results from the final test data using models trained on 600,000 iterations.

4 Conclusion and Future Work

We developed Fast-cWDM, a fast and memory-efficient framework for cross-modality 3D MRI synthesis, contributing to the BraTS 2025 BraSyn Challenge (Task 8) [13–16, 19–21]. By integrating reduced-step Fast-DDPM sampling with wavelet-based decomposition, our method synthesizes missing modalities with high image quality and low computational cost. Our models achieved competitive performance on image quality metrics and yielded strong tumor segmentation results, as shown in Table 2. In this stage, we cannot compare our results to the leader board on validation phase as we are not sure if other teams' segmentation scores were based on nnUnet. These results highlight the practical value of our approach in enabling robust downstream analysis in incomplete imaging scenarios for both clinical uses and AI based diagnosis. From Table 1, we can see Fast-cWDM models for T1 and T2 achieved better image evaluation scores compared to other two modalities' models. Our models, trained for 600,000 iterations, were evaluated by the BraSyn 2025 team on the final test data, and they reported that our submissions achieved **third place** in this year's challenge. Although the SSIM scores for all groups of the tumors in the final test data, it seems the segmentation dice scores were the best in the glioma brain tumors, as shown in Table 4.

Table 1. Evaluation scores for synthesis MRI images for 250 examples in the BraSyn validation dataset. Number of iterations = 74,500, timesteps = 100, validation test conducted 4 times. * Refers to the same models that trained with number of iterations = 200,000. ** Refers to the same models that trained with number of iterations = 600,000.

Model	MSE ($\times 10^{-3}$)	PSNR (dB)	SSIM
T1	2.140 ± 1.690	27.74 ± 2.90	0.9386 ± 0.0234
T1c	3.189 ± 2.743	25.93 ± 2.69	0.9175 ± 0.0234
T2	2.665 ± 1.515	27.35 ± 3.15	0.9344 ± 0.0293
FLAIR	2.532 ± 3.970	26.58 ± 2.24	0.9145 ± 0.0203
T1*	1.976 ± 1.690	28.25 ± 3.12	0.9399 ± 0.0224
T1c*	2.947 ± 2.440	26.32 ± 2.83	0.9159 ± 0.0246
T2*	2.540 ± 3.834	27.71 ± 3.32	0.9366 ± 0.0306
FLAIR*	2.336 ± 1.385	26.90 ± 2.18	0.9124 ± 0.0214
T1**	1.910 ± 1.630	28.38 ± 3.09	0.9391 ± 0.0243
T1c**	2.994 ± 2.443	26.23 ± 2.81	0.9097 ± 0.0251
T2**	2.672 ± 4.231	27.58 ± 3.37	0.9351 ± 0.0307
FLAIR**	2.322 ± 1.436	26.98 ± 2.27	0.9126 ± 0.0226

Table 2. nnUnet Segmentation dice scores for the three Brain tumor regions in the BraSyn validation dataset using synthesis generated images for random missing modality. The last row shows the segmentation dice scores for all real MRI modalities.

Model	WT	ET	TC
Fast-cWDM: 100 timesteps, 74,500 iterations	0.869	0.635	0.724
Fast-cWDM: 100 timesteps, 200,000 iterations	0.872	0.677	0.762
Fast-cWDM: 100 timesteps, 600,000 iterations	0.877	0.667	0.769
All MRI modalities are real	0.897	0.778	0.851

To further enhance our results, we propose training on smaller image patches and experimenting with different timestep schedules, including optimized timestep sampling strategies. In the third column of Fig. 3, we can see the absolute difference maps between the synthesized T1-weighted MRI slices and the corresponding ground truth images. These heatmaps highlight the spatial distribution of reconstruction errors across the brain slice. Notably, larger differences are observed around structural boundaries and tumor regions, where intensity variations and complex textures increase the modeling challenge. In contrast, homogeneous tissue regions exhibit lower reconstruction errors, reflecting the model's ability to capture smoother anatomical patterns. This qualitative evaluation helps identify specific areas where synthesis performance could be further improved, such as enhancing boundary precision and tumor representation. However,

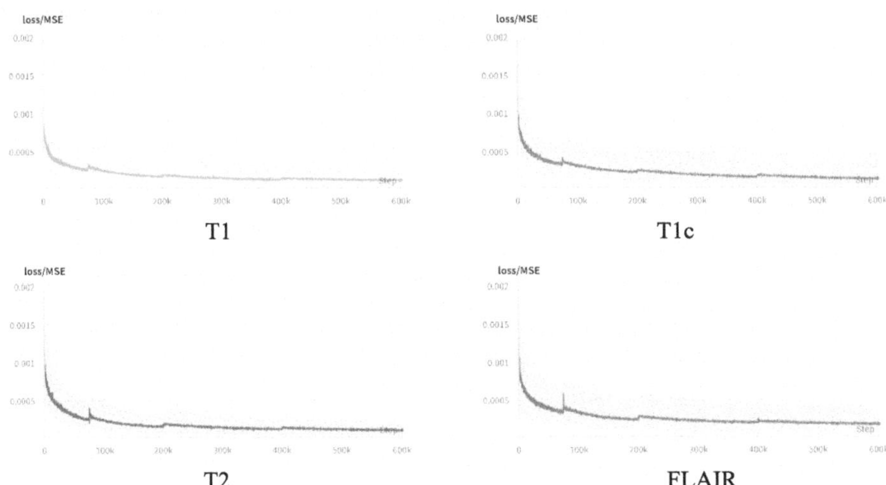

Fig. 3. Train/validation loss curves. Each curve is for a specific Fast-cWDM missing MRI modality: T1 (Orange), T1c (Green), T2 (Red), and FLAIR (Purple).

Table 3. Training time (600,000 iterations) and average inference time/modality for the four Fast-cWDM MRI missing modalities.

	T1	T1c	T2	FLAIR
Training time	89 h	89 h	89 h	89 h
Inference time	42 s	41 s	67 s	67 s

Flair modality does not show any large differences in the tumor region. Based on the above, we suggest as future work to integrate attention mechanisms to better focus on tumor regions and boundaries, combine synthesis with segmentation using multi-task learning, and use perceptual or adversarial losses to improve detail. Exploring multi-scale architecture or patch-based refinement may also help capture both global and local features for more accurate synthesis. In addition, we plan to explore alternative mother wavelets, such as Daubechies-2 (db2) and Daubechies-4 (db4), which may improve performance over the currently used Haar wavelet. Unlike Haar, which tends to aggressively downsample and emphasize sharp edges, Daubechies wavelets have longer support and smoother basis functions, allowing them to capture more contextual information. This may be particularly beneficial for encoding texture and soft transitions in anatomical structures, potentially enhancing both synthesis quality and downstream segmentation performance.

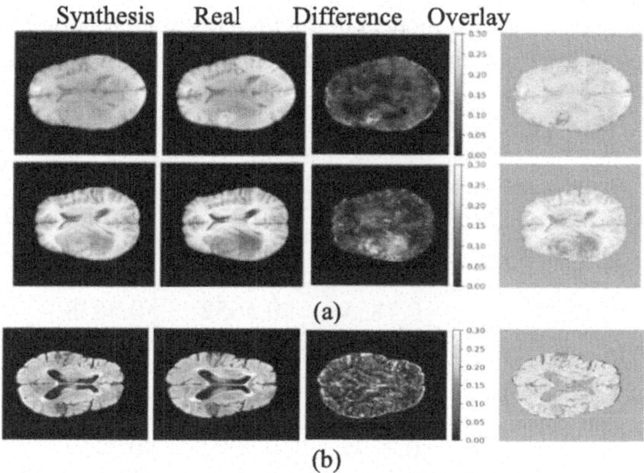

Fig. 4. Qualitative comparison of: (a) synthesized T1-weighted MRI and corresponding real image (slice 80) of sample BraTS-GLI-00001-000 (top), and sample BraTS-GLI-00001-001 (bottom); (b) synthesized Flair MRI and corresponding real image (slice 80) of sample BraTS-MET-00207-000.

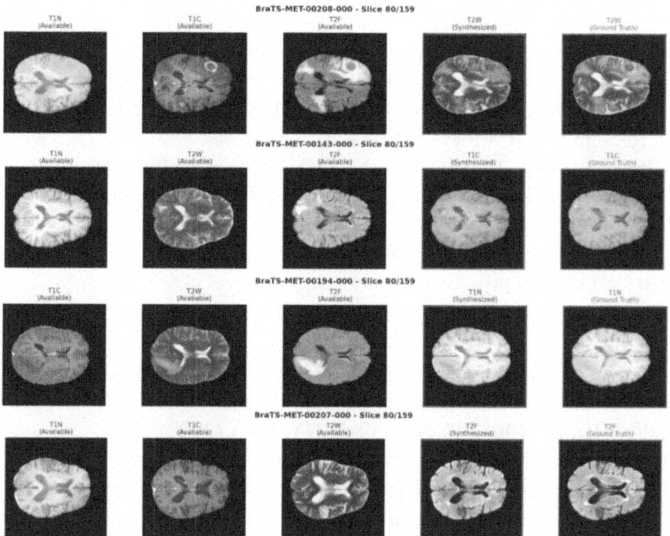

Fig. 5. Results from validation dataset.

Table 4. Performance of Fast-cWDM models in the final test data reported by BraTS 2025-Task 8 (achieving third place in the challenge). GLI: Glioma, MEN: Meningioma.

Group	Type	Dice_ET	Dice_TC	Dice_WT	NSD_0.5 ET	NSD_0.5 TC	NSD_0.5 WT	SSIM
GLI	Mean	0.7443	0.8073	0.9168	0.5312	0.4685	0.5006	0.9304
GLI	Std	0.2866	0.2746	0.0985	0.2887	0.2944	0.1923	0.0510
MEN	Mean	0.7210	0.7349	0.7855	0.5652	0.5638	0.5424	0.9279
MEN	Std	0.3836	0.3753	0.3341	0.3513	0.3539	0.2866	0.0223
ALL	Mean	0.7253	0.7730	0.8609	0.5326	0.4931	0.5011	0.9291
ALL	Std	0.3251	0.3179	0.2295	0.3094	0.3160	0.2317	0.0427

References

1. Hussain, S., et al.: Modern diagnostic imaging technique applications and risk factors in the medical field: a review. Biomed. Res. Int. **2022**, 5164970 (2022)
2. Cen, L.P. et al. : Automatic detection of 39 fundus diseases and conditions in retinal photographs using deep neural networks. Nat. Commun. 2021;12(1):4828. (2021)
3. Rahman, A., Valanarasu, J.M.J., Hacihaliloglu, I., Patel, V.M.: Ambiguous medical image segmentation using diffusion models. In: 2022 IEEE/CVF Conference on Computer Vision and Pattern Recognition (CVPR) (2022)
4. Konz, N., Chen, Y., Dong, H., Mazurowski, M.A.: Anatomically-controllable medical image generation with segmentation-guided diffusion models. In: Lecture Notes in Computer Science, pp. 88–98 (2024)
5. Khader, F., et al.: Denoising diffusion probabilistic models for 3D medical image generation. Sci. Rep. **13**(1), 7303 (2023)
6. Skandarani, Y., Jodoin, P., Lalande, A.: GANS for medical image synthesis: an empirical study. J. Imaging. **9**(3), 69 (2023)
7. Zhang, H.W., Lu, H., Won, D., Yoon, S.W.: Medical image synthesis with generative adversarial networks for tissue recognition. In: 2018 IEEE International Conference on Healthcare Informatics (ICHI), pp. 199–207, New York, NY, USA (2022)
8. Bonato, B., Nanni, L., Bertoldo, A.: Advancing precision: a comprehensive review of MRI segmentation datasets from BraTS challenges (2012–2025). Sensors. **25**, 1838 (2025)
9. Conte, G.M., et al.: Generative adversarial networks to synthesize missing T1 and FLAIR MRI sequences for use in a multisequence brain tumor segmentation model. Radiology. **299**(2), 313–323 (2021)
10. Jiang, H., et al.: Fast-DDPM: fast Denoising diffusion probabilistic models for medical image-to-image generation. IEEE J. Biomed. Health Inform., 1–11 (2025)
11. Ho, J., Jain, A., Abbeel, P.: Denoising diffusion probabilistic models. 34th international conference on neural information processing Systemsm 2020. Art. **574**, 6840–6851 (2020)
12. Friedrich, P., Durrer, A., Wolleb, J., Cattin, P.C.: CWDM: Conditional Wavelet Diffusion Models for cross-modality 3D medical image synthesis. arXiv.org. https://arxiv.org/abs/2411.17203. (2024)
13. Li, H.B., et al.: The Brain Tumor Segmentation (BRATS) Challenge 2023: Brain MR Image Synthesis for Tumor Segmentation (BrASYN). arXiv.org. https://arxiv.org/abs/2305.09011. (2023)

14. Baid, U., et al.: The RSNA-ASNR-MICCAI BraTS 2021 benchmark on brain tumor segmentation and radiogenomic classification. arXiv preprint arXiv, 2107.02314 (2021)
15. Moawad, A.W., et al.: The Brain Tumor Segmentation - Metastases (BraTS-METS) Challenge 2023: Brain Metastasis Segmentation on Pre-treatment MRI. ArXiv, arXiv, 2306.00838v3 (2024)
16. LaBella, D. et al.: Analysis of the BRATS 2023 intracranial meningioma segmentation challenge. The journal of machine learning for biomedical Imaging 3:38–58 (2025), Machine Learn. Biomed. Imag.
17. Friedrich, P., Wolleb, J., Bieder, F., Durrer, A., Cattin, P.C.: WDM: 3D wavelet diffusion models for high-resolution medical image synthesis. In: Mukhopadhyay, A., Oksuz, I., Engelhardt, S., Mehrof, D., Yuan, Y. (eds.) Deep Generative Models. DGM4MICCAI 2024 Lecture Notes in Computer Science, vol. 15224. Springer, Cham (2025)
18. Weitzel, D., et al.: The National Research Platform: stretched, multi-tenant, scientific Kubernetes cluster. In Practice and Experience in Advanced Research Computing 2025, the Power of Collaboration (PEARC '25). Association for Computing Machinery, New York, NY, USA, Article 69, 1–5. (2025)
19. Menze, B.H., Jakab, A., Bauer, S., Kalpathy-Cramer, J., Farahani, K., Kirby, J., et al.: The multimodal brain tumor image segmentation benchmark (BRATS). IEEE Trans. Med. Imaging. **34**(10), 1993–2024 (2015)
20. Bakas, S., et al.: Advancing the cancer genome atlas glioma MRI collections with expert segmentation labels and radiomic features. Sci. Data. **4** (2017)
21. Verdier, M.C., et al.: The 2024 Brain tumor segmentation (BraTS) challenge: glioma segmentation on post-treatment MRI. ArXiv, abs, 2405.18368 (2024)

SLaM-DiMM: Shared Latent Modeling for Diffusion Based Missing Modality Synthesis in MRI

Bhavesh Sandbhor[1], Bheeshm Sharma[2], and Balamurugan Palaniappan[2](✉)

[1] Department of MEMS, IIT Bombay, Mumbai, India
22b2446@iitb.ac.in
[2] Department of IEOR, IIT Bombay, Mumbai, India
{bheeshmsharma,balamurugan.palaniappan}@iitb.ac.in

Abstract. Brain MRI scans are often found in four modalities, consisting of T1-weighted with and without contrast enhancement (T1ce and T1w), T2-weighted imaging (T2w), and Flair. Leveraging complementary information from these different modalities enables models to learn richer, more discriminative features for understanding brain anatomy, which could be used in downstream tasks such as anomaly detection. However, in clinical practice, not all MRI modalities are always available due to various reasons. This makes missing modality generation a critical challenge in medical image analysis. In this paper, we propose SLaM-DiMM, a novel missing modality generation framework that harnesses the power of diffusion models to synthesize any of the four target MRI modalities from other available modalities. Our approach not only generates high-fidelity images but also ensures structural coherence across the depth of the volume through a dedicated coherence enhancement mechanism. Qualitative and quantitative evaluations on the BraTS-Lighthouse-2025 Challenge dataset demonstrate the effectiveness of the proposed approach in synthesizing anatomically plausible and structurally consistent results. Code is available at this link.

Keywords: Brain MRI Synthesis · Diffusion Models · Medical Imaging

1 Introduction

Missing modality generation [4] in brain MRI has emerged as a critical research area due to its impact on the training and performance of deep learning models used for anatomical localization and pixel-level annotation. Brain MRI data is typically acquired in multiple modalities, including T1-weighted imaging with and without contrast enhancement (T1ce and T1w), T2-weighted imaging (T2w), and Flair, each capturing distinct tissue properties and pathological features. While deep learning models have achieved strong performance in anomaly detection and analysis tasks, their effectiveness is often compromised in clinical

S. Bakas et al. (Eds.): MICCAI 2025, LNCS 16377, pp. 66–78, 2026.
https://doi.org/10.1007/978-3-032-16370-7_6

settings where one or more modalities may be missing due to protocol differences or other reasons. The absence of modalities limits the model's access to complementary information crucial for accurate detection and characterization of anomalous regions.

To address the challenge, we propose SLaM-DiMM: Shared Latent Modeling for Diffusion Based Missing Modality Synthesis in MRI. SLaM-DiMM is a novel framework designed to synthesize any target brain MRI modality from other available input modalities, enabling robust and flexible cross-modal image generation. Our architecture follows an encoder-decoder paradigm, in which a shared encoder maps the multi-channel input into a compact shared latent representation. This latent representation is then refined through a Latent Diffusion Model (LDM) [21]-based bottleneck. The enhanced latent representation is subsequently decoded by modality-specific decoders to generate high-fidelity outputs in the target MRI modality. Furthermore, we introduce a coherence enhancement network (CEn) that explicitly enforces 3D spatial consistency across depth, improving volumetric smoothness in the reconstructed 3D volumes. Synthesis results obtained using SLaM-DiMM on BraTS-Lighthouse 2025 Challenge dataset [16], highlight its superior ability to preserve fine textures and tissue contrast across diverse imaging modalities.

2 Related Work

Dar et al. [8] proposed pGAN and cGAN architectures to synthesize missing modalities using adversarial learning for multi-contrast MRI translation, and Dalmaz et al. introduced ResViT [7], a transformer-based model that integrates convolutional and vision transformer blocks for realistic synthesis. In 3D wavelet diffusion model (WDM), a diffusion model is directly applied on wavelet-decomposed images to preserve high-frequency details while enabling full-resolution image generation [10]. Further conditional Wavelet Diffusion Model (cWDM) extends the WDM architecture by conditioning on the available modalities to enable effective cross-modality MRI synthesis [9]. Recently, HF-GAN [6] was used as a baseline to synthesize 2D MR images, incorporating a hybrid fusion encoder, a channel attention-based feature fusion module, a modality infuser, and a CNN decoder; additionally, a 3D U-Net-based refiner was used to enhance the quality of the synthesized slices by leveraging volumetric context [5]. SwinUNETR [11], a hybrid architecture combining Swin Transformers and CNNs, was also applied to MRI synthesis and showed strong performance [20]. UNETR, where convolutional encoders are replaced with transformers to model long-range spatial dependencies in 3D segmentation, has achieved state-of-the-art results on multiple benchmarks, and enhances the quality of 3D MRI by capturing global contextual information during synthesis [5].

Recently, diffusion models [13] have gained popularity for medical image generation, with successful applications in segmentation and anomaly detection [23]. Denoising Diffusion Probabilistic Models (DDPMs) [13] have demonstrated strong performance in image synthesis tasks; however, they are computationally expensive due to their operation in high-dimensional pixel space. To address this, Rombach et al. [21] introduced Latent Diffusion Models (LDMs), which operate in a learned latent space to reduce training cost while preserving high image quality. LDMs can also be used for paired image-to-image translation, such as MRI sequence conversion. These prior works form the basis for our proposed method, which integrates 2D intensity-based generation and 3D volumetric enhancements, minimizes slice-based artifacts and improves 3D consistency, resulting in enhanced segmentation performance.

3 SLaM-DiMM Methodology

This section contains the discussion of our proposed model SLaM-DiMM which includes missing modality generation (MMG) and coherence enhancement (CEn). Our approach is inspired by recent advances in deep generative modeling, particularly Latent Diffusion Models (LDMs) [21] and Variational Autoencoders (VAEs) [14].

3.1 Missing Modality Generation (MMG)

Our MMG architecture consists of a shared encoder, a Latent Diffusion Model (LDM)-inspired bottleneck, and four modality-specific decoders, as illustrated in Fig. 1. This design enables the model to learn a unified latent representation that captures high-level semantic features common across different MRI modalities while still allowing for modality-specific reconstruction through dedicated decoding. By learning a shared, modality-invariant latent space, the architecture facilitates flexible and accurate cross-modal synthesis, enabling the generation of any target modality from other available input modalities. A 3D brain MRI volume is represented as $X_m \in \mathbb{R}^{H \times W \times D}$, where H, W, D denote the height, width, depth of volume, respectively. Each volume X_m is associated with a specific imaging modality $m \in \{\text{T1w}, \text{T1ce}, \text{Flair}, \text{T2w}\}$.

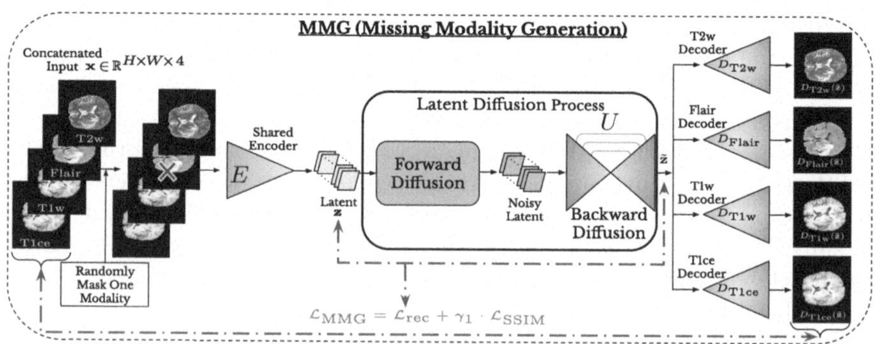

Fig. 1. SLaM-DiMM architecture for multi-modality synthesis.

For computational efficiency during training, we operate on 2D axial slices extracted from the 3D volumes. Specifically, we process individual slices $X_m^f \in \mathbb{R}^{H\times W}$ independently, where $f \in \{1, 2, ..., D\}$ denotes the slice index within a volume. This 2D-slice based approach significantly reduces memory consumption and training time while still preserving the diagnostic quality of the data. During inference, the model progressively processes all slices, generating the corresponding reconstructed 2D slice outputs, which are then concatenated along the depth dimension to reconstruct the full 3D MRI volume.

Encoding Stage: The encoder serves as the first stage of the pipeline, which extracts a lower-dimensional latent representation from the input 2D slices. It takes as input a 4-channel tensor $\mathbf{x} \in \mathbb{R}^{H\times W\times 4}$, where each channel corresponds to one of the four MRI modalities. During training, we simulate missing modalities by randomly masking one of the four input channels with zeros (see Fig. 1). This forces the model to learn robust, shared representations that can infer the missing modality based on the context provided by the remaining three.

The encoder maps the input to a lower-dimensional latent representation $\mathbf{z} = E(\mathbf{x}) \in \mathbb{R}^{h\times w\times d}$ where $E(\cdot)$ denotes the encoder function, and $\mathbf{z}$ is a latent feature map of reduced spatial dimensions $h \times w$ and channel depth d. The encoder follows the design of the downsampling path of the OpenAI UNet [19].

Latent Diffusion Bottleneck Stage: Once the latent $\mathbf{z}$ is obtained, it is passed through a Latent Diffusion Model (LDM) [21]-inspired diffusion-based bottleneck. This bottleneck plays a critical role in refining the latent representation by introducing a stochastic transformation that enhances the semantic richness and generalization capability of the shared latent space across all imaging modalities.

The forward diffusion process, gradually corrupts the latent features $\tilde{\mathbf{z}}_0 = \mathbf{z}$ with Gaussian noise, producing $\tilde{\mathbf{z}}_t$ over a series of time steps $t = 1, \ldots, T$, using: $q(\tilde{\mathbf{z}}_t|\tilde{\mathbf{z}}_{t-1}) = \mathcal{N}\left(\tilde{\mathbf{z}}_t; \sqrt{1-\beta_t}\tilde{\mathbf{z}}_{t-1}, \beta_t\mathbf{I}\right)$, where β_t controls the variance of the noise at timestep t. The full forward process from $\tilde{\mathbf{z}}_0$ to $\tilde{\mathbf{z}}_t$ can then be expressed in closed form as $q(\tilde{\mathbf{z}}_t|\tilde{\mathbf{z}}_0) = \mathcal{N}\left(\tilde{\mathbf{z}}_t; \sqrt{\bar{\alpha}_t}\tilde{\mathbf{z}}_0,\ (1-\bar{\alpha}_t)\mathbf{I}\right)$, where $\alpha_t = 1 - \beta_t$ and $\bar{\alpha}_t = \prod_{s=1}^{t} \alpha_s$. This allows us to directly sample $\tilde{\mathbf{z}}_t$ from $\tilde{\mathbf{z}}_0$ without computing intermediate steps. After T steps, $\tilde{\mathbf{z}}_T$ becomes approximately pure Gaussian noise $\mathcal{N}(0, \mathbf{I})$.

The reverse diffusion process aims to reconstruct the original latent features by learning to iteratively denoise the corrupted representation. It is defined as $p_\theta(\tilde{\mathbf{z}}_{t-1}|\tilde{\mathbf{z}}_t) = \mathcal{N}\left(\tilde{\mathbf{z}}_{t-1}; \mu_\theta(\tilde{\mathbf{z}}_t, t), \Sigma_\theta(\tilde{\mathbf{z}}_t, t)\right)$, where the mean μ_θ and covariance Σ_θ are parameterized by a neural network (OpenAI UNet [19]), with parameters θ. The network is conditioned on the time step t, enabling it to learn distinct denoising behaviors at different stages of the process. This process results in refined, shared latent space features $\tilde{\mathbf{z}}$, which capture modality-invariant features useful for reconstructing all four MRI modalities.

Modality-specific Decoding Stage: To reconstruct different modalities from the shared latent representation $\tilde{\mathbf{z}}$, we employ four independent decoders corresponding to the four modalities T1w, T1ce, Flair, and T2w. These decoders allow the model to preserve modality-specific characteristics while still benefiting from a shared modality-invariant latent representation. For each modality $m \in \{\text{T1w}, \text{T1ce}, \text{Flair}, \text{T2w}\}$, the corresponding decoder $D_m(\cdot)$ maps the shared latent representation back to the image domain: $\widehat{\mathbf{x}}_m = D_m(\tilde{\mathbf{z}}) \in \mathbb{R}^{H \times W}$ where $\widehat{\mathbf{x}}_m$ is the reconstructed output for modality m. The decoders follow the upsampling path of the OpenAI UNet architecture, without skip connections, to ensure that the model relies solely on the shared latent features for reconstruction.

Training and Inference: To ensure accurate reconstruction of all four MRI modalities while preserving the integrity of the latent representation, we define a composite reconstruction loss that includes both image-space and latent-space components as:

$$\mathcal{L}_{\text{rec}} = \underbrace{\sum_{m=1}^{4} \|(\widehat{\mathbf{x}}_m - \mathbf{x}_m) \cdot (1 + \lambda_1 \cdot \mathbf{S})\|_2^2}_{\text{Spatially weighted Image-space reconstruction loss}} + \underbrace{\lambda_2 \cdot \|\tilde{\mathbf{z}} - \mathbf{z}\|_2^2}_{\text{Latent-space consistency loss}}$$

where $\widehat{\mathbf{x}}_m = D_m(U(E(\mathbf{x})))$, $E(\cdot)$ denotes the shared encoder, $U(\cdot)$ represents the latent diffusion bottleneck, $D_m(\cdot)$ denotes the modality-specific decoder for MRI modality $m \in \{\text{T1w}, \text{T1ce}, \text{Flair}, \text{T2w}\}$, and $\|\cdot\|_2^2$ denotes the element-wise squared L2 loss.

The first term defines the spatially weighted image-space reconstruction loss. $\mathbf{S} \in \{0, 1\}^{H \times W}$ is a binary segmentation mask given in the dataset as the ground truth, which highlights regions of interest (anomalous regions). This mask is used to spatially weigh the reconstruction loss, placing higher emphasis on anomalous regions where accurate reconstruction is most vital. λ_1 is a hyperparameter that controls the degree of importance placed on these anomalous regions. Note that the ground truth mask $\mathbf{S}$ is only used in training; during inference, ground truth mask is not necessary.

The second term introduces a latent-space consistency loss to regularize the diffusion bottleneck and prevent excessive information loss during the stochastic refinement process. In the second term, $\mathbf{z} = E(\mathbf{x})$ is the initial latent representation obtained from the encoder, $\tilde{\mathbf{z}}$ is the refined latent representation after passing through the diffusion bottleneck, λ_2 controls the strength of the constraint on latent information preservation. This term ensures that the diffusion process enhances, rather than distorts, the meaningful content of the latent space.

To further improve the perceptual quality of the generated images, we incorporate an SSIM-based loss. This loss measures the structural similarity between the generated outputs and the corresponding ground truth slices: $\mathcal{L}_{\text{SSIM}} = \sum_{m=1}^{4} (1 - \text{SSIM}(\widehat{\mathbf{x}}_m, \mathbf{x}_m))$. This term helps preserve anatomical structures of the synthesized images, especially in complex regions such as anomalies or tissue boundaries.

The total training objective is a weighted combination of the above two losses: $\mathcal{L}_{\text{MMG}} = \mathcal{L}_{\text{rec}} + \gamma_1 \cdot \mathcal{L}_{\text{SSIM}}$, where γ_1 is a hyperparameter that balances the contributions of the SSIM loss component. This composite loss ensures that the model learns to reconstruct missing modalities accurately while maintaining high structural fidelity.

3.2 Coherence Enhancement (CEn)

Following the generation of 2D MRI slices across all modalities and their subsequent concatenation into a 3D volume, we observed a degradation in volumetric coherence. Figure 2 shows an example of an original Glioma slice and an MMG-generated slice from the coronal and sagittal views, where the lack of coherence is observable. This is primarily due to the frame-level training paradigm, which does not explicitly model spatial dependencies between adjacent slices. As a result, the reconstructed volumes may exhibit inter-slice intensity mismatches, structural discontinuities, and loss of anatomical consistency along the depth axis.

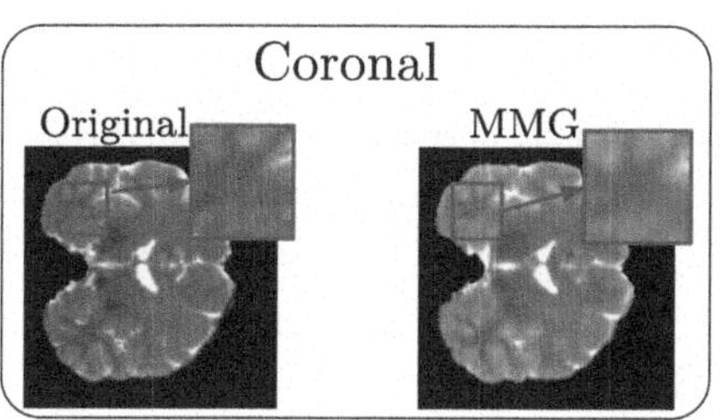

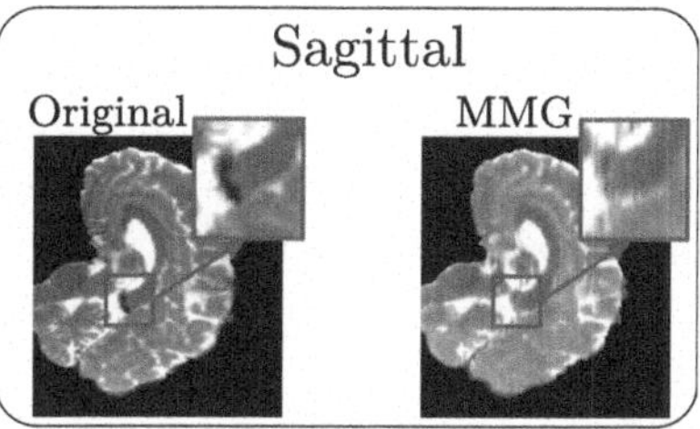

Fig. 2. An example of MMG-generated slices from the coronal plane and sagittal plane views. A comparison between the original and MMG-generated samples reveals inter-slice inconsistencies, evident as vertical blurry lines in the MMG-generated slices, which become more pronounced upon zooming out.

To address this limitation, motivated by [5], we introduce a Coherence Enhancement Network (CEn) based on the 3D-UNETR [12], which integrates transformer-based self-attention mechanisms with a 3D-UNet backbone, enabling it to capture long-range contextual dependencies in 3D space. This enables the network to effectively reduce artifacts and improve anatomical consistency throughout the reconstructed volume.

In our CEn training setup, we utilize the initial reconstructed volume $\widehat{\mathbf{V}}_m \in \mathbb{R}^{H\times W\times D}$, from MMG for each modality m, where H, W, D are the spatial dimensions. The network processes the volume in a fully volumetric manner, refining the inter-slice transitions and aligning anatomical structures across the depth dimension. To manage computational complexity, the synthesized 3D volume of size $H \times W \times D$ is divided into overlapping sub-volumes of size $H \times W \times \frac{D}{s}$, where s is a positive integer referred to as the subvolume factor. This factor controls the depth of each sub-volume. A sliding-window approach with a stride $\frac{D}{2s}$ along the depth dimension is employed to ensure sufficient overlap between adjacent sub-volumes.

The CEn model is trained using a composite reconstruction loss that combines both pixel-wise similarity and perceptual similarity (captured using SSIM),

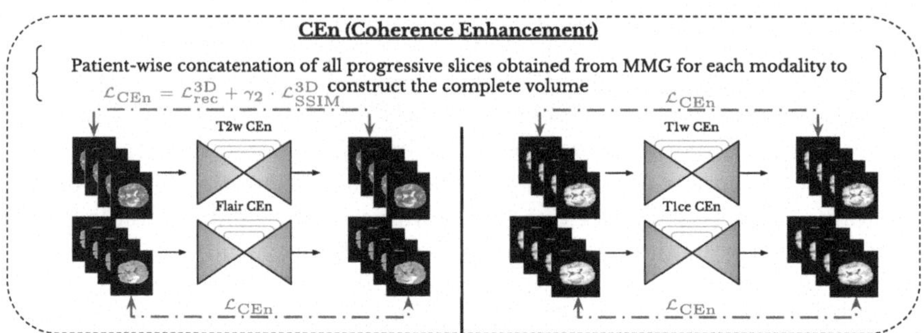

Fig. 3. CEn architecture designed to enhance inter-slice consistency in reconstructed 3D MRI volumes.

between the 3D sub-volumes. The overall CEn loss is defined as a weighted combination: $\mathcal{L}_{\text{CEn}} = \mathcal{L}^{3D}_{\text{rec}} + \gamma_2 \cdot \mathcal{L}^{3D}_{\text{SSIM}}$ where $\gamma_2 \in [0, 1]$ balances the contribution of the SSIM loss component.

4 Experimental Details and Results

4.1 Experimental Setup

All experiments were conducted on an NVIDIA RTX A6000 GPU with 48 GB of memory, using the PyTorch framework. In the MMG model, we employ a configuration of 3 blocks for encoders and decoders in E, D_m, and U, with each block comprising 5 residual sub-blocks. For the diffusion process, time steps are uniformly sampled from the interval $[1, T]$ during training, where $T = 1000$. During inference, we used DDPM sampling with a fixed time step $t_{\text{test}} = \frac{T}{2} = 500$. A linear noise schedule is applied for β_t, ranging from 1×10^{-4} to 2×10^{-2}. The MMG model is trained for a maximum of 1600 epochs, where each epoch consists of processing 500 randomly selected image slices. Optimization is performed using the Adam optimizer with a learning rate of 10^{-4} and a batch size of 4. The reconstruction loss combines multiple components, weighed by hyperparameters $\lambda_1 = 4$ and $\lambda_2 = 2$. To select the optimal value for hyperparameter γ_1, we evaluated the MMG model performance using the SSIM metric with values $\gamma_1 \in \{0.1, 0.25, 0.5, 0.75\}$. The corresponding SSIM scores were 94.59, 94.66, 94.78, and 94.51, respectively. The highest SSIM was achieved at $\gamma_1 = 0.5$, which was therefore used in all experiments.

For the CEn network, a subvolume factor $s = 10$ is used to extract 16-slice subvolumes from each 3D volume, with a stride of $\frac{D}{2s} = 8$ along the depth axis. Training is performed for up to 250 epochs with a batch size of 2, and each epoch includes 100 randomly sampled 3D volumes. Similarly, we conducted experiments to tune γ_2 over the same set of values: $\{0.1, 0.25, 0.5, 0.75\}$. The obtained SSIM scores were 94.84, 94.18, 94.44, and 94.24, respectively. Based on these results, $\gamma_2 = 0.1$ yielded the best performance and was selected for the final model.

4.2 Dataset Details and Preprocessing

The BraSyn-2025 dataset [1–3,16–18,22] is derived from a combination of three publicly available datasets: BraTS-GLI 2023, BraTS-METS 2023, and BraTS-MENINGIOMA. It represents a retrospective multi-institutional collection of brain tumor multi-parametric MRI (mpMRI) scans acquired under standard clinical conditions. These scans vary significantly in image quality and characteristics due to differences in scanner hardware, imaging protocols, and institutional practices, thereby introducing realistic clinical heterogeneity. Expert neuroradiologists have manually reviewed and validated the ground truth annotations for all tumor sub-regions, ensuring high-quality segmentation masks.

The training dataset consists of 1,251 glioma patient volumes and 238 metastasis patient volumes. For validation, the dataset includes 219 glioma and 31 metastasis cases. Each volume contains four MRI modalities: T1-weighted (T1w), T2-weighted (T2w), Flair, and contrast-enhanced T1-weighted (T1ce). Training dataset further contains ground-truth segmentation masks. During training, complete sets of all four modalities are provided in BraSyn-2025 data. In contrast, for validation and testing, one of the modalities is randomly omitted in each sample to evaluate the model's ability to synthesize the missing modality.

Prior to training, we apply intensity normalization by clipping values to the range between the 0.5th and 99.5th percentiles to mitigate outliers. The top and bottom 15 axial slices are removed, and the remaining 3D volumes are decomposed into 2D axial slices, which are saved as individual images for training.

4.3 Quantitative Results

The quantitative performance of the proposed MMG (Missing Modality Generation) and MMG+CEn (MMG with Coherence Enhancement) models is evaluated on the BraSyn2025 validation dataset, which includes 219 Glioma and 31 Metastasis patient volumes. Each model is tasked with synthesizing one of the four MRI modalities (T1w, T2w, Flair, T1ce). The performance metric used is the Structural Similarity Index Measure (SSIM), computed across the entire 3D volume for each modality synthesis task.

Table 1. SSIM (%) comparison of MMG and MMG+CEn for missing modalities. The symbol × indicates missing modality, and ✓ represents available modality.

Modality				**Glioma**		**Metastasis**	
T1w	T2w	Flair	T1ce	MMG	MMG+CEn	MMG	MMG+CEn
×	✓	✓	✓	94.96	94.81	91.61	91.97
✓	×	✓	✓	93.82	93.86	89.61	90.39
✓	✓	×	✓	91.75	91.94	89.41	90.29
✓	✓	✓	×	92.44	92.26	89.67	89.98

Table 2. Dice and HD95 scores for MMG and MMG+CEn methods on Glioma and Metastasis datasets across labels.

	Glioma				Metastasis			
	MMG		MMG+CEn		MMG		MMG+CEn	
	Dice↑	HD95↓	Dice↑	HD95↓	Dice↑	HD95↓	Dice↑	HD95↓
Tumor Core	0.7601	3.6651	0.7301	4.0226	0.5571	11.3043	0.5046	11.9173
Whole Tumor	0.8993	2.1149	0.8876	2.4600	0.8211	10.7675	0.8155	5.1284
Enhancing Tumor	0.7873	3.3372	0.7702	3.6991	0.7912	13.6090	0.7836	7.9839

The results for the MMG and MMG+CEn models are summarized in Table 1, where for the MMG model, the highest SSIM scores are observed for T1w synthesis in Glioma cases (94.96%), and the lowest for Flair in Metastasis cases (89.41%). On average, both MMG and MMG+CEn perform slightly better on Glioma samples compared to Metastasis across all modalities, likely due to the larger number of Glioma samples in the training set. The MMG+CEn model further refines the output of MMG model by enforcing spatial coherence and structural fidelity of the synthesized volume across the depth axis. The results show a marginal improvement in SSIM scores for Metastasis cases compared to the MMG model.

Further, Table 2 presents the Dice and HD95 distance scores for individual segmentation labels (Tumor Core (TC), Whole Tumor (WT), Enhancing Tumor (ET)) on the validation dataset. The segmentation inference is performed using pseudo-labels produced by the BraTS orchestrator model [15], on generated data where, for each sample, one modality is randomly masked and reconstructed using both the MMG and MMG+CEn models. The results show that for Label 3 (ET), both MMG and MMG+CEn achieve comparable performance across the Glioma and Metastasis datasets. For Label 2 (WT), there is a slight performance dip in the Metastasis dataset compared to Glioma. However, for Label 1 (TC),

Table 3. Quantitative results on Test Dataset: Mean and standard deviation in terms of Dice, NSD (0.5), and SSIM scores for Glioma (GLI), Meningioma (MEN), and Combined (ALL).

	Type	Dice ↑			NSD (0.5) ↑			SSIM ↑
		ET	TC	WT	ET	TC	WT	
Glioma	Mean	0.7414	0.8142	0.9168	0.5356	0.4731	0.4885	0.9238
	std dev	0.3032	0.2755	0.0915	0.2893	0.2919	0.1947	0.0516
Meningioma	Mean	0.7150	0.7373	0.7774	0.5638	0.5657	0.5309	0.9331
	std dev	0.3916	0.3775	0.3354	0.3535	0.3522	0.2906	0.0231
ALL	Mean	0.7215	0.7778	0.8572	0.5347	0.4965	0.4899	0.9255
	std dev	0.3375	0.3201	0.2307	0.3105	0.3139	0.2338	0.0448

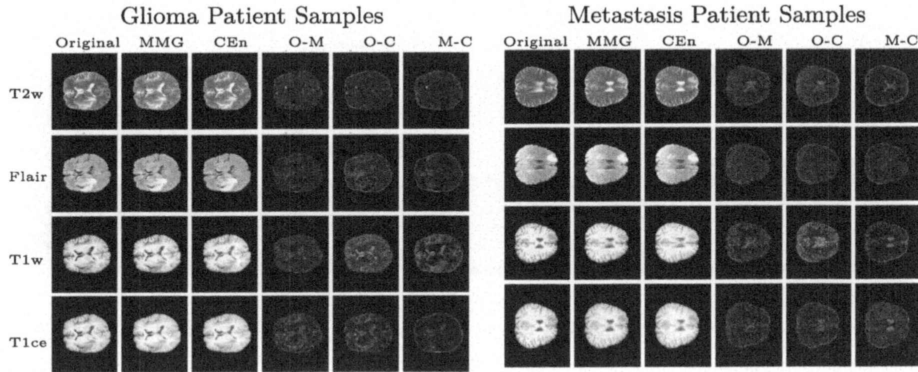

Fig. 4. Qualitative comparison between MMG and MMG+CEn. Columns "O–M", "O–C" and "M–C" denote difference maps between the original and MMG-generated slices, the original and MMG+CEn-generated slices, and the MMG and MMG+CEn generated slices, respectively. These maps highlight the structural modifications introduced by each model.

there is a more significant drop in performance between the two datasets, suggesting that generating or segmenting tumor core is more challenging in metastasis cases.

Table 3 presents the quantitative results of MMG model on the test dataset, as provided by the competition organizers. These results demonstrate the MMG model's strong segmentation performance across both Glioma (GLI) and Meningioma (MEN) cases. The table also reports the combined (ALL) results, which indicate that the MMG model generalizes well across tumor types, obtaining better scores in terms of both Dice (0.86 ± 0.23 for WT) and SSIM (0.93 ± 0.04). Overall, the MMG model performs more consistently on the Glioma dataset while still exhibiting robust cross-domain generalization when evaluated on the other datasets. However it is to be noted that the model can be improved to better the performance in terms of Normalized Surface Distance score (with tolerance 0.5), as demonstrated in the NSD (0.5) results in Table 3. We will take this up as a future work towards improving the model.

4.4 Qualitative Results

Figure 4 presents a qualitative comparison of the synthesized MRI modalities for patients from glioma (left) and metastasis (right) abnormalities. To evaluate generation quality and structural fidelity, difference maps are provided as "O–M", "O–C" and "M–C" in Fig. 4, visualizing pixel-wise deviations between the synthesized results and the ground truth. The "O–M" map (Original vs. MMG) reveals only minor discrepancies across all modalities, indicating that MMG achieves high anatomical consistency and preserves fine structural details with minimal distortion. In contrast, the "O–C" map (Original vs. MMG+CEn) exhibits larger intensity differences in the T1w modality, suggesting that the

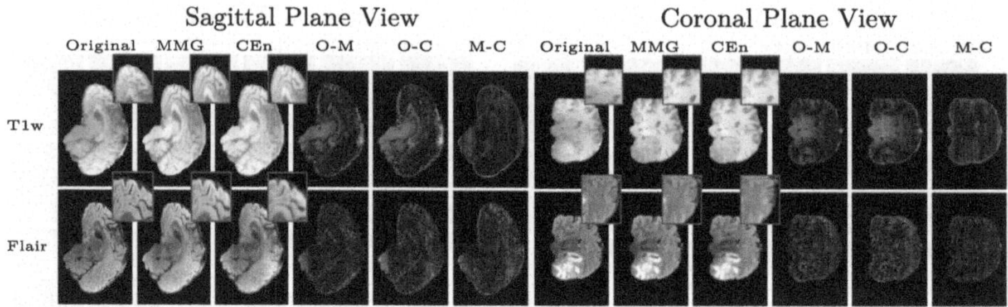

Fig. 5. Qualitative comparison of coronal and sagittal plane views illustrating inter-slice inconsistency present in MMG-generated slices, which is effectively resolved in MMG+CEn-generated slices. Specifically, the "M–C" map highlights the removal of vertical blurry artifacts caused by inter-slice inconsistency.

CEn module induces more noticeable changes relative to the original anatomical structure. The "M–C" map (MMG vs. MMG+CEn) further illustrates these model-level differences. While reconstructions for T2w, Flair, and T1ce remain largely consistent between the two variants, T1w shows higher residual, reflecting significant modifications introduced by the coherence enhancement component.

These changes may arise due to the CEn module training to enhance 3D coherence across slices, addressing potential misalignments or artifacts caused by slice-wise (2D) generation in the MMG model (see Fig. 5). This demonstrates that while MMG excels in per-slice synthesis quality, MMG+CEn prioritizes spatial coherence across depth, making it more suitable for applications where 3D structural integrity is essential.

5 Conclusion

In this paper, we present SLaM-DiMM, a missing brain MRI modality generation framework comprising MMG and CEn modules. MMG built on a diffusion-based architecture, helps learn shared latent representations across modalities, resulting in flexible generation of a desired target MRI modality. The CEn network improves inter-slice structural consistency in the generated 3D volumes, crucial for downstream 3D segmentation tasks. Together, these components enable robust and anatomically plausible modality synthesis, offering a promising solution for medical imaging scenarios with incomplete multimodal data.

Acknowledgment. We gratefully acknowledge Technocraft Centre of Applied Artificial Intelligence (TCAAI), IIT Bombay, for their support through generous funding.

References

1. Baid, U., et al.: The RSNA-ASNR-MICCAI BraTS 2021 Benchmark on Brain Tumor Segmentation and Radiogenomic Classification (2021). https://arxiv.org/abs/2107.02314
2. Bakas, S., et al.: Advancing the cancer genome atlas glioma MRI collections with expert segmentation labels and radiomic features. Sci. Data **4**(1), 1–13 (2017)
3. Bakas, S., et al.: Segmentation labels for the pre-operative scans of the TCGA-LGG collection. Cancer Imaging Archive (2017)
4. Baltruschat, I.M., Janbakhshi, P., Lenga, M.: BraSyn 2023 challenge: missing MRI synthesis and the effect of different learning objectives. In: Brain Tumor Segmentation, and Cross-Modality Domain Adaptation for Medical Image Segmentation: MICCAI Challenges, BraTS 2023 and CrossMoDA 2023, Held in Conjunction with MICCAI 2023, Vancouver, BC, Canada, October 12 and 8, 2024, Proceedings. Springer-Verlag, Berlin, Heidelberg (2023)
5. Cho, J., Park, S., Park, J.: Two-stage approach for brain MR image synthesis: 2D image synthesis and 3D refinement. arXiv preprint arXiv:2410.10269 (2024)
6. Cho, J., Woo, J., Park, J.: A unified framework for synthesizing multisequence brain MRI via hybrid fusion. arXiv preprint arXiv:2406.14954 (2024)
7. Dalmaz, O., Yurt, M., Çukur, T.: ResViT: residual vision transformers for multimodal medical image synthesis. IEEE Trans. Med. Imaging **41**(10), 2598–2614 (2022)
8. Dar, S.U., Yurt, M., Karacan, L., Erdem, A., Erdem, E., Cukur, T.: Image synthesis in multi-contrast MRI with conditional generative adversarial networks. IEEE Trans. Med. Imaging **38**(10), 2375–2388 (2019)
9. Friedrich, P., Durrer, A., Wolleb, J., Cattin, P.C.: cWDM: conditional wavelet diffusion models for cross-modality 3D medical image synthesis. arXiv preprint arXiv:2411.17203 (2024)
10. Friedrich, P., Wolleb, J., Bieder, F., Durrer, A., Cattin, P.C.: WDM: 3D wavelet diffusion models for high-resolution medical image synthesis. In: Deep Generative Models: 4th MICCAI Workshop. DGM4MICCAI 2024, Held in Conjunction with MICCAI 2024, Marrakesh, Morocco, October 10, 2024, Proceedings, pp. 11–21. Springer-Verlag, Berlin, Heidelberg (2024)
11. Hatamizadeh, A., Nath, V., Tang, Y., Yang, D., Roth, H.R., Xu, D.: Swin UNETR: swin transformers for semantic segmentation of brain tumors in MRI images. In: Brainlesion: Glioma, Multiple Sclerosis, Stroke and Traumatic Brain Injuries: 7th International Workshop, BrainLes 2021, Held in Conjunction with MICCAI 2021, Virtual Event, September 27, 2021, Revised Selected Papers, Part I. Springer-Verlag, Berlin, Heidelberg (2021)
12. Hatamizadeh, A., Yang, D., Roth, H.R., Xu, D.: UNETR: transformers for 3D medical image segmentation. In: 2022 IEEE/CVF Winter Conference on Applications of Computer Vision (WACV) (2021)
13. Ho, J., Jain, A., Abbeel, P.: Denoising diffusion probabilistic models. In: Proceedings of the 34th International Conference on Neural Information Processing Systems (NIPS) (2020)
14. Kingma, D.P., Welling, M.: An introduction to variational autoencoders. Found. Trends® Mach. Learn. **12**(4), 307–392 (2019). https://doi.org/10.1561/2200000056
15. Kofler, F., et al.: BraTS orchestrator : democratizing and disseminating state-of-the-art brain tumor image analysis (2025). https://arxiv.org/abs/2506.13807

16. Li, H.B., et al.: The Brain Tumor Segmentation (BraTS) Challenge 2023: Brain MR Image Synthesis for Tumor Segmentation (BraSyn) (2024). https://arxiv.org/abs/2305.09011
17. Menze, B.H., et al.: The multimodal brain tumor image segmentation benchmark (BRATS). IEEE Trans. Med. Imaging **34**(10), 1993–2024 (2014)
18. Moawad, A.W., et al.: Bend: the brain tumor segmentation (BraTS-METS) Challenge 2023: Brain Metastasis Segmentation on Pre-treatment MRI (2024). https://arxiv.org/abs/2306.00838
19. Nichol, A., Dhariwal, P.: Improved denoising diffusion probabilistic models. In: ICML (2021)
20. Pang, H., Guo, W., Ye, C.: Multi-modal brain MRI synthesis based on Swin-UNETR. arXiv preprint arXiv:2506.02467 (2025)
21. Rombach, R., Blattmann, A., Lorenz, D., Esser, P., Ommer, B.: High-resolution image synthesis with latent diffusion models. In: 2022 IEEE/CVF Conference on Computer Vision and Pattern Recognition (CVPR) (2021)
22. Spyridon, B., et al.: Segmentation labels and radiomic features for the pre-operative scans of the TCGA-GBM collection. Cancer Imaging Archive (2017)
23. Wyatt, J., Leach, A., Schmon, S.M., Willcocks, C.G.: AnoDDPM: anomaly detection with denoising diffusion probabilistic models using simplex noise. In: Proceedings of the IEEE/CVF Conference on Computer Vision and Pattern Recognition (2022)

Controllable Diffusion-Based Generation for MRI

Haoran Zhang[1] and Wesley Tansey[2](✉)

[1] University of Texas at Austin, Austin, TX 78712, USA
hz6453@utexas.edu
[2] Memorial Sloan Kettering Cancer Center, New York, NY 10065, USA
tanseyw@mskcc.org

Abstract. Magnetic resonance imaging (MRI) provides spatial, multi-channel volumetric data, where each channel captures complementary features of underlying anatomy or pathology. However, in practice, one or more of these channels can be missing due to time constraints and motion artifacts. This limits the applicability of current MRI-based diagnosis pipelines and motivates the need for robust MRI synthesis. In this work, we trained a unified diffusion framework (DiffuseMRI) for controllable MRI sequence synthesis based on DiffuseTME, designed to handle high-dimensional, spatially aligned volumetric data with complex inter-channel relationships. Our model features two key components: (1) a hierarchical feature injection mechanism that enables multi-resolution conditioning on spatially aligned observed MRI sequences, and (2) channel-wise attention modules to model the dependencies across MRI sequences. To generalize across arbitrary missing sequences, we train the model using a random masking strategy, allowing DiffuseMRI to reconstruct any missing sequences while preserving anatomical consistency. Our framework is evaluated on the BraSyn benchmark, part of BraTS challenge in MICCAI 2025, which standardizes the evaluation of MRI synthesis methods for downstream brain tumor segmentation.

Keywords: Diffusion model · Conditional generation · Amortized training

1 Introduction

Magnetic Resonance Imaging (MRI) is widely used in brain tumor diagnosis and treatment planning, offering non-invasive and high-soft-contrast imaging across multiple tissue types. It is an indispensable tool in clinical workflows, providing information for the detection, characterization, and monitoring of brain tumors. Multiple MRI signals, such as non-contrast T1-weighted (T1N), contrast-enhanced T1 (T1CE), T2-weighted (T2W), and T2-weighted fluid attenuated inversion recovery (FLAIR), capture complementary information about tumor structure, edema, and infiltration. However, in practice, some

S. Bakas et al. (Eds.): MICCAI 2025, LNCS 16377, pp. 79–88, 2026.
https://doi.org/10.1007/978-3-032-16370-7_7

MRI modalities may not be available due to patient motion, scan time constraints, or acquisition artifacts [3]. The missing channel issue limits downstream clinical assessments, such as tumor segmentation, which typically rely on the complete set of MRI sequences for optimal performance.

To address the challenge of missing MRI sequences, accurate and clinically reliable synthesis methods are required. The goal is to generate a missing MRI sequence from the observed ones. This task has gained increasing attention through the Brain MRI Synthesis for BraTS (BraSyn), a track of the BraTS challenge [3]. The BraSyn task specifically focuses on synthesizing one missing sequence (e.g., T1CE) given the remaining three (T1N, T2W, FLAIR), to generate missing MRI data that can support downstream clinical tasks such as tumor segmentation. Recent methods based on convolutional neural networks (CNNs), Transformers, and generative adversarial networks (GANs) have demonstrated promising results in missing MRI sequence generation [4,7,12]. However, current approaches face several key limitations:

1. While MRI sequences are spatially aligned, the correlations between them are complex, reflecting the heterogeneous composition of brain tissue, especially in tumor regions. These inter-channel relationships can be sparse, nonlinear, and asymmetric, driven by varying biophysical contrast mechanisms across channels. Capturing these structured dependencies is important for reliable synthesis, yet existing methods often overlook these interchannel relationships.
2. Most existing methods train a separate model for each condition-target sequence combination (e.g., T1N+T1CE+T2W to FLAIR), requiring four distinct models to impute the standard four-sequence MRI protocol. This setup is not only inefficient, but the number of models needed also scales linearly with the number of source-target sequence combinations. It significantly limits the ability to generalize to more MRI sequences, such as diffusion-weighted imaging (DWI), diffusion-tensor imaging (DTI), and perfusion-weighted imaging (PWI), which offer richer physiological or vascular information.
3. These modality-specific models assume fixed condition-target combinations, and thus cannot adapt to scenarios where an arbitrary subset of modalities is missing. This reduces their clinical applicability, where missingness patterns vary between patients or more than one sequence is missing.

Recently, diffusion models have emerged as a powerful class of generative models capable of generating high-quality natural images with spatial conditions [14] and show great potential in medical and biological imaging [13]. In this work, we adapt the controllable diffusion-based generative framework from DiffuseTME [13] to tackle the problem of missing-sequence MRI synthesis, which was initially developed for high-dimensional biological imaging data (e.g., spatial proteomics).

Our model (DiffuseMRI) is designed to handle arbitrary combinations of observed and missing MRI channels while preserving spatial fidelity and modeling inter-channel relationships. Unlike prior works that treat modalities as fixed input-output mappings, our approach enables training a single model that generalizes to all MRI sequences. To achieve this, DiffuseMRI inherits three key components from DiffuseTME designed for controllable generation on high-dimensional data: (1) a hierarchical feature injection mechanism that injects the multi-resolution spatial features learnt from the observed signals to the synthesis network, (2) two versions of channel attention modules to model semantic relationships between channels explicitly, and (3) a random masking training strategy that amortizes over the conditional space and enables dynamic test time conditioning. Together, these components allow our model to generate MRI data with high fidelity on different target sequences within a unified diffusion framework. Our model achieves state-of-the-art results in both structural similarity and segmentation benchmarks.

2 Method

DiffuseMRI builds upon our prior work on controllable diffusion-based generation for multi-channel biological imaging data (DiffuseTME) [13]. DiffuseTME developed a flexible generative model capable of handling high-dimensional biological image data, like imaging mass cytometry, with complex inter-channel dependencies and spatial alignment. Here, we adopt the same framework and architectural components to address the challenge of missing MRI sequence synthesis. While the MRI data differ from spatial proteomic data in the number of channels (4 in MRI vs. 20–64 in proteomics), both domains share key structural features: (1) channels represent distinct but spatially aligned views of the same underlying sample; (2) arbitrary subsets of channels can be missing; and (3) inter-channel correlations are sparse, nonlinear, and often context-dependent. Therefore, the DiffuseTME framework is naturally suited to this domain with minimal adaptation.

2.1 Model Architecture

We retain the core backbone architecture and condition injection mechanisms introduced in DiffuseTME. The model is based on the EDM diffusion framework [8] with an additional spatial condition branch, where observed sequences serve as spatially aligned conditioning signals to guide the synthesis of missing MRI modalities.

To synthesize missing MRI sequences from arbitrary observed subsets, the model must (1) preserve spatial alignment between observed conditions and synthesis outputs, and (2) adaptively model the semantic relationships across modalities. We address these requirements through two key architectural components: hierarchical feature injection and channel attention.

Hierarchical feature injection We condition the diffusion generation by injecting features learned from the observed sequences at multiple resolutions by an auxiliary conditional branch. The observed MRI signals are first encoded through a sequence of UNet blocks of decreasing latent dimensions, producing multi-scale feature maps. These features are then injected into the corresponding decoder blocks of the main denoising branch through additive connections with channel-specific weights. Such injections preserve the spatial alignment between the observed and synthesized modalities through the pixel-wise addition. This multi-scale conditioning also allows the model to incorporate both low-level textures and high-level structures from the available inputs.

MRI sequences exhibit structured but asymmetric dependencies: for instance, FLAIR and T2W are often redundant in peritumoral regions but differ in signal characteristics elsewhere. To capture such context-dependent relationships, we apply the two styles of channel attention modules.

Soft channel attention Inspired by the Squeeze-and-Excitation (SE) network [6], DiffuseTME introduced the lightweight attention mechanism. Given a latent feature map $z \in \mathbb{R}^{D \times H \times W}$, we compute

$$\begin{aligned} \alpha &= \mathrm{GAP}(z) \\ w &= \sigma\left(W_2 \cdot \phi(W_1 \cdot \alpha)\right) \\ z' &= w \cdot z \end{aligned} \tag{1}$$

where ϕ is a non-linearity (e.g., ReLU), GAP stands for global average pooling, and σ is the sigmoid function. This mechanism learns global feature weights and injects spatial conditions adaptively into the hierarchical feature injection mechanism.

Full channel attention Following the standard attention mechanism that attends over pixels, DiffuseTME modified it and attends over different channels and captures inter-channel relationships,

$$\begin{aligned} &x_{\text{flat}} \in \mathbb{R}^{D \times N}, \quad N = H \times W, \\ &Q = x_{\text{flat}} W_Q, \quad K = x_{\text{flat}} W_K, \quad V = x_{\text{flat}} W_V \end{aligned} \tag{2}$$

$$A = \mathrm{softmax}\left(\frac{QK^\top}{\sqrt{d}}\right), \quad x'_{\text{flat}} = AV\,. \tag{3}$$

2.2 Uniform Random Masking

We follow the random masking training strategy from DiffuseTME to enable flexible conditioning and test-time generalization. In the original formulation, channels are masked by independent Bernoulli random variables, and the model was trained to reconstruct all channels. This amortized training approach allows a single model to learn conditional generation over the entire power set of channel configurations and minimizes the amortized loss

$$\mathbb{E}_{c \sim P(c)} \mathbb{E}_{t, x_0, \epsilon}\left[||\epsilon - \epsilon_\theta(x_t, t, c)||^2\right] \tag{4}$$

However, brain MRI typically consists of only four input sequences: T1N, T1CE, T2W, and FLAIR. Using independent Bernoulli random variables to determine masking introduces a high variance in the conditional distribution $P(c)$, resulting in uneven coverage of the conditioning space during training. This problem can degrade learning and stability. On the other hand, in the BraTS synthesis setting, the test-time task always involves exactly one missing modality, with the other three available.

Therefore, DiffuseMRI replaces the Bernoulli random masking with a uniform categorical masking strategy Algorithm 1: during training, we randomly select one of the four MRI channels to mask uniformly and use the remaining three as conditioning input.

Algorithm 1 Uniform random masking strategy for missing MRI sequence synthesis in DiffuseMRI.

Require: Full data $x \in \mathbb{R}^{4\times H\times W}$, masking prob. p

1: **for** each training iteration **do**

2: Sample masked channel $M \sim Uni(\{0,\ldots,C\})$

3: Construct condition c such that

$$c_i = \begin{cases} x_i, & \text{if } i \neq M \\ 0, & \text{if } i = M \end{cases}$$

4: Diffusion step with target x and condition c

5: **end for**

2.3 Training Strategy

The model takes the 4-channel MRI data as conditional input and is trained to reconstruct all four MRI sequences, as well as the associated tumor segmentation mask, producing five output channels in total.

This design offers several advantages:

1. It aligns the training and test-time distributions, reducing generalization mismatch.
2. It maintains the flexibility of the diffusion framework while avoiding unnecessary complexity in the conditioning space.
3. Predicting the segmentation mask as an auxiliary target guides the model to learn latent representations that are semantically aligned with tumor regions, which improves sample quality and provides free segmentation output during inference.

By combining uniform random masking with joint prediction of modalities and segmentation, we ensure DiffuseMRI focuses on clinically relevant features such as tumor boundaries, while maintaining generalization to different missing-sequence conditions in a controlled and amortized fashion.

Loss function. DiffuseMRI uses the diffusion denoising loss in Eq. (4). The four MRI modalities and the tumor mask are stacked as a 5-channel output tensor. One of the four MRI modalities is randomly masked during training, and the model jointly reconstructs all five channels under the same diffusion loss. Importantly, the segmentation mask is not part of the conditioning input, and no separate segmentation loss is used.

Preprocessing. Following BraTS protocols, all MR images were skull-stripped, registered in a common atlas, and resampled to a 1 mm isotropic resolution. The MRI signal is clipped at the 99.5-percentile and linearly normalized to the range $[-1, 1]$. All signals in the masked-out channels are set to 0, according to the random masking procedure in algorithm 1.

Training setup. The model was trained for 50 epochs with a batch size of 32 using the Adam optimizer ($lr = 1 \times 10^{-4}, \beta_1 = 0.9, \beta_2 = 0.999$). Training was performed on four NVIDIA A100 GPUs and completed in around 12 hours.

3 Results

We evaluate our model on the BraSyn2025 dataset [9], consisting of MRI samples from both glioma [1,2,10] and metastases patients. Specifically, for each sample, we randomly drop one modality using the `dropout_modality.py` script provided in the official tutorial, and we use the remaining three MRI sequences to synthesize the missing one Fig. 1. We compare our performance against pix2pix [7], HF-GAN [4], and SwinUNETR [12] Table 1.

3.1 Metrics

Structural similarity To quantify the accuracy of the generated MRI volumes, we compute the Structural Similarity Index (SSIM) between the synthesized and ground truth sequences. We note that the global SSIM can be artificially inflated in 3D MRI due to the dominance of background voxels. To address this, we report three SSIM metrics for each sample:

1. $\text{SSIM}_{\text{global}}$ computed across the full 3D volume.
2. $\text{SSIM}_{\text{tissue}}$ computed only within the brain tissue region, which is defined as the union of all non-zero voxels across the four sequences in ground truth.
3. $\text{SSIM}_{\text{tumor}}$ computed within the tumor region, which is defined by the binarized ground truth segmentation mask.

Segmentation-based metric To assess the clinical utility of the synthesized MRI sequence, we compare the pathologist's tumor segmentation annotation with the segmentation results based on the synthesized sequence combined with the observed ones. Segmentation accuracy is quantified using the DICE coefficient for three tumor sub-regions: enhancing tumor (ET), whole tumor (WT), and tumor core (TC). The segmentation masks used in DICE calculation are determined by GliGAN [5] and SegResNet [11] for glioma and metastases respectively; both methods are implemented in the `brats` package. Since the ground truth tumor segmentation is not available in the validation set, the benchmarks in Table 1 are calculated on a held-out set from the training set that consists of an equal number of samples from both the Glioma and Metastases datasets ($n = 50$).

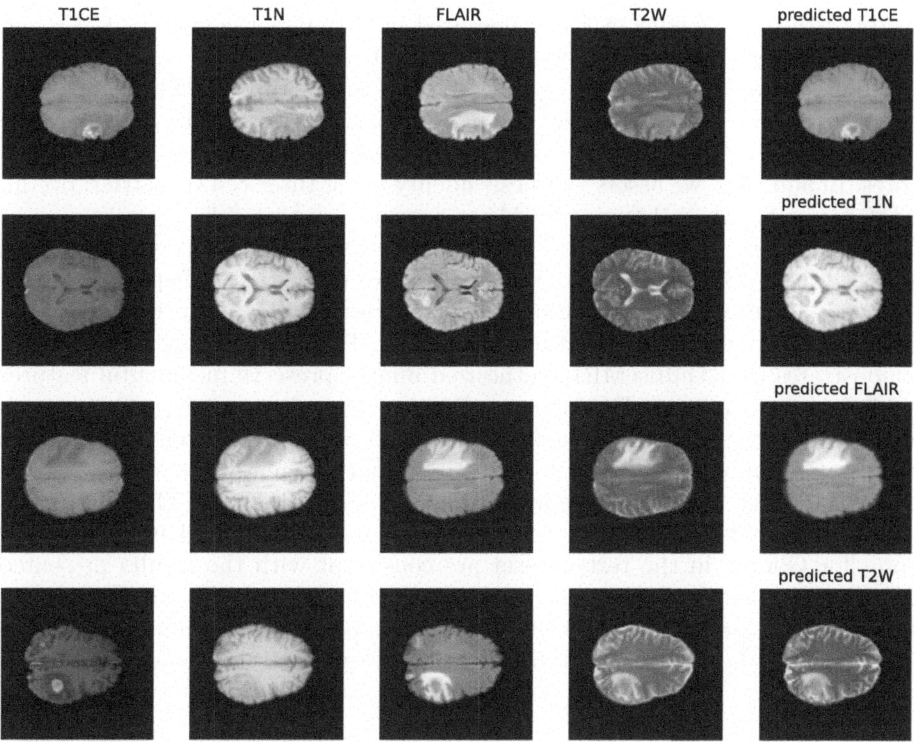

Fig. 1. Visualization of missing modality imputation results for each MRI channel (T1N, T1CE, T2W, and FLAIR). Each row shows the ground truth observations of a slice from a sample, together with the synthesis result. In inference, the corresponding target sequence is masked out.

Table 1. Comparison of segmentation accuracy and structural similarity across different synthesis methods. Our method outperforms adversarial baselines (pix2pix), as well as the winner (HF-GAN) and runner-up (SwinUNETR) of BraSyn 2024 and achieves the best DICE and SSIM scores across tumor, tissue, and global regions.

Method	DICE ↑	$\text{SSIM}_{\text{tumor}}$ ↑	$\text{SSIM}_{\text{health}}$ ↑	$\text{SSIM}_{\text{tissue}}$ ↑	$\text{SSIM}_{\text{global}}$ ↑
pix2pix	0.549	0.719	0.570	0.583	0.807
HF-GAN	0.714	0.761	0.604	0.615	0.919
SwinUNETR	0.709	0.759	0.628	0.637	0.916
DiffuseMRI	**0.738**	**0.774**	**0.631**	**0.643**	**0.928**

3.2 Performance

We compare the performance of our model against three representative baselines in the BraSyn synthesis setting: pix2pix [7], HF-GAN [4], and SwinUNETR [12].

Pix2pix is a conditional GAN baseline used in the official demo. HF-GAN and SwinUNETR are the winner and runner-up of BraSyn2024.

All models are evaluated using the same test-time setup: given three observed modalities, the model synthesizes the missing one. The synthesized volumes are then used as inputs for downstream segmentation, and evaluated using DICE scores. In addition, we assess synthesis fidelity using three SSIM metrics: overall SSIM, tissue SSIM, and tumor SSIM, as described in sect. 3.1.

Table 1 shows the benchmark results. DiffuseMRI outperforms all baselines across all three SSIM metrics and the DICE score. While HF-GAN performs competitively, DiffuseMRI shows improvement in tissue SSIM, reflecting the accuracy in fine-grained tissue structures generation. The improvement in $\mathrm{SSIM}_{\mathrm{tumor}}$ demonstrates that DiffuseMRI-synthesized images preserve meaningful features for clinical segmentation. For further validation for each tumor type, we also calculate the class-specific (Glioma vs. Metastases) SSIM of each missing sequence in the validation dataset Table 2. Since the tumor segmentation is not available in the validation set, we only report $\mathrm{SSIM}_{\mathrm{global}}$ and $\mathrm{SSIM}_{\mathrm{tissue}}$. The test performance on the hidden test dataset is reported as in Table 3. The DICE and SSIM scores for Glioma in the test dataset are consistent with the results presented in Table 1, further confirming the robustness of our method. On the other hand, the scores for Meningioma, which is not included in the training set, remain comparable to those for Glioma, highlighting the generalizability of DiffuseMRI.

Table 2. Class-specific SSIM on the synthesis results for Glioma and Metastases

		$\mathrm{SSIM}_{\mathrm{global}} \uparrow$	$\mathrm{SSIM}_{\mathrm{tissue}} \uparrow$
Metastases	T1N	0.932	0.657
	T1CE	0.931	0.664
	T2W	0.933	0.668
	FLAIR	0.932	0.669
Glioma	T1N	0.959	0.784
	T1CE	0.963	0.791
	T2W	0.965	0.798
	FLAIR	0.959	0.766

4 Discussion

We presented DiffuseMRI, a diffusion-based generative model for MRI sequence imputation, evaluated on the BraTS 2025 missing sequence synthesis benchmark. DiffuseMRI demonstrates strong performance in both structural similarity and segmentation accuracy, as measured by DICE and SSIM scores, outperforming prior state-of-the-art models, such as HF-GAN and SwinUNETR. Notably, our

Table 3. Test performance (Mean and Std) of DiffuseMRI for Glioma (GLI), Meningioma (MEN), and the combined cohort (ALL).

Group	Type	$DICE_{ET}$	$Dice_{TC}$	$DICE_{WT}$	$NSD_{0.5_{ET}}$	$NSD_{0.5_{TC}}$	$NSD_{0.5_{WT}}$	SSIM
GLI	Mean	0.7312	0.7956	0.9101	0.5186	0.4582	0.4738	0.9239
GLI	Std	0.3013	0.2848	0.1008	0.2951	0.2980	0.1935	0.0503
MEN	Mean	0.7060	0.7146	0.7655	0.5560	0.5546	0.5209	0.9280
MEN	Std	0.3995	0.3928	0.3480	0.3552	0.3585	0.2942	0.0149
ALL	Mean	0.7125	0.7594	0.8505	0.5219	0.4838	0.4777	0.9249
ALL	Std	0.3386	0.3298	0.2375	0.3142	0.3197	0.2341	0.0410

generated modalities not only visually resemble the ground truth but also yield superior segmentation outcomes, highlighting the clinical utility of our model.

A key distinction between our method and prior work lies in its unified architecture. Existing approaches typically require training four separate models, one for each missing modality (T1N, T1CE, T2W, FLAIR). In contrast, our model is trained only once to handle arbitrary missing-sequence combinations and produces high-quality outputs across all target channels simultaneously. Furthermore, our model is trained jointly with a segmentation head, enabling it to directly produce tumor segmentations alongside synthesized MRI volumes, which further simplifies the workflow.

Looking forward, a promising extension is to incorporate emerging advanced MRI sequences, such as perfusion-weighted imaging (PWI) and diffusion tensor imaging (DTI). These modalities are not widely available in clinical setups due to scan time and technological limitations. Future projects that train the model to synthesize such sequences from standard MRI modalities (T1, T1CE, T2, FLAIR) could significantly enhance the diagnostic power of routine MRI scans and further establish diffusion-based synthesis as a flexible and general framework for modality completion in medical imaging.

References

1. Baid, U., et al.: The RSNA-ASNR-MICCAI BraTS 2021 benchmark on brain tumor segmentation and radiogenomic classification (2021). https://arxiv.org/abs/2107.02314
2. Bakas, S., et al.: Advancing the cancer genome atlas glioma MRI collections with expert segmentation labels and radiomic features. Sci. Data **4**(1), 170117 (2017)
3. Baltruschat, I.M., Janbakhshi, P., Lenga, M.: BraSyn 2023 challenge: missing MRI synthesis and the effect of different learning objectives (2024). https://arxiv.org/abs/2403.07800
4. Cho, J., Park, S., Park, J.: Two-stage approach for brain MR image synthesis: 2d image synthesis and 3D refinement (2024). https://arxiv.org/abs/2410.10269
5. Ferreira, A., et al.: How we won brats 2023 adult glioma challenge? just faking it! enhanced synthetic data augmentation and model ensemble for brain tumour segmentation (2024). https://arxiv.org/abs/2402.17317

6. Hu, J., Shen, L., Sun, G.: Squeeze-and-excitation networks. In: Proceedings of the IEEE Conference on Computer Vision and Pattern Recognition, pp. 7132–7141 (2018)
7. Isola, P., Zhu, J.Y., Zhou, T., Efros, A.A.: Image-to-image translation with conditional adversarial networks. In: Proceedings of the IEEE conference on computer vision and pattern recognition, pp. 1125–1134 (2017)
8. Karras, T., Aittala, M., Aila, T., Laine, S.: Elucidating the design space of diffusion-based generative models. In: Advances in Neural Information Processing Systems (2022)
9. Li, H.B., et al.: The brain tumor segmentation (BraTS) challenge 2023: brain MR image synthesis for tumor segmentation (BraSyn) (2024). https://arxiv.org/abs/2305.09011
10. Menze, B.H., et al.: The multimodal brain tumor image segmentation benchmark (BRATS). IEEE Trans. Med. Imaging **34**(10), 1993–2024 (2015). https://doi.org/10.1109/TMI.2014.2377694
11. Myronenko, A., Yang, D., He, Y., Xu, D.: Automated 3d segmentation of kidneys and tumors in MICCAI KiTS 2023 challenge (2023). https://arxiv.org/abs/2310.04110
12. Pang, H., Guo, W., Ye, C.: Multi-modal brain MRI synthesis based on SwinUNETR (2025). https://arxiv.org/abs/2506.02467
13. Zhang, H., Zhou, M., Tansey, W.: Controllable diffusion-based generation for multi-channel biological data (2025). https://arxiv.org/abs/2507.02902
14. Zhang, L., Rao, A., Agrawala, M.: Adding conditional control to text-to-image diffusion models. In: ICCV (2023)

Challenge 9 – BraTS-Inpainting

A Biophysically-Conditioned Generative Framework for 3D Brain Tumor MRI Synthesis

Valentin Biller[1], Lucas Zimmer[1,2], Can Erdur[1], Sandeep Nagar[1], Daniel Rückert[1,2,3], Niklas Bubeck[1,2], and Jonas Weidner[1,2](✉)

[1] Technical University of Munich, Munich, Germany
{valentin.biller,niklas.bubeck,j.weidner}@tum.de
[2] Munich Center for Machine Learning (MCML), Munich, Germany
[3] Imperial College London, London, UK

Abstract. Magnetic resonance imaging (MRI) inpainting supports numerous clinical and research applications. We introduce the first generative model that conditions on voxel-level, continuous tumor concentrations to synthesize high-fidelity brain tumor MRIs. For the BraTS 2025 Inpainting Challenge[1](Profil-ID:3504517), we adapt this architecture to the complementary task of healthy tissue restoration by setting the tumor concentrations to zero. Our latent diffusion model conditioned on both tissue segmentations and the tumor concentrations generates 3D spatially coherent and anatomically consistent images for both tumor synthesis and healthy tissue inpainting. For healthy inpainting, we achieve a PSNR of 18.5, and for tumor inpainting, we achieve 17.4. Our code is available at: https://github.com/valentin-biller/ldm.git

Keywords: Medical Generative Model · 3D Diffusion Model · Latent Diffusion Model · Conditional Diffusion Model · Brain MRI · Brain Tumor Generation · Healthy Brain Generation · Medical Image Inpainting

1 Introduction

A wide range of automated analysis tools for brain MRI is available for clinical decision support. However, these tools often assume healthy anatomy, limiting their reliability when applied to pathological images. For brain tumor patients, this mismatch is particularly relevant, as MRI typically commences post-diagnosis when lesions are already present. This limits the effectiveness of algorithms that depend on healthy anatomical priors, such as parcellation, tissue segmentation, or brain extraction. Data-driven generative models can synthesize healthy tissue by inpainting or reconstructing resection cavities while preserving surrounding anatomical structures. These models can also be leveraged to

N. Bubeck and J. Weidner—Equal contribution.

S. Bakas et al. (Eds.): MICCAI 2025, LNCS 16377, pp. 91–101, 2026.
https://doi.org/10.1007/978-3-032-16370-7_8

generate anatomically consistent tumorous images. To generate realistic healthy tissue, establishing a method for tumor synthesis supports a unified framework that benefits from learning both tasks. As tumor synthesis has been studied more extensively, it serves as a logical starting point for reviewing prior work before addressing inpainting as a downstream application.

Early efforts in tumor image synthesis relied on 2D generation or the use of convolutional architectures [21,24]. Diffusion models have recently emerged as state-of-the-art for high-fidelity image synthesis. Operating the diffusion process in a compressed latent space further improves efficiency and memory footprint [18]. While most medical implementations remain restricted to 2D slices, recent work demonstrates fully 3D diffusion for volumetric CT and MRI [4]. Building on these advances, we employ a 3D latent diffusion framework that preserves inter-slice consistency, avoiding the misalignment artifacts reported for slice-wise approaches [14].

Most generative approaches for brain tumors rely on discrete tumor segmentation masks [8,21]. While effective for defining gross tumor geometry, these masks lack biological realism, treating tumor regions as uniformly dense and failing to capture infiltrative growth. Since gliomas often extend beyond MRI-visible margins, biophysical tumor growth modeling provides a means to reveal this hidden infiltration and reduces reliance on standard uniform treatment margins, which do not account for patient-specific tumor spread [3,22]. By conditioning our models on continuous tumor concentrations generated through such growth modeling, we overcome the limitations of discrete masks [2,3,5,9,22,23]. These scalar fields encode spatially varying tumor density, capturing both the visible tumor bulk and subtle infiltration into surrounding tissue, while providing fine-grained control over lesion appearance. By leveraging biophysically grounded priors, our approach better aligns with clinical reality.

We evaluate our method on the Brain MR Image Inpainting Challenge [13] by setting the tumor concentration to zero, effectively asking the model to remove the lesion. Quantitative and qualitative results confirm that the same network can act as a controllable tumor generator and an anatomically aware inpainting tool.

Our contributions are threefold:

- We developed the first 3D generative brain tumor MRI model, which is conditioned on continuous tumor concentrations generated by biophysical tumor growth models.
- We show that the same model excels at healthy brain inpainting under the zeroed condition.
- Our pipeline can easily be extended to further modalities like different MRI sequences or PET.

2 Method

Our proposed method, illustrated in Fig. 1, is a two-stage 3D latent diffusion framework designed for anatomically consistent brain tumor MRI synthesis and inpainting. We condition a latent diffusion model on both the tissue segmentations and a continuous tumor concentration, which encodes spatially varying tumor cell density and is generated by a biophysical growth model. This scalar field enables fine-grained control over lesion appearance, allowing the model to synthesize realistic tumor-bearing images or, by setting the concentration to zero, perform healthy tissue inpainting.

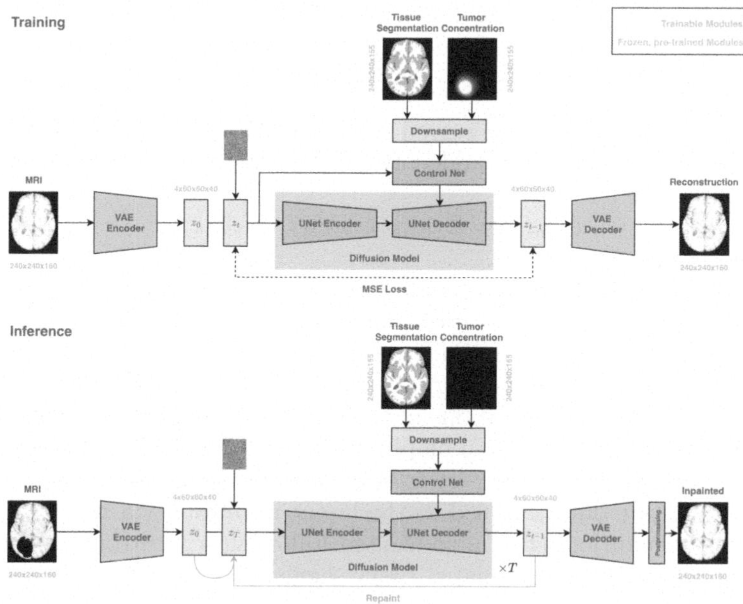

Fig. 1. For the training of our model, we input the tissue segmentations and tumor concentrations as conditions to the latent diffusion model. During inference, we set the tumor concentration to 0 to inpaint the voided regions as healthy brain tissue.

2.1 Overview

Autoencoder. To efficiently represent high-resolution 3D brain MR images, we adopt the pretrained variational autoencoder (VAE) from the MAISI framework [10] to map input T1-weighted volumes into a compact latent space. Formally, given an input image volume $\mathbf{x} \in \mathbb{R}^{240\times240\times155}$, the encoder network E_ϕ produces a latent distribution $q_\phi(\mathbf{z}|\mathbf{x})$, parameterized by a mean and variance, from which a latent code $\mathbf{z} \in \mathbb{R}^{4\times60\times60\times40}$ is sampled via the reparameterization trick. This compression reduces the spatial resolution by a factor of 4 in each dimension while preserving semantically relevant anatomical features. The decoder network D_θ reconstructs the image from the latent representation, yielding $\hat{\mathbf{x}} = D_\theta(\mathbf{z})$. The VAE used in our pipeline is a pretrained model, trained independently of the inpainting task. Its parameters (ϕ, θ) are kept fixed throughout all stages of our method. This latent encoding significantly reduces computational cost and memory footprint during training and inference.

Latent Diffusion. We employ a generative model based on the Denoising Diffusion Probabilistic Models (DDPM) framework [11], which learns to reverse a forward diffusion process defined over latent variables. The forward process progressively perturbs a clean latent sample z_0 into a sequence of noisy versions $\{z_t\}_{t=1}^{T}$ according to the marginal distribution:

$$q(z_t \mid z_0) = \mathcal{N}(\sqrt{\bar{\alpha}_t} z_0, (1 - \bar{\alpha}_t)\mathbf{I}), \tag{1}$$

where $\{\bar{\alpha}_t\}_{t=1}^{T}$ is the level of preserved signal. A 3D U-Net $\epsilon_\theta(z_t, t)$ is trained to estimate the noise component ϵ added at each timestep, minimizing the following objective:

$$\mathcal{L}_{\text{gen}}(z) = \mathbb{E}_{z_0,\epsilon,t}\left[\|\epsilon_\theta(z_t, t) - \epsilon\|_2^2\right]. \tag{2}$$

Tissue and Tumor Conditioning. Anatomical conditioning is provided via one-hot encoded tissue segmentations for cerebrospinal fluid (CSF), gray matter (GM), and white matter (WM), obtained through atlas-based registration using the `gbm_bench`[1] framework. Additionally, a continuous scalar field denoting voxel-wise tumor concentrations in the range $[0, 1]$ is used to encode relative tumor cell density, derived from a biophysical growth model [22]. For inpainting, these tumor concentrations are set to zero to indicate lesion absence. All conditioning inputs are downsampled to the latent resolution via nearest-neighbor interpolation. Conditioning is implemented following a ControlNet-style architecture [25], where the concatenated tissue segmentations and tumor concentrations are processed by a separate convolutional branch and fused with the diffusion U-Net through feature-wise addition at multiple layers, enabling structured spatial guidance during generation. This design enables the model to synthesize tumors in accordance with the provided tumor concentrations while ensuring that the surrounding anatomy remains consistent with the underlying tissue segmentations.

2.2 Inference

To leverage the strong theoretical foundations and principled probabilistic modeling, we adopt the Denoising Diffusion Probabilistic Models (DDPM) sampling strategy [11] in the latent space. The latent update at timestep $t-1$ is given by:

$$\begin{aligned} z_{t-1} =& \sqrt{\bar{\alpha}_{t-1}}\left(\frac{x_t - \sqrt{1-\bar{\alpha}_t}\epsilon_\theta(z_t, t, c^*)}{\sqrt{\bar{\alpha}_t}}\right) \\ &+ \sqrt{1 - \bar{\alpha}_{t-1} - \sigma_t^2} \cdot \epsilon_\theta(z_t, t, c^*) + \sigma_t \epsilon_t, \end{aligned} \tag{3}$$

[1] https://github.com/LMZimmer/gbm_bench.

where c^* corresponds to the conditioning information encoding anatomical tissue segmentations and tumor concentrations, $\epsilon_t \sim \mathcal{N}(0, \mathbf{I})$ is noise and σ_t is the timestep-dependent variance.

Known Region Injection for Inpainting. In the inpainting task, reconstruction is guided through a process commonly referred to as known region injection. At each diffusion timestep t, voxels corresponding to regions with known ground truth values are injected back into the model's current denoised latent estimate to enforce spatial consistency. Formally, the denoised latent $\hat{z}_t$ at timestep t is partially overwritten by a noisy version of the ground truth latent, where the noise level matches the current timestep. This noisy ground truth latent z_t^{GT} is sampled from the forward diffusion process as

$$z_t^{GT} \sim \mathcal{N}\left(\sqrt{\bar{\alpha}_t} z_0^{GT}, (1 - \bar{\alpha}_t)\mathbf{I}\right),$$

with z_0^{GT} representing the clean ground truth latent. The injection is implemented as

$$\hat{z}_t \leftarrow M \odot z_t^{GT} + (1 - M) \odot \hat{z}_t,$$

where M is a binary mask indicating known voxel locations and $\odot$ denotes element-wise multiplication. This procedure ensures that the known regions remain consistent with the original data distribution throughout the reverse diffusion process, while allowing the model to synthesize plausible content in the unknown regions. As the noise level decreases over timesteps, the injected regions converge to their true values, thereby facilitating accurate and spatially coherent inpainting of the missing tissue. Notably, the mask used during this process was a slightly expanded version of the unknown region, obtained by applying one iteration of binary dilation to $1 - M$. This helps ensure a smoother transition between known and unknown regions, supporting more realistic tissue reconstruction.

Repainting Mechanism. While known region injection enforces consistency, it introduces discontinuities at the boundary between known and unknown regions. This naïve injection causes disharmony, as the model cannot smoothly blend generated and fixed content - it lacks visibility into how its outputs interact with the static known regions over time. To address this, we use the RePaint algorithm by Lugmayr et al. [15] that refines boundary regions through targeted re-noising and resampling. In each denoising step, the content for the known region (x_{t-1}^{known}) is sampled using the known pixels in the given image $m \odot x_0$, while the content for the unknown region (x_{t-1}^{unknown}) is sampled from the model, given the previous iteration x_t. These components are then composited using a binary mask m to form the complete latent for the next step, as described by the equation:

$$x_{t-1} = m \odot x_{t-1}^{\text{known}} + (1 - m) \odot x_{t-1}^{\text{unknown}}$$

To improve harmony between these regions, a resampling technique is used, which involves taking steps both backward and forward in diffusion time. This allows the model to iteratively re-contextualize and harmonize the generated content with the known image information, improving overall coherence and semantic plausibility without disturbing known regions.

Image-Space Postprocessing. To improve visual coherence at the boundaries between inpainted and known regions, we apply image-space postprocessing composed of poisson blending [17] and histogram equalization [12]. Poisson blending refines low-level transitions by harmonizing gradient fields across region boundaries, mitigating visible seams caused by pixel discontinuities. Complementarily, histogram equalization aligns intensity distributions between the synthesized region and the known context. This is computed using non-black voxels from both the generated output and the corresponding ground truth, ensuring normalization focuses on anatomically relevant structures. Together, these techniques enhance both the perceptual smoothness and photometric consistency of the inpainted images.

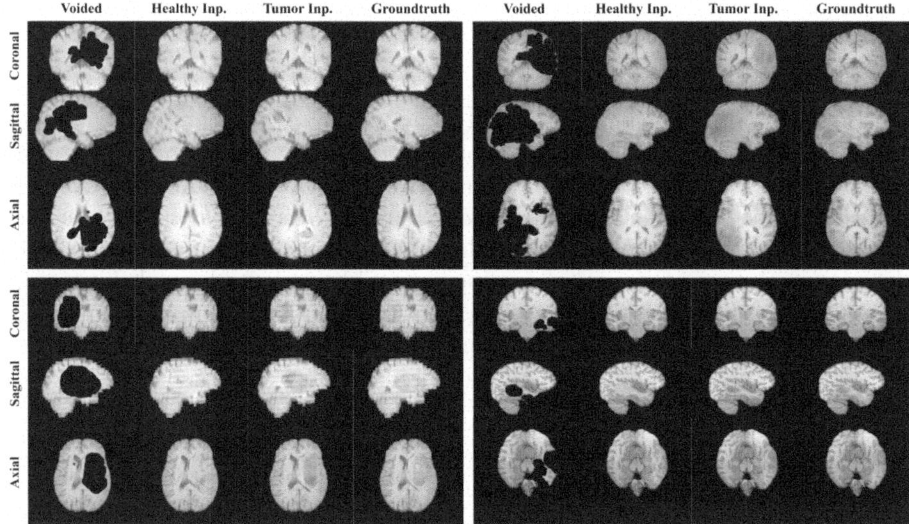

Fig. 2. Qualitative inpainting results are presented for four representative subjects across the coronal, sagittal, and axial views. We showcase our ability to reconstruct missing regions in a 3D spatially coherent and anatomically consistent manner, both for tumor reconstruction and healthy tissue, with a single model.

3 Experiments

Dataset. We employed the publicly available BraTS 2021 dataset [1] in conjunction with several additional private and public datasets (ucsf-pdgm, tcga-gbm, tcga-lgg, Rembrandt) [6,16,19,20], collectively comprising MRI scans of brain tumor patients. The aggregated cohort consists of 3,602 subjects, partitioned into 80% for training (2,881 subjects) and 20% for validation (721 subjects). All volumes were spatially normalized via co-registration to a standardized anatomical template, resampled to an isotropic voxel resolution of 1 mm^3, and subjected to skull-stripping to remove non-brain tissues. For the purpose of this study, only the T1-weighted MRI modality was utilized. Each volume was intensity-normalized to the range $[0, 1]$, zero-padded to a uniform size of $240 \times 240 \times 160$, and subsequently cropped back to $240 \times 240 \times 155$ post-generation to preserve the original brain region.

Implementation Details. The diffusion model is trained with a linear noise schedule, where β_t increases from 1×10^{-4} to 0.02 over 1,000 timesteps. For inference, we adopt the sampling schedule from the RePaint algorithm by Lugmayr et al. [15], which uses 250 timesteps and incorporates their resampling strategy with a jump length of 10 and 10 resampling steps. The model architecture is implemented using the MONAI framework [7].

Training Details. Training was conducted using PyTorch Lightning on 2 NVIDIA H100 GPUs (94 GB each) with a batch size of 2 over a duration of approximately 2.5 weeks. Optimization employed the AdamW algorithm with weight decay of 0.01 and an initial learning rate of 1×10^{-4}, modulated by a cosine annealing scheduler. The noise prediction U-Net and the ControlNet modules were trained jointly differing from the original ControlNet scheme.

Healthy Tissue Inpainting. To evaluate the performance of tissue inpainting, we adopted the BraTS-based inpainting dataset generation protocol[2]. For each subject, the volumetric MRI data were masked in two regions: one containing the tumor and another selected randomly from healthy tissue, simulating missing regions. To rigorously assess inpainting accuracy, quantitative performance metrics - including SSIM, PSNR, MAE, MSE, RMSE, and MSLE - were computed exclusively within the masked healthy region, as ground truth data are available only for that area.

Tumor Inpainting. The same dataset and masking protocol were used for evaluating tumor inpainting. In this case, performance metrics were computed in both the healthy and tumorous regions, as ground truth information is available for both areas. Unlike in the healthy tissue evaluation, the tumor concentrations were not zeroed out but retained as provided in the dataset. A detailed description of this representation is provided in Sect. 2.1.

4 Results

Quantitative Results. The quantitative metrics reported in Table 1 demonstrate that the proposed inpainting model achieves moderate to high performance across structural, perceptual, and reconstruction-based evaluation criteria for both healthy tissue and tumor inpainting tasks. The distribution of these

[2] https://github.com/BraTS-inpainting/2023_challenge.

Table 1. Quantitative values for both healthy tissue (a) and tumor (b) inpainting.

Metric	Mean	Median	Std
SSIM ↑	0.754	0.746	0.134
PSNR ↑	18.542	18.140	3.121
MAE ↓	0.088	0.084	0.032
MSE ↓	0.017	0.015	0.011
RMSE ↓	0.123	0.121	0.040
MSLE ↓	0.007	0.006	0.005

(a) Healthy Tissue Inpainting

Metric	Mean	Median	Std
SSIM ↑	0.578	0.576	0.090
PSNR ↑	17.360	17.664	2.262
MAE ↓	0.104	0.095	0.041
MSE ↓	0.022	0.017	0.024
RMSE ↓	0.141	0.131	0.047
MSLE ↓	0.009	0.007	0.011

(b) Tumor Inpainting

Table 2. Ablation study results for both healthy tissue (a) and tumor (b) inpainting comparing no postprocessing (I), histogram equalization (HE), and poisson blending (PB).

I	HE	PB	SSIM ↑	PSNR ↑	MAE ↓	MSE ↓	RMSE ↓	MSLE ↓
✓			0.715	14.615	0.153	0.045	0.198	0.016
✓	✓		0.735	17.514	0.097	0.021	0.138	0.009
✓	✓	✓	0.754	18.542	0.088	0.017	0.123	0.007

(a) Healthy Tissue Inpainting

I	HE	PB	SSIM ↑	PSNR ↑	MAE ↓	MSE ↓	RMSE ↓	MSLE ↓
✓			0.549	13.864	0.175	0.054	0.217	0.019
✓	✓		0.555	16.767	0.110	0.025	0.151	0.010
✓	✓	✓	0.578	17.360	0.104	0.022	0.141	0.009

(b) Tumor Inpainting

metrics, visualized through violin plots in Fig. 3, reveals a concentrated central tendency with a pronounced tail of lower-performing cases—particularly in SSIM and RMSE. These outliers suggest the presence of challenging anatomical or masking conditions to which the model may be particularly sensitive, highlighting the need for further stratified or case-specific analysis. In Table 4, we show our results at the BraTS challenge.

Qualitative Results. The qualitative examples shown in Fig. 2 illustrate that the proposed inpainting model is capable of generating anatomically plausible reconstructions, exhibiting spatial coherence across coronal, sagittal, and axial planes. The reconstructed regions generally preserve structural continuity and align well with surrounding anatomical features. However, in certain cases, subtle texture inconsistencies and imperfect transitions between the original and inpainted regions are observable, particularly near region boundaries. These artifacts suggest limitations in the model's ability to fully harmonize edge details,

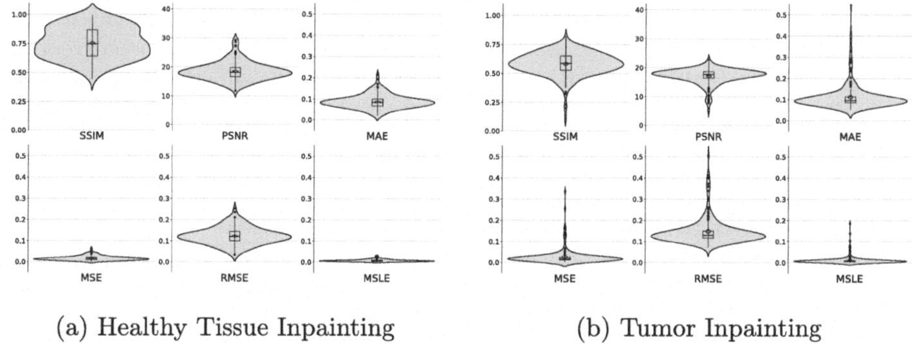

(a) Healthy Tissue Inpainting (b) Tumor Inpainting

Fig. 3. Violin plots of quantitative metrics for healthy (a) and tumor (b) inpainting. Median performance is indicated by a thick horizontal line, mean performance by a rhombus. The box bounds represent the first and third quartiles, and density is shown by the violin plot.

I	HE	PB	SSIM ↑	PSNR ↑	MAE ↓	MSE ↓	RMSE ↓	MSLE ↓
✓			0.715	14.615	0.153	0.045	0.198	0.016
✓	✓		0.735	17.514	0.097	0.021	0.138	0.009
✓	✓	✓	0.754	18.542	0.088	0.017	0.123	0.007

(a) Healthy Tissue Inpainting

I	HE	PB	SSIM ↑	PSNR ↑	MAE ↓	MSE ↓	RMSE ↓	MSLE ↓
✓			0.549	13.864	0.175	0.054	0.217	0.019
✓	✓		0.555	16.767	0.110	0.025	0.151	0.010
✓	✓	✓	0.578	17.360	0.104	0.022	0.141	0.009

(b) Tumor Inpainting

Fig. 4. Quantitative values for validation and test datasets of the BraTS Inpainting Challenge.

indicating potential areas for improvement in boundary refinement and texture blending mechanisms.

Ablation Study. An ablation study, detailed in Table 2, was conducted to evaluate the contribution of individual postprocessing components on the final output. The results clearly demonstrate the efficacy of a sequential enhancement pipeline. The baseline model without any postprocessing yields the lowest performance across all metrics. The introduction of histogram equalization provides a substantial improvement, most notably increasing the PSNR from 14.615 to 17.514 and reducing the MAE from 0.153 to 0.097. The subsequent application of poisson blending provides a further, albeit more modest, refinement, improving the

PSNR to 18.542 and the MAE to 0.088. This incremental enhancement underscores the value of both steps: histogram equalization is critical for correcting the overall intensity distribution, while poisson blending is effective in seamlessly integrating the inpainted patch, which directly addresses the boundary artifacts mentioned in the qualitative assessment.

5 Discussion and Conclusion

We present a unified neural network that performs 3D MRI inpainting for both brain tumors and healthy tissue. The model is conditioned on brain tissue segmentations and continuous tumor concentrations. Qualitative evaluation shows anatomically coherent reconstructions in every spatial direction and stable image quality at tissue boundaries, while the quantitative results confirm the model's strong performance.
Conditioning on tissue segmentations and tumor concentrations enables fine control over pathological and healthy tissue generation. The known region injection strategy preserves anatomical integrity in known areas while enabling robust inpainting in unknown ones.
Despite promising results, our system has certain limitations. Despite the advantages of latent diffusion, the training remains computationally intensive. Further, the repetitive repainting steps result in costly and time-consuming inference. Visual artifacts may still differentiate inpainted areas from original tissues in some outlier cases.
Future work will explore VAE fine-tuning, integration of additional MRI modalities, and dynamic tumor simulation for clinical decision support or tumor growth prediction. In the longer term, we aim to visualize an entire tumor trajectory by combining physics-based simulations with generative models, which enhances treatment planning, explainability and outcome forecasting.

References

1. Baid, U., et al.: The rsna-asnr-miccai brats 2021 benchmark on brain tumor segmentation and radiogenomic classification. arXiv preprint arXiv:2107.02314 (2021). https://arxiv.org/abs/2107.02314
2. Balcerak, M., et al.: Physics-regularized multi-modal image assimilation for brain tumor localization. Adv. Neural. Inf. Process. Syst. **37**, 41909–41933 (2024)
3. Balcerak, M., et al.: Individualizing glioma radiotherapy planning by optimization of a data and physics-informed discrete loss. Nat. Commun. **16**(1), 5982 (2025)
4. Bohnenberger, T.K., Ulrich, M., Albarqouni, S.: Diffusion models for fully 3d medical image synthesis. Med. Image Anal. **90**, 102907 (2024)
5. Bortfeld, T., Buti, G.: Modeling the propagation of tumor fronts with shortest path and diffusion models–implications for the definition of the clinical target volume. Phys. Med. Biology **67**(15), 155014 (2022)
6. Calabrese, E., et al.: The university of california san francisco preoperative diffuse glioma MRI (ucsf-pdgm) dataset. Radiol. Artifi. Intell. **4**(6), e220058 (2022). https://doi.org/10.1148/ryai.220058

7. Cardoso, M.J., et al.: Monai: an open-source framework for deep learning in healthcare. arXiv preprint arXiv:2211.02701 (2022)
8. Dorjsembe, Z., Pao, H.K., Odonchimed, S., Xiao, F.: Conditional diffusion models for semantic 3d brain MRI synthesis. IEEE J. Biomed. Health Inform. **28**(7), 4084–4093 (2024)
9. Ezhov, I., et al.: Learn-morph-infer: a new way of solving the inverse problem for brain tumor modeling. Med. Image Anal. **83**, 102672 (2023)
10. Guo, P., et al.: Maisi: medical AI for synthetic imaging. In: 2025 IEEE/CVF Winter Conference on Applications of Computer Vision (WACV), pp. 4430–4441. IEEE (2025)
11. Ho, J., Jain, A., Abbeel, P.: Denoising diffusion probabilistic models. Adv. Neural. Inf. Process. Syst. **33**, 6840–6851 (2020)
12. Kim, Y.T.: Contrast enhancement using brightness preserving bi-histogram equalization. IEEE Trans. Consum. Electron. **43**(1), 1–8 (1997)
13. Kofler, F., et al.: The brain tumor segmentation (brats) challenge 2023: local synthesis of healthy brain tissue via inpainting. arXiv preprint arXiv:2305.08992 (2023)
14. Liu, Q., et al.: Treatment-aware diffusion probabilistic model for longitudinal MRI generation and diffuse glioma growth prediction. IEEE Transactions on Medical Imaging (2025)
15. Lugmayr, A., et al.: Repaint: inpainting using denoising diffusion probabilistic models. In: Proceedings of the IEEE/CVF conference on computer vision and pattern recognition, pp. 11461–11471 (2022)
16. Pedano, N., et al.: The cancer genome atlas low grade glioma collection (tcga-lgg) (version 3) (2016). https://doi.org/10.7937/K9/TCIA.2016.L4LTD3TK
17. Pérez, P., Gangnet, M., Blake, A.: Poisson image editing. In: Seminal Graphics Papers: Pushing the Boundaries, Volume 2, pp. 577–582 (2023)
18. Rombach, R., Blattmann, A., Lorenz, D., Esser, P., Ommer, B.: High resolution image synthesis with latent diffusion models. In: Proceedings of the IEEE Conference on Computer Vision and Pattern Recognition, pp. 10684–10695 (2022)
19. Scarpace, L., Flanders, A.E., Jain, R., Mikkelsen, T., Andrews, D.W.: Data from rembrandt (2019). https://doi.org/10.7937/K9/TCIA.2015.588OZUZB
20. Scarpace, L., et al.: The cancer genome atlas glioblastoma multiforme collection (tcga-gbm) (version 5) (2016). https://doi.org/10.7937/K9/TCIA.2016.RNYFUYE9
21. Truong, N.C., et al.: Synthesizing 3d multicontrast brain tumor mris using tumor mask conditioning. In: Medical Imaging 2024: Imaging Informatics for Healthcare, Research, and Applications. vol. 12931, pp. 116–120. SPIE (2024)
22. Weidner, J., et al.: Spatial brain tumor concentration estimation for individualized radiotherapy planning. arXiv preprint arXiv:2412.13811 (2024)
23. Weidner, J., et al.: A learnable prior improves inverse tumor growth modeling. IEEE Transactions on Medical Imaging (2024)
24. Wolleb, J., Sandkühler, R., Bieder, F., Cattin, P.C.: The swiss army knife for image-to-image translation: Multi-task diffusion models. arXiv preprint arXiv:2204.02641 (2022)
25. Zhang, L., Rao, A., Agrawala, M.: Adding conditional control to text-to-image diffusion models. In: Proceedings of the IEEE/CVF international conference on computer vision. pp. 3836–3847 (2023)

Robust 3D Brain MRI Inpainting with Random Masking Augmentation

Juexin Zhang, Ying Weng(✉), and Ke Chen

University of Nottingham Ningbo China, Ningbo 315100, China
{juexin.zhang,ying.weng,ke.chen2}@nottingham.edu.cn

Abstract. The ASNR-MICCAI BraTS-Inpainting Challenge was established to mitigate dataset biases that limit deep learning models in the quantitative analysis of brain tumor MRI. This paper details our submission to the 2025 challenge, a novel deep learning framework for synthesizing healthy tissue in 3D scans. The core of our method is a U-Net architecture trained to inpaint synthetically corrupted regions, enhanced with a random masking augmentation strategy to improve generalization. Quantitative evaluation confirmed the efficacy of our approach, yielding an SSIM of 0.873 ± 0.004, a PSNR of 24.996 ± 4.694, and an MSE of 0.005 ± 0.087 on the validation set. On the final online test set, our method achieved an SSIM of 0.919 ± 0.088, a PSNR of 26.932 ± 5.057, and an RMSE of 0.052 ± 0.026. This performance secured first place in the BraTS-Inpainting 2025 challenge and surpassed the winning solutions from the 2023 and 2024 competitions on the official leaderboard.

Keywords: Healthy Tissue Synthesis · BraTS 2025 · Inpainting · MRI

1 Introduction

The quantitative analysis of brain tumors, particularly high-grade gliomas, from multi-modal Magnetic Resonance Imaging (MRI) is a cornerstone of modern neuro-oncology. It provides critical information for diagnosis, surgical planning, radiotherapy guidance, and monitoring treatment response. In recent years, deep learning models have achieved state-of-the-art performance on well-defined tasks such as tumor segmentation. However, the performance and generalizability of these models are intrinsically dependent on access to large, diverse, and accurately annotated datasets. This dependency reveals a fundamental challenge: the very pathology we aim to analyze introduces significant biases into the data and the standard computational workflows used to process it.

A fundamental challenge in neuro-oncological image analysis stems from a critical data void: for any given patient, a corresponding "healthy" scan from a pre-pathological state is almost never available. Patients typically undergo their first MRI only after the onset of symptoms, meaning their anatomical baseline is already compromised. This lack of a patient-specific, ground-truth healthy reference is the root cause of the "pathology bias" that confounds downstream

S. Bakas et al. (Eds.): MICCAI 2025, LNCS 16377, pp. 102–109, 2026.
https://doi.org/10.1007/978-3-032-16370-7_9

algorithms. Without this reference, it is difficult to accurately quantify the true extent of anatomical deformation or to train models that can robustly differentiate pathological changes from normal inter-subject variability.

However, this challenge also illuminates a powerful new opportunity for generative modeling. If one could accurately synthesize the missing healthy anatomy for a patient, it would create a pristine digital canvas. This "anatomical canvas" would not only serve as an ideal reference for tasks like registration but would also enable a paradigm-shifting approach to data augmentation: generative pathology transplantation. This goes far beyond simple geometric transformations. By first inpainting the original tumor to create a healthy proxy, one can then programmatically synthesize and implant different tumors—of varying types, sizes, and growth patterns—onto the same patient's unique anatomical substrate.

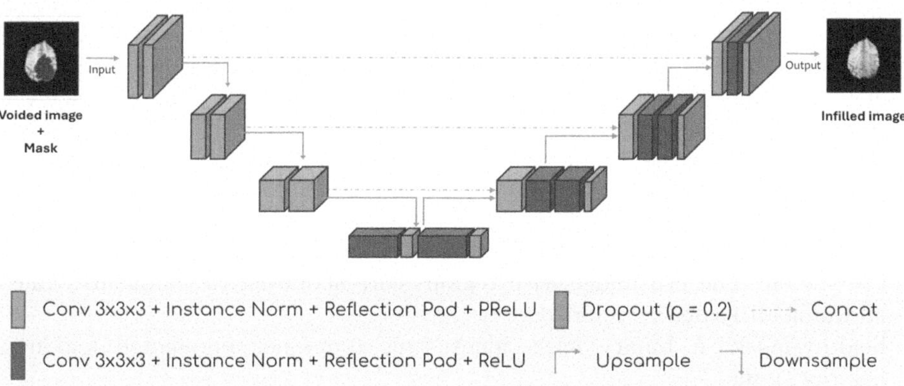

Fig. 1. The figure illustrates the architecture of our U-Net model.

Consider a real-world clinical scenario: a dataset may be rich in cases of ring-enhancing glioblastoma but contain very few examples of diffuse, non-enhancing astrocytomas. A model trained on this biased data will naturally perform poorly on the rarer subtype. Using our proposed framework, we can take a scan of a patient with a glioblastoma, computationally "resect" the tumor via inpainting to generate a healthy version of their brain, and then synthetically "graft" a realistic, non-enhancing astrocytoma into the same location. This process generates a highly valuable, perfectly co-registered data pair: a specific patient's anatomy with two different, clinically relevant pathologies. By repeating this process, we can synthetically enrich datasets with rare disease manifestations, creating highly controlled counterfactuals that are essential for developing next-generation AI models that are not only accurate but also robustly generalizable across the entire spectrum of disease expression.

As our contribution to the ASNR-MICCAI BraTS Local Synthesis of Tissue via Inpainting (BraTS-Inpainting) Challenge, we propose a method to synthesize a subject-specific, "healthy" anatomical proxy from pathological MRI scans using a deep learning model with a U-Net backbone. The remainder of this paper is structured as follows: The BraTS dataset and the methodologies related to the U-Net like model are described in Sect. 2. Section 3 presents the experimental methods of the proposed model, and the paper is concluded in Sect. 4.

2 Methods

2.1 Dataset

Our dataset extends the methodology of the BraTS-Local-Inpainting dataset [2] to create a more comprehensive training resource. The dataset is built from 1251 T1-weighted MRI scans from the BraTS-GLI 2023 collection [1], each featuring tumor annotations approved by expert neuroradiologists.

A key distinction of our work is the generation of five unique healthy tissue masks for each source image. We first identified healthy brain tissue spatially separated from the tumor using the algorithm from [2]. These masks were then augmented through random mirroring and rotation to create five distinct versions per scan, aiming to improve model generalization. All MRI volumes and masks were standardized to dimensions of $240 \times 240 \times 155$. Each training sample consists of the following five components:

- t1n: The original ground truth T1-weighted image.
- t1n-voided: The t1n image with regions corresponding to the healthy-mask and unhealthy-mask occluded.
- healthy-mask: A binary mask identifying a unique, augmented region of healthy tissue.
- unhealthy-mask: The binary mask of the expert-annotated tumor region.
- mask: A combined binary mask representing the union of the healthy-mask and unhealthy-mask.

2.2 Pre-processing

We began with the BraTS 2021 GLI dataset, which had already undergone standard pre-processing: co-registration to a common anatomical template, resampling to a uniform $1\,\text{mm}^3$ isotropic resolution, and skull-stripping. We then applied our own processing pipeline. First, we normalized the images in two stages, scaling them to a $[0, 1]$ range by dividing by their maximum intensity value, and subsequently to a $[-1, 1]$ range. Following normalization, all MRI scans and masks were cropped to a size of $208 \times 208 \times 144$. Finally, to generate the output, our model's predictions on these cropped patches are stitched together with the original T1-weighted MRI.

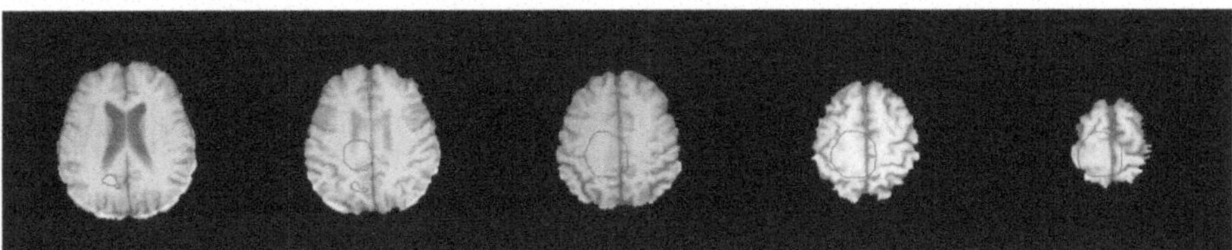

(a) BraTS-GLI-00114-000 (best): SSIM 0.999069, PSNR 38.939751, MSE 0.000128

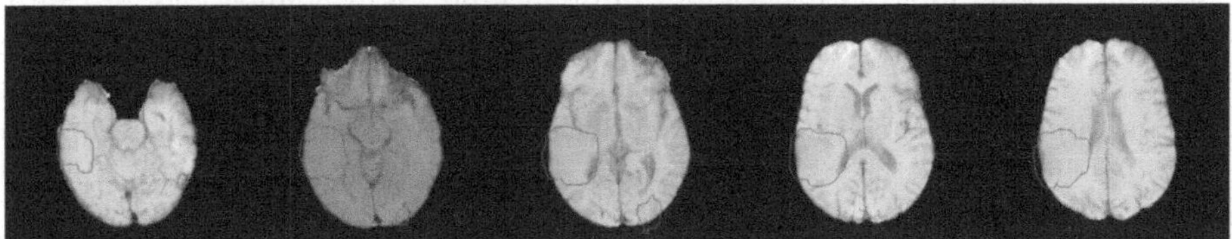

(b) BraTS-GLI-01773-000 (median): SSIM 0.906654, PSNR 22.563231, MSE 0.005542

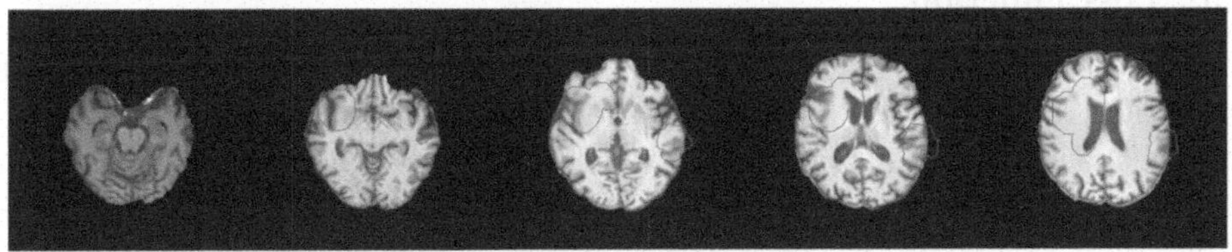

(c) BraTS-GLI-00467-000 (worst): SSIM 0.709323, PSNR 16.336607, MSE 0.023246

Fig. 2. Qualitative results of our model's infilling performance on validation MRI scans, showcasing the best (Fig. 2(a)), median (Fig. 2(b)), and worst (Fig. 2(c)) cases. The green masks indicate the inpainted regions, which contained both healthy and unhealthy tissues as these were not explicitly labeled. (Color figure online)

2.3 Data Augmentation

To address the common issue of overfitting in high-capacity deep learning models and improve generalization to unseen data, we employ a robust data augmentation strategy. As mentioned above, we generate five unique healthy tissue masks using the algorithm described in [2] for each MRI scan. These masks are created by applying a set of random transformations, including mirroring and rotation. Specifically, mirroring is applied independently to each dimension with a probability of 50%, while random rotations between 0° and 360° are performed on both the XY and YZ planes. Although some overlap between the five masks for a given scan is expected, the resulting variability in mask shape, location, and size is crucial for training a more robust and generalized model.

2.4 Network Architecture

For the task of synthesizing healthy tissue, we propose a model based on the U-Net architecture [3]. As depicted in Fig. 1, the network utilizes an encoder-decoder structure comprising three downsampling blocks, a central bridge block, and three upsampling blocks.

Each block contains two 3D convolutional layers with a $3 \times 3 \times 3$ kernel. We employ Parametric ReLU (PReLU) as the activation function in the downsampling and upsampling blocks, while the standard ReLU is used in the bridge. Instance normalization is applied after each convolutional layer to stabilize training. The number of feature channels starts at 32, doubling with each downsampling step and halving with each upsampling step. Skip connections are integrated to pass features from the encoder stages to their corresponding decoder stages, preserving low-level details. To mitigate overfitting, dropout with a rate of 0.2 is applied in the bridge and upsampling blocks. The model accepts a t1n-voided image and its associated mask as input, and it outputs an infilled image.

2.5 Loss Function

The model is trained using a composite loss function, which is a weighted sum of the Mean Absolute Error (MAE) and the Structural Similarity Index Measure (SSIM) [4]. This hybrid design was motivated by our observation that SSIM alone performs poorly in preserving masked regions and can introduce artifacts at mask boundaries. To address this, the MAE component is calculated exclusively on the healthy regions of the ground truth (GT) and the generated image (I), while the SSIM component is computed on the entire images to maintain overall structural coherence.

The loss functions are formulated as follows:

$$MAE(x, y) = \frac{1}{m} \sum_{i=1}^{m} |y_i - f(x_i)| \tag{1}$$

$$SSIM(x, y) = \frac{(2\mu_x\mu_y + c_1)(2\sigma_{xy} + c_2)}{(\mu_x^2 + \mu_y^2 + c_1)(\sigma_x^2 + \sigma_y^2 + c_2)} \tag{2}$$

$$Loss(I, GT) = \lambda_1 \cdot MAE(I, GT) + \lambda_2 \cdot SSIM(I, GT) \tag{3}$$

3 Experiment Results

3.1 Evaluation Metrics

The performance of our model is quantitatively assessed by comparing the generated healthy regions to the ground truth data. We use three standard metrics for this evaluation: Structural Similarity Index Measure (SSIM), Peak-Signal-to-Noise-Ratio (PSNR), and Mean-Square-Error (MSE). Notably, this evaluation is performed only on the healthy regions defined by the ground truth masks.

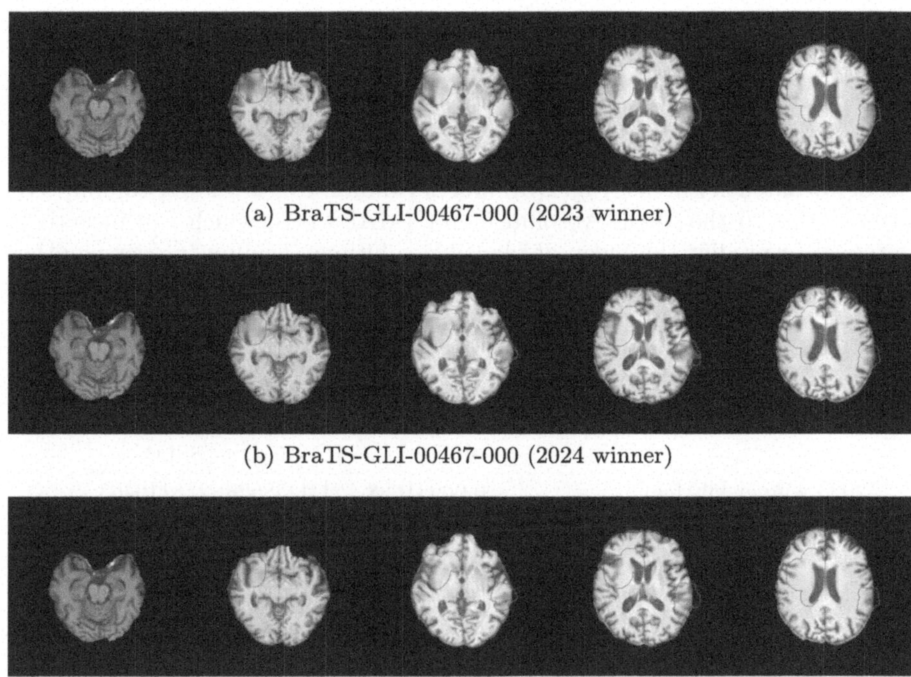

(a) BraTS-GLI-00467-000 (2023 winner)

(b) BraTS-GLI-00467-000 (2024 winner)

(c) BraTS-GLI-00467-000 (ours)

Fig. 3. Qualitative comparison of our method's worst-performing case against the winning methods of the BraTS 2023 and 2024 challenges.

3.2 Experiment Settings

We utilized 5-fold cross-validation to select hyperparameters. Models were trained for a maximum of 500 epochs, and for each fold, we saved the checkpoint corresponding to the lowest validation loss. We employed the Adam optimizer with an initial learning rate of 1×10^{-4} and betas of $(0.9, 0.999)$. The loss weights λ_1 and λ_2 were both set to 1. During the validation phase, the healthy mask region of the ground truth image is normalized to a $[0, 1]$ range based on the maximum intensity value across both healthy and unhealthy regions.

3.3 Validation Phase

Table 1 summarizes the quantitative performance of our method on the BraTS-Local-Inpainting validation dataset, benchmarked against the winning solutions of the 2023 [5] and 2024 challenges [6]. All metrics were computed using the official Sage Bionetworks Synapse online evaluation platform. To complement this analysis, Fig. 2 provides qualitative results, illustrating the best, median, and worst inpainting cases from the validation set. The evaluation protocol has two key constraints: 1) the ground truth is withheld, precluding direct visual comparison, and 2) scoring is confined to healthy tissue, although inpainting masks cover both healthy and pathological regions.

Visually, our model effectively captures fine-grained textures and generates plausible tissue structures that integrate well with the surrounding context. However, the inpainted regions exhibit some blurriness, an artifact most prominent in low-intensity areas (Fig. 2(b), fourth column; Fig. 2(c), first column). We attribute this to the Mean Absolute Error (MAE) loss, which can incentivize the model to predict the mean of plausible solutions, leading to oversmoothed textures. We also illustrate the worst-performing case of our method against the winner solution of 2023 and 2024 in Fig. 3.

Table 1. Online validation data results.

		MSE	PSNR	SSIM
2023 winner [5]	Mean	0.00931688	21.4458628	0.8119463
	Standard deviation	0.00645289	3.44400102	0.11350122
	25 quantile	0.00489901	18.4753408	0.69751903
	Median	0.00815745	20.8844547	0.82023758
	75 quantile	0.01239707	23.689291	0.89072207
2024 winner [6]	Mean	0.00650362	23.3814246	0.84116632
	Standard deviation	0.00466064	4.26449611	0.10317845
	25 quantile	0.00278909	20.3874092	0.75842395
	Median	0.00579681	22.3681049	0.84412175
	75 quantile	0.00914667	25.5454702	0.92018622
Ours	Mean	**0.00476023**	**24.9959218**	**0.87300897**
	Standard deviation	0.00360885	4.69427685	0.08699671
	25 quantile	0.00188717	21.7267790	0.80683365
	Median	0.00405384	23.9213314	0.87929922
	75 quantile	0.00671933	27.2419672	0.94228190

3.4 Test Phase

We present our model's overall performance on the test set in Table 2. Due to restricted access, the organizers executed the inference runs, which prevents us from providing visualizations of the infilled images. Despite this lack of visual evidence, the quantitative results confirm our model's robust performance and strong generalization capabilities.

Table 2. Performance Metrics on the Test Set.

	SSIM	PSNR	RMSE
Mean	0.91928125	26.9321548	0.05162604
Standard deviation	0.08843877	5.0565417	0.02610840

4 Conclusion

In this paper, we presented a novel deep learning framework for synthesizing healthy brain tissue in pathological MRI scans, our winning submission to the ASNR-MICCAI BraTS-Inpainting 2025 Challenge. Our method, centered on a U-Net architecture enhanced with a random masking augmentation strategy, demonstrated state-of-the-art performance. The quantitative results, achieving an SSIM of 0.919, a PSNR of 26.932, and an RMSE of 0.052 on the final test set, not only secured first place but also surpassed the winning entries from previous years. While our qualitative analysis identified minor blurriness as an area for improvement, the overall success underscores the model's robustness and its potential to mitigate pathology-induced data bias. This work represents a significant step forward in generating high-fidelity anatomical proxies, opening new possibilities for data augmentation and the development of more generalizable AI models in neuro-oncological image analysis.

Acknowledgments. This work was supported by Ningbo Major Science & Technology Project under Grant 2022Z126.

References

1. Baid, U., et al.: The RSNA-ASNR-MICCAI BraTS 2021 benchmark on brain tumor segmentation and radiogenomic classification. arXiv preprint arXiv:2107.02314 (2021)
2. Kofler, F., et al.: The brain tumor segmentation (BraTS) challenge 2023: local synthesis of healthy brain tissue via inpainting. arXiv preprint arXiv:2305.08992 (2023)
3. Ronneberger, O., Fischer, P., Brox, T.: U-Net: convolutional networks for biomedical image segmentation. In: Navab, N., Hornegger, J., Wells, W.M., Frangi, A.F. (eds.) MICCAI 2015. LNCS, vol. 9351, pp. 234–241. Springer, Cham (2015). https://doi.org/10.1007/978-3-319-24574-4_28
4. Wang, Z., Bovik, A.C., Sheikh, H.R., Simoncelli, E.P.: Image quality assessment: from error visibility to structural similarity. IEEE Trans. Image Process. **13**(4), 600–612 (2004)
5. Zhang, J., Chen, K., Weng, Y.: Synthesis of healthy tissue within tumor area via U-Net. In: Baid, U., et al. (eds.) Brain Tumor Segmentation, and Cross-Modality Domain Adaptation for Medical Image Segmentation, pp. 233–240. Springer Nature Switzerland, Cham (2024)
6. Zhang, J., Weng, Y., Chen, K.: U-Net based healthy 3d brain tissue inpainting. arXiv preprint arXiv:2507.18126 (2025)

Local2Global: UNet with Hierarchical Attention Mechanisms for Improved MR Image Inpainting

Erdi Sarıtaş[1(✉)], İlkay Öksüz[1], and Hazım Kemal Ekenel[1,2]

[1] Department of Computer Engineering, Istanbul Technical University, Istanbul, Türkiye
{saritas21,oksuzilkay,ekenel}@itu.edu.tr
[2] Division of Engineering, NYU Abu Dhabi, Abu Dhabi, UAE
he2244@nyu.edu

Abstract. The BraTS Inpainting Challenge aims to synthesize healthy brain tissue to replace tumor-affected regions, which are localized with masks, on 3D magnetic resonance imaging. This effort supports clinical and research applications by generating anatomically plausible reconstructions. In this paper, we propose Local2Global, a novel UNet-like architecture combining convolutional and multiple attention mechanisms to synthesize anatomically coherent healthy brain tissue. Our model comprises four encoder stages, where each stage is designed to progressively capture distinct levels of context from local patterns with the convolution stage to global context with full attention. This local-to-global strategy enables the network to leverage the advantages of each layer type while reducing the computational burden associated with processing 3D volumes. Experimental results on the BraTS Inpainting dataset demonstrate the effectiveness of our approach. The proposed model was evaluated during the challenge. Our model achieved an SSIM of 0.768 and a PSNR of 20.548 on the validation set, whereas an SSIM of 0.844 and a PSNR of 21.954 on the testing set. The code is available on https://github.com/ThEnded32/Local2Global.

Keywords: Convolution · Attention · Transformer · UNet · Inpainting

1 Introduction

The Brain Tumor Segmentation (BraTS) challenge, organized annually by the Medical Image Computing and Computer-Assisted Intervention Society (MICCAI), has become an essential benchmark for evaluating segmentation algorithms on multiparametric magnetic resonance imaging (MRI) scans affected by gliomas [1–5]. Over the years, BraTS has evolved from focusing solely on tumor segmentation to encompassing tasks such as synthesizing healthy brain tissue via image inpainting [6]. Image inpainting reconstructs missing or corrupted areas of an image for visual coherence. In medicine, it refers to restoring healthy brain

S. Bakas et al. (Eds.): MICCAI 2025, LNCS 16377, pp. 110–122, 2026.
https://doi.org/10.1007/978-3-032-16370-7_10

tissue in tumor-affected areas by replacing the void with synthesized normal tissue [6]. This technique is vital for identifying pathological regions and aiding in surgical planning. Although inpainting has been extensively researched for general 2D images [7], volumetric brain MRI applications pose challenges due to the dimensionality and anatomical variability.

Brain MRI inpainting can be categorized by the generative modeling approaches used, primarily Generative Adversarial Networks (GANs) [8] and diffusion models [9], often employing UNet-like encoder-decoder architectures [10]. These architectures vary, with some using only convolutional layers and others incorporating transformer [11] components. A trade-off exists between local fidelity and global coherence. CNNs excel at capturing local features but struggle with long-range dependencies. Conversely, transformer architectures model global context effectively but face challenges in computational intensity and need for long training time with a large dataset to converge, especially in 3D medical imaging due to limited datasets and high memory costs.

To leverage the strengths of both CNNs and transformers while mitigating their drawbacks, we propose a hybrid UNet-like architecture called Local2Global with a staged processing design. Transitioning from local to global feature processing, the encoder includes four stages with different feature extractors: a standard convolutional block, a shifted-window attention [12], a grid attention transformer block [13], and a full attention block [14] as the bottleneck. The decoder mirrors the encoder and uses skip connections to preserve spatial details and incorporate multiscale context. We compared our architecture with baseline models and conducted several ablation experiments, including using an atlas image as auxiliary input, applying two data augmentation strategies, and testing different model configurations. Our top model achieved an SSIM of 0.768 and a PSNR of 20.548 on the validation dataset of the BraTS Inpainting Challenge, as well as an SSIM of 0.844 with a PSNR of 21.954 on the challenge testing set.

2 Related Works

Medical image analysis has advanced rapidly due to deep learning [15], enabling automated interpretations of complex radiological data. The Brain Tumor Segmentation (BraTS) challenge is a key benchmark that has driven innovation by offering standardized multi-parametric MRI datasets and clearly defined tasks, initially focusing on glioma sub-region segmentation [1–5] and later expanding to specialized challenges, such as tumor-affected region inpainting [6].

2.1 Brain MRI Inpainting

In the Brain Tumor Segmentation (BraTS) challenge, image inpainting aims to restore tumor-affected brain regions with synthetic healthy tissue, facing challenges due to the complexity of 3D MRI data and the need for structural coherence. Techniques such as GAN-based models [16–18] and diffusion-based models [19–21] have demonstrated effectiveness in generating realistic content, often utilizing UNet-like architectures. Zhang, J. et al. [22] synthesized healthy 3D brain tissue from pathological MRI scans using a UNet-like model. Zeineldin, R. A., and Mathis-Ullrich, F. [17] combined transformer and CNN architectures with a 3D Pix2Pix GAN. Liu, X. et al. [23] introduced symmetry-constrained strategy global perception inference, along with patch-based reconstruction guided by anatomical symmetry. Modifications to the standard 3D Pix2Pix model [18] have improved structural detail preservation. DiffKAN-Inpainting [21] combines the Kolmogorov-Arnold Network [24] with diffusion sampling for high-quality healthy tissue representation. Other diffusion models [19,20] have been developed for multitask inpainting. Zhu, R. et al. [16] explored adapting 2D inpainting techniques for 3D brain MRI.

2.2 Attention Mechanisms in Computer Vision

Attention mechanisms are essential in medical image analysis for modeling long-range dependencies in 3D data. Transformers [11] have been adapted for imaging tasks such as the Vision Transformer (ViT) [14]. The Swin Transformer [12] utilizes shifted window-based attention to lower computational costs, while models like MaxViT [13] combine local and global receptive fields with grid attention. These mechanisms are applied in medical imaging to enhance spatial coherence and semantic consistency [25,26]. Moreover, hybrid approaches blend the precision of CNNs with the contextual capabilities of transformers [15]. Our proposed architecture incorporates convolution and various attention mechanisms within a hierarchical design, using different mechanisms for each feature extraction stage to maintain simplicity without complex attention relations.

3 Methodology

The proposed UNet-like architecture combines convolutional and attention-based mechanisms in a hierarchical manner, allowing the model to maintain anatomical consistency and produce visually coherent reconstructions. The architecture is illustrated in Fig. 1. The explanations of the stages are as follows;

- **Convolutional stage:** This stage uses ResNet-like [27] convolution blocks that consist of 3D convolutional layers. These layers extract essential low-level spatial features from textures and anatomical details, which are crucial for accurate inpainting near structural boundaries.
- **Shifted window attention stage:** This stage utilizes transformer blocks with non-overlapping windows and a shifting mechanism between layers [12]. These layers effectively understand mid-range relations while ensuring computational efficiency.
- **Grid attention stage:** To approximate the global context with lower computational requirements, this stage uses transformer blocks featuring grid attention [13]. These layers model suboptimal global relationships without processing the whole volume.

– **Full attention stage:** Serving as the bottleneck of the network, this stage employs a classical/full attention mechanism [14] to capture the global context throughout the 3D volume. These layers enable the model to infer information about the entire brain structure.

The network starts with a stem block that processes the input MRI volume through two 3D convolution layers with a kernel size of 5, transforming it into a feature space. The decoder mirrors the encoder's four stages in reverse, allowing for symmetric reconstruction. Skip connections between the encoder and decoder stages enable the fusion of high-resolution spatial information with deep features. The output layer refines these features into the inpainted 3D brain MRI volume, consisting of two convolutional layers with kernel sizes of 3 and 1, followed by a tanh layer. Downsampling occurs between encoding stages with a $2 \times 2 \times 2$ convolution (stride 2), while upsampling with transposed convolutions happens between decoding stages. The upsampled output from the previous stage is concatenated with the skip connection features before being processed through a $1 \times 1 \times 1$ convolution to effectively fuse the information.

4 Experimental Setup

We conducted our experiments using the BraTS 2023 Local-Inpainting dataset [6], which includes 1,251 T1-weighted brain MRI scans. Each scan com-

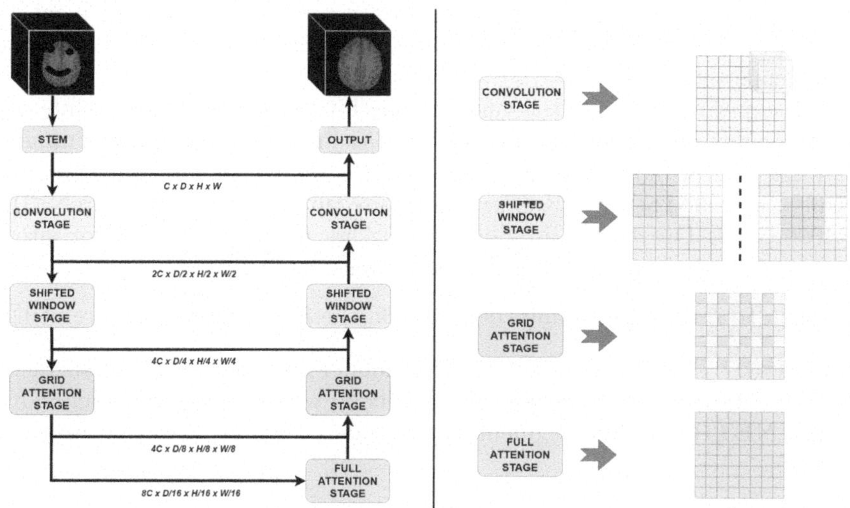

Fig. 1. Visualization of the network on the left. The network architecture includes an encoder with four stages: convolutional, shifted-window attention, grid attention, and full attention. The decoder mirrors the encoder and uses skip connections for multiscale contextual information. On the right, the stages are illustrated, with colors indicating sampling/grouping strategies; features with the same color are used for processing information. From top to bottom, processing progresses from local to global context.

prises expert-verified annotations of tumor regions and is accompanied by synthetic inpainting masks that indicate healthy and pathological tissues. The MRI volumes are preprocessed to a uniform size of $240 \times 240 \times 155$ voxels, with an isotropic resolution of $1mm^3$. For model training, the volumes are further randomly cropped into sub-volumes of $128 \times 128 \times 96$, ensuring that they include inpainting mask regions, and normalized to the range of $[-1, 1]$. For the evaluations, a center crop is taken with the volume of $208 \times 208 \times 144$.

To evaluate the inpainted regions, we used the Structural Similarity Index Measure (SSIM), which assesses perceptual similarity by comparing luminance, contrast, and structural patterns. For pixel-wise fidelity, we employed both the Peak Signal-to-Noise Ratio (PSNR), a logarithmic measure of reconstruction error relative to signal strength, and the Mean Absolute Error (MAE), which directly averages the absolute intensity differences. All metrics are computed only within the healthy inpainting mask regions.

4.1 Training Configuration

The training procedures follow the official BraTS Inpainting Challenge codebase, which adopts a paired GAN-based framework with additional $L1$ and SSIM losses. The total objective is defined as

$$L_{Total} = \lambda_{GAN} \times L_{GAN} + \lambda_{L1} \times L_{L1} + \lambda_{SSIM} \times L_{SSIM}, \quad (1)$$

where λ_{L1} is 10 and λ_{GAN} and λ_{SSIM} are set to one. Full implementation details can be found in the official GitHub repository, which closely follows the 2023 challenge setup [6].

For all experiments, only the generator architecture is modified, while other hyperparameters remain consistent with the baseline configuration. Training uses a batch size of 2 for most models, except Pix2Pix3D, which employs a batch size of 4. Unless specified otherwise, experiments are run on a server with an NVIDIA RTX 4090 GPU. The dataset is split into 80% for training and 20% for internal validation, distinct from the official validation set used for challenge reporting.

Baselines. To set a performance benchmark, the following models are utilized:

- **Pix2Pix3D**: The standard 3D Pix2Pix model provided by the challenge [6].
- **Pix2Pix3DL**: A larger variant of Pix2Pix3D with doubled channel width.
- **SwinUNETR**: A 3D segmentation model adapted for the inpainting task [26].

Architecture Evolution. The proposed network is developed progressively with continuous enhancements to achieve its final architecture, which is described in Sect. 3. These improvements primarily focus on the decoder structure and the strategies for downsampling and upsampling. To minimize the time and resources spent on model evolution, these experiments were conducted with a short training time of 10 epochs.

- **V1**: Employs fixed channel sizes. Downsampling and upsampling are performed using max-pooling and nearest-neighbor interpolation, respectively, with a purely convolutional decoder.
- **V2**: Introduces channel scaling to increase feature dimensionality across encoder stages. Strided convolutions are used for downsampling, and transposed convolutions are used for learned upsampling.
- **V3 (Local2Global)**: Adopts a symmetric decoder structure. This model is the proposed model, which is explained in Sect. 3.

4.2 Ablations

Atlas Image Usage. An atlas image is generated by taking the arithmetic mean of the T1-weighted MRI scans (without any registration) from the training dataset. This atlas is combined with the input volume channels, acting as a prior to guide the inpainting process.

Data Augmentation. Two augmentation strategies were applied during training. The first, called *Degradation*, introduces variations such as Gaussian blur, intensity drift, Gaussian noise, and occasional dropout artifacts to increase data diversity. The second, called *More Mask*, enlarges the masked areas by randomly adding rectangular or elliptical regions (with varying radius or edge length) outside the original healthy mask. This increases the overall masked volume and makes the task more challenging. Example outputs are shown in Fig. 2: noise artifacts appear in the fourth column for the *Degradation* case, while the last two columns illustrate additional masked regions from the *More Mask* strategy. To fully leverage these augmentations, models were trained for 200 epochs with augmentations applied on-the-fly.

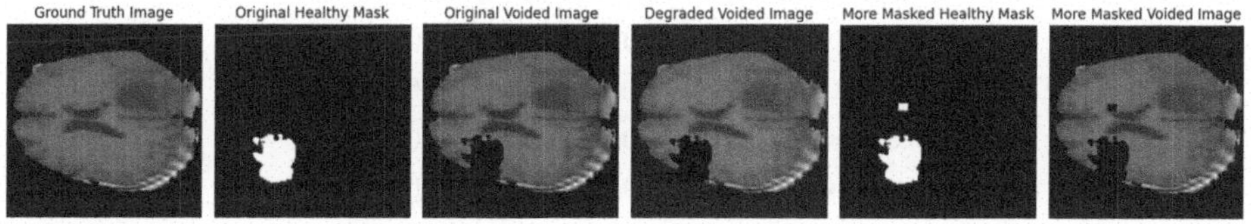

Fig. 2. Augmentation sample visuals. The original ground truth image, its mask, and the original masked image are displayed in the first three columns. *Degradation* augmentation applied to the image is in the fourth column. *More Mask* augmentation is applied to the mask, and its masked image version is in the last two columns.

Model Size. The proposed model's default setup is $48/2-2-2-3$, meaning an initial channel size of 48 and a sequence of block counts across the four stages. With access to an A100 GPU, larger model variants were also trained. To ensure fairness, all variants were trained on a single A100 GPU for 80 epochs with a batch size of 4, and the learning rate was doubled following the scaling rule [28].

5 Results

Table 1 presents the results of evaluating the progressive modifications introduced across the three architectural variants of the proposed Local2Global model. V3 achieved the best performance among all variants, with an SSIM of 0.684, a PSNR of 16.552, and an MAE of 0.119. Table 1 highlights the benefits of employing a symmetric decoder structure. For the latter part of the manuscript, Local2Global will refer to the V3 architecture.

Table 1. Analysis of Local2Global Network Versions.

Model	SSIM↑	PSNR↑	MAE↓
V1	0.658	14.980	0.135
V2	0.666	14.556	0.148
V3	**0.684**	**16.552**	**0.119**

Table 2 provides a comparative evaluation of the proposed Local2Global model against other methods, including Pix2Pix3D (and its larger version) and SwinUNETR. Across both training durations, Local2Global outperforms the baselines in terms of PSNR and SSIM. Local2Global trained 200 epochs achieves 0.755 SSIM, 19.519 PSNR, and 0.075 MAE scores. When analyzing the impact of training time, it is evident that longer training periods significantly enhance performance.

Table 2. Comparison of Proposed and Baseline Models versus Training Time.

Model	Epoch	SSIM↑	PSNR↑	MAE↓
Pix2Pix3D	10	0.651	14.817	0.143
SwinUNETR	10	0.655	14.997	0.144
Local2Global	10	**0.684**	**16.552**	**0.119**
Pix2Pix3D	200	0.731	17.558	0.095
Pix2Pix3DL	200	0.744	17.786	0.094
SwinUNETR	200	0.727	18.437	0.085
Local2Global	200	**0.755**	**19.519**	**0.075**

A visual comparison of the models' inpainting results is presented in Fig. 3, which displays three anatomical views (axial, coronal, and sagittal). The Local2Global model, comparing the other baselines, generates anatomically consistent structures better with sharper boundaries and less perceptual distortion, particularly in areas with complex brain geometry. In contrast, Pix2Pix3D and Pix2Pix3DL often suffer from over-smoothed textures or incomplete boundary closure. SwinUNETR, despite yielding worse scores, produced plausible outputs similar to those of our model.

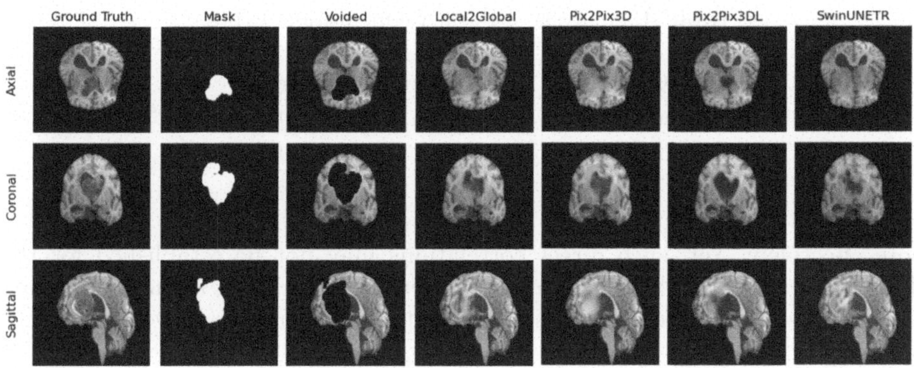

Fig. 3. Sample inpainting results. For each axis, the mid-slice is taken to display. Models trained for 200 epochs are selected.

5.1 Ablations

Atlas Image Usage. Table 3 displays the results with the atlas image used. The results indicate that the atlas image has a varying impact on models. For both epoch numbers, SSIM scores are better for Pix2Pix3D, while PSNR scores are better for Local2Global models. Moreover, MAE scores better when the models are trained longer. The Local2Global trained 200 epochs with the atlas image performed better than Local2Global without the atlas image in terms of PSNR.

Table 3. Analysis of Atlas Image Used Models versus Training Time.

Model	Epoch	SSIM↑	PSNR↑	MAE↓
Pix2Pix3D	10	0.670	14.153	0.146
Local2Global	10	0.657	15.005	0.132
Pix2Pix3DL	200	0.754	18.982	0.078
Local2Global	200	0.752	19.825	0.076

Data Augmentation. Table 4 shows the result of models trained with data augmentation. We can see that applying synthetic degradations, such as blur or noise, diminishes the performance for all metrics. However, employing the "More Mask" strategy helped the model achieve the best PSNR and MAE scores among previous trials, while maintaining a matching SSIM score.

Model Size. Table 5 exhibits the results of trials conducted on an A100 GPU. As both batch sizes and training times differ, the previous results are not directly comparable. We can see from the results that widening the model helps achieve better PSNR scores, while increasing the number of layers improves the SSIM

Table 4. Analysis of Data Augmentation Types.

Augmentation Type	SSIM↑	PSNR↑	MAE↓
Degradation	0.742	18.675	0.089
More Mask	0.755	19.997	0.071

more effectively. Yet, such direct correlations may not be established for the MAE scores. Rather than expanding the feature dimension upon lengthening the model, adding more layers results in better performance on average.

Table 5. Analysis of Greater Model Configurations.

Model	Configuration	SSIM↑	PSNR↑	MAE↓
Default	$48/2-2-2-3$	0.697	17.440	0.094
Long	$48/3-4-4-6$	0.716	17.013	0.102
Longer	$48/4-4-4-8$	0.736	17.819	0.094
Large	$96/2-2-2-3$	0.681	17.543	0.094
Big	$96/2-4-4-4$	0.699	17.813	0.092

5.2 Submission

The Local2Global model with default configuration from Table 2 was continued to train with vanilla setting (no atlas image or augmentation is used) on an RTX 4090 GPU server for 500 epochs and then fine-tuned on an A100 GPU server for 20 epochs on test-time resolution ($208 \times 208 \times 144$).. This model achieved an SSIM of 0.758, a PSNR of 20.170, and an MAE of 0.063 on the validation split on the training dataset, and an SSIM of 0.768 and a PSNR of 20.548 on the challenge validation set. Moreover, our proposed model yields an SSIM of 0.844 and a PSNR of 21.954 on the challenge test set.

6 Discussion

6.1 Model Complexity and Efficiency

To evaluate the tradeoff between performance and complexity, base models were tested with an input of random values of batch size 1. The results, shown in Table 6, highlight Pix2Pix3D as the most lightweight and efficient model, with the smallest size and fastest throughput. Among larger models, Pix2Pix3DL has the highest parameter count and GPU memory requirement, but its inference speed is moderate. SwinUNETR has fewer parameters but is still memory-intensive with slightly lower throughput. Local2Global is the most computationally intensive and slowest, despite lower memory usage.

Table 6. Comparison of Model Complexity and Efficiency at Train/Test Input Resolutions.

	Metric	Pix2Pix3D	Pix2Pix3DL	SwinUNETR	Local2Global
	Params (M)	4.43	17.7	15.7	15.6
Train	FLOPs ($\times 10^{11}$)	2.90	11.5	1.50	16.0
	Throughput (imgs/s)	32.9	15.6	16.0	8.0
	GPU Mem. (MB)	1461	2938	2503	2058
Test	FLOPs ($\times 10^{11}$)	11.9	47.2	7.62	73.5
	Throughput (imgs/s)	7.9	3.8	3.3	1.5
	GPU Mem. (MB)	5751	11464	10771	8966

Disclaimer: The slower runtime of Local2Global may comes from how its attention layers are implemented. Instead of using efficient kernel-fused window/grid operations, the code applies full attention separately to each window or grid cell. This extra repetition may remove the speed advantage of sparse attention and add overhead, making the model slower. Even so, the network still converges easily despite being largely composed of transformer-based blocks.

The Local2Global architecture effectively combines convolutional layers with transformer-based attention mechanisms. Comparative evaluations show its superior performance in perceptual similarity and reconstruction accuracy against the other baselines. Ablation studies highlight the advantages of using an atlas image and targeted data augmentation strategies, particularly the "More Mask" approach. These studies also stress the importance of model depth and width balance. However, larger models were not extensively tested over extended training epochs due to time constraints. Future work should explore the model's performance across various tasks and domains to validate its generalizability and address implementation inefficiencies.

7 Conclusion

In this work, we proposed a hybrid UNet-like architecture for 3D brain MRI inpainting, combining convolutional layers with multiple attention mechanisms to progressively capture from local to global context. Our design follows a four-stage pipeline, starting with convolutional blocks and advancing through shifted-window-based, grid-based, and full attention modules, enabling effective representation learning from local textures to holistic anatomical structures. Through extensive experiments, we demonstrated that the symmetric decoder and hierarchical attention design make significant contributions and improve reconstruction quality. The proposed Local2Global model consistently outperformed baseline methods, including Pix2Pix3D, its larger variant, and SwinUNETR, across both quantitative metrics and qualitative evaluation. Ablation studies emphasize the importance of architectural choices, atlas image integration, and targeted data augmentation in enhancing model performance. Our extensive experiments validate the effectiveness of the proposed Local2Global model. On the challenge validation set, the model achieved an SSIM of 0.768 and a PSNR of 20.548. Further, on the challenge testing set, it reached an SSIM of 0.844 and a PSNR of 21.954.

Acknowledgements. The paper benefited from ITU BAP research funds (Project ID: 47363). This study also benefited from funding from the Health Institutes of Turkiye (TUSEB) 2022-EKG-01 Program (Project No. : 20101) and TUBITAK bilateral research grant (Project No.: 124N419). Computing resources used in this work were provided by the National Center for High Performance Computing of Turkey (UHeM) under grant number 4023702025.

References

1. Baid, U., et al.: The RSNA-ASNR-MICCAI BraTS 2021 benchmark on brain tumor segmentation and radiogenomic classification (2021). arXiv:2107.02314
2. Menze, B.H., Jakab, A., Bauer, S., Kalpathy-Cramer, J., Farahani, K., Kirby, J., et al.: The multimodal brain tumor image segmentation benchmark (BRATS). IEEE Trans. Med. Imaging **34**(10), 1993–2024 (2015). https://doi.org/10.1109/TMI.2014.2377694
3. Bakas, S., Akbari, H., Sotiras, A., Bilello, M., Rozycki, M., Kirby, J.S., et al.: Advancing the cancer genome atlas glioma MRI collections with expert segmentation labels and radiomic features. Nature Scientific Data **4**, 170117 (2017). https://doi.org/10.1038/sdata.2017.117
4. Bakas, S., Akbari, H., Sotiras, A., Bilello, M., Rozycki, M., Kirby, J., et al.: Segmentation labels and radiomic features for the pre-operative scans of the TCGA-GBM collection. Cancer Imaging Archive (2017). https://doi.org/10.7937/K9/TCIA.2017.KLXWJJ1Q
5. Bakas, S., Akbari, H., Sotiras, A., Bilello, M., Rozycki, M., Kirby, J., et al.: Segmentation labels and radiomic features for the pre-operative scans of the TCGA-LGG collection. Cancer Imaging Archive (2017). https://doi.org/10.7937/K9/TCIA.2017.GJQ7R0EF
6. Kofler, F., et al.: The brain tumor segmentation (BRATS) challenge 2023: local synthesis of healthy brain tissue via inpainting (2023). arXiv preprint arXiv:2305.08992
7. Rombach, R., Blattmann, A., Lorenz, D., Esser, P., Ommer, B.: High-resolution image synthesis with latent diffusion models. In: Proceedings of the IEEE/CVF Conference on Computer Vision and Pattern Recognition, pp. 10684–10695 (2022)
8. Goodfellow, I.J., et al.: Generative adversarial nets. Adv. Neural Inf. Process. Syst. **27** (2014)
9. Ho, J., Jain, A., Abbeel, P.: Denoising diffusion probabilistic models. Adv. Neural. Inf. Process. Syst. **33**, 6840–6851 (2020)
10. Ronneberger, O., Fischer, P., Brox, T.: U-Net: convolutional networks for biomedical image segmentation. In: Navab, N., Hornegger, J., Wells, W.M., Frangi, A.F. (eds.) MICCAI 2015. LNCS, vol. 9351, pp. 234–241. Springer, Cham (2015). https://doi.org/10.1007/978-3-319-24574-4_28
11. Vaswani, A., et al.: Attention is all you need. Adv. Neural Inf. Process. Syst. **30** (2017)

12. Liu, Z., et al.: Swin transformer: hierarchical vision transformer using shifted windows. In: Proceedings of the IEEE/CVF International Conference on Computer Vision, pp. 10012–10022 (2021)
13. Tu, Z., et al.: Maxvit: Multi-axis vision transformer. In: European Conference on Computer Vision, pp. 459–479. Cham: Springer Nature Switzerland (2022)
14. Dosovitskiy, A., et al.: An Image is Worth 16x16 Words: transformers for image recognition at scale. In: International Conference on Learning Representations (2020)
15. Yazıcı, Z.A., Öksüz, İ, Ekenel, H.K.: GLIMS: attention-guided lightweight multiscale hybrid network for volumetric semantic segmentation. Image Vis. Comput. **146**, 105055 (2024)
16. Zhu, R., Zhang, X., Pang, H., Xu, C., Ye, C.: Advancing brain tumor inpainting with generative models (2024). arXiv preprint arXiv:2402.01509
17. Zeineldin, R.A., Mathis-Ullrich, F.: Ensemble learning and 3D Pix2Pix for comprehensive brain tumor analysis in multimodal MRI. In: International Challenge on Cross-Modality Domain Adaptation for Medical Image Segmentation, pp. 24–34. Cham, Springer Nature Switzerland (2023)
18. Sadique, M.S., Rahman, M.M., Farzana, W., Glandon, A., Temtam, A., Iftekharuddin, K.M.: Local synthesis of healthy brain tissue using an enhanced 3D Pix2Pix model for medical image inpainting. In: International Challenge on Cross-Modality Domain Adaptation for Medical Image Segmentation, pp. 312–321. Cham, Springer Nature Switzerland (2023)
19. Rouzrokh, P., Khosravi, B., Faghani, S., Moassefi, M., Vahdati, S., Erickson, B.J.: Multitask brain tumor inpainting with diffusion models: a methodological report (2022). arXiv preprint arXiv:2210.12113
20. Durrer, A., Cattin, P.C., Wolleb, J.: Denoising diffusion models for inpainting of healthy brain tissue. In: International Challenge on Cross-Modality Domain Adaptation for Medical Image Segmentation, pp. 35–45. Cham, Springer Nature Switzerland (2023)
21. Tao, T., Wang, Z., Zhang, H., Arvanitis, T. N., Zhang, L.: DiffKAN-Inpainting: KAN-based diffusion model for brain tumor inpainting. In: 2025 IEEE 22nd International Symposium on Biomedical Imaging (ISBI), pp. 1–4. IEEE (2025)
22. Zhang, J., Chen, K., Weng, Y.: Synthesis of healthy tissue within tumor area via u-net. In: International Challenge on Cross-Modality Domain Adaptation for Medical Image Segmentation, pp. 233–240. Cham, Springer Nature Switzerland (2023)
23. Liu, X., Xing, F., Yang, C., Kuo, C.C.J., El Fakhri, G., Woo, J.: Symmetric-constrained irregular structure inpainting for brain mri registration with tumor pathology. In: Brainlesion: Glioma, Multiple Sclerosis, Stroke and Traumatic Brain Injuries: 6th International Workshop, BrainLes 2020, Held in Conjunction with MICCAI 2020, Lima, Peru, October 4, 2020, Revised Selected Papers, Part I 6, pp. 80–91 (2021). Springer International Publishing
24. Liu, Z., et al.: Kan: Kolmogorov-Arnold Networks (2024). arXiv preprint arXiv:2404.19756
25. Khan, A. R., Khan, A.: MaxViT-UNet: Multi-axis attention for medical image segmentation (2023). arXiv preprint arXiv:2305.08396
26. Hatamizadeh, A., Nath, V., Tang, Y., Yang, D., Roth, H. R., Xu, D.: Swin UNETR: Swin transformers for semantic segmentation of brain tumors in MRI images. In: International MICCAI Brain Lesion Workshop, pp. 272–284 (2021)

27. He, K., Zhang, X., Ren, S., Sun, J.: Deep residual learning for image recognition. In: Proceedings of the IEEE Conference on Computer Vision and Pattern Recognition, pp. 770–778 (2016)
28. Goyal, P., et al.: Accurate, large minibatch sgd: Training imagenet in 1 hour (2017). arXiv preprint arXiv:1706.02677

Achieving Over 10 × Faster Sample Generation with Conditional Denoising Diffusion

André Ferreira[1,2,6,7](✉), Gijs Luijten[2,5,9], Behrus Hinrichs-Puladi[6,7], Jens Kleesiek[2,3,4,8,10], Victor Alves[1], and Jan Egger[2,3,5,9,10]

[1] Center Algoritmi / LASI, University of Minho, Braga 4710-057, Portugal
[2] Institute for Artificial Intelligence in Medicine (IKIM), Essen University Hospital (AöR), University of Duisburg-Essen, Essen, Germany
[3] Cancer Research Center Cologne Essen (CCCE), West German Cancer Center, University Hospital Essen (AöR), Essen, Germany
[4] Partner site University Hospital Essen (AöR), German Cancer Consortium (DKTK), Essen, Germany
[5] Institute of Computer Graphics and Vision, Graz University of Technology, Inffeldgasse 16, Graz 8010, Austria
[6] Institute of Medical Informatics, University Hospital RWTH Aachen, Aachen, Germany
[7] Department of Oral and Maxillofacial Surgery, University Hospital RWTH Aachen, Aachen, Germany
id10656@alunos.uminho.pt
[8] Department of Physics, TU Dortmund University, Dortmund, Germany
[9] Center for Virtual and Extended Reality in Medicine (ZvRM), University Hospital Essen (AöR), Essen, Germany
[10] Faculty of Computer Science, University of Duisburg-Essen, Essen, Germany

Abstract. This paper presents our solutions for Task 8 and 9 of BraTS 2025, which respectively involve the generation of a missing MRI modality and inpainting a missing region. Task 8 aims to solve the problem of missing a MRI modality for cases which acquisition is infeasible or the quality is not good enough for analysis. Task 9 seeks to produce pathology-free cases which would allow the analysis of healthy brains. We use denoising diffusion models to solve both tasks in a unified framework. Since regular diffusion models require 1000 steps or more for inference, we propose a solution to speed up inference while obtaining competitive results while keeping a low computational footprint. Compared to our solution from BraTS 2024, our new solution achieves better results with over 10 times faster processing. We obtain Dice scores of 0.80, 0.83, and 0.88 for ET, TC, and WT, respectively, along with an SSIM of 0.95 on Task 8 test set. On the Task 9 test set, we achieve an RMSE of 0.053, a PSNR of 26.77, and an SSIM of 0.918. The code will be released following the conclusion of the challenge.

Keywords: Conditional Denoising Diffusion · IDDPM · Synthetic Data Generation · MRI Reconstruction · Computational Efficiency · Image Inpainting

S. Bakas et al. (Eds.): MICCAI 2025, LNCS 16377, pp. 123–132, 2026.
https://doi.org/10.1007/978-3-032-16370-7_11

1 Introduction

Generative models have been the a predominant topic in AI research in the last years. Ranging from text-based models to image and multi-modality models, the quality of the synthetic generation has been improving, to a point where is nearly impossible to distinguish from real information [5].

For image generation, Generative Adversarial Networks (GANs) and Denoising Diffusion Probabilistic Models (DDPM) have shown unprecedented realism, making possible to image editing or even real full image creation [18]. However, in the medical field such technology still lacks deep study, due to the sensibility of the data and the limitation of data sharing. Medical data is restrict by data protection laws that difficult or even do not allow the sharing of the data, even for research purposes [6,13]. The BraTS challenge has advanced research on this topic by providing large pre-processed datasets for different tasks and a platform for comparing methods. This enables multiple researchers to access their methods in a simple and reliable way and evaluate them against other researchers' solutions [1,10–12,15]. We propose a solution for Task 8 - Brain MR Image Synthesis Challenge (BraSyn) and Task 9 - BraTS Local Synthesis of Tissue via Inpainting of 2025 edition, which aim at two different tasks but have one common aspect - the generation of missing data.

Task 8 [12] aims to find the best solution for the problem of missing modalities of daily routines. Automatic brain tumor segmentation methods usually really on four MRI modalities, i.e. T1n (T1-weighted), T1c (T1-weighted with contrast), T2w (T2-weighted) and T2f (FLAIR). However, in clinical practice, some of these modalities might be missing due to the lack of quality or by the lack of time. An algorithm capable of generating the missing modality would allow a better automatic segmentation of patient cases from centers with less extensive imaging protocols or for analyzing legacy datasets. The purpose is to recover the performance of models trained on four modalities (T1, T1-Gd, T2 and FLAIR) for brain tumor segmentation by hallucinating the missing modality.

Task 9 [10] seeks solutions to completely replace the unhealthy part of the brain with healthy tissue. This is particularly important for algorithms that have only been trained on healthy brains, such as brain extraction, tissue segmentation and brain anatomy parcellation algorithms. It is also important to monitor the expected progression of the brain tumor during treatment and to study biomarkers by comparing the healthy and unhealthy brain in other diseases such as Alzheimer's.

2 State-of-the-Art

Modality generation and inpaing tasks were introduced as part of the BraTS 2023 competition. Since then, several different solutions have been proposed.

The winners from modality generation task in 2023, Baltruschat et al. [3] proposed the use of a 2.5D U-Net generator with PatchGAN. In addition to the adversarial loss, Mean Absolute Error (MAE), Structural Similarity Index Measure (SSIM), perceptual were also used. Histogram standardization was applied and linear normalization between [0:1]. Axial, sagittal and coronal planes were used for training, and random cropping random horizontal flipping and random rations were applied. A network is trained for each modality. In 2024 edition, Ferreira et al. [7] proposed the use of conditional diffusion models, more concretely the 3DWDM [8]. The loss function is composed by the Mean-Square-Error (MSE) between the modality to generate and the ground truth and the MSE of the tumor region. 3000 sampling steps were used for the generation of each missing modality, which made this method slow.

Kofler et al. [10] present winning solutions of 2023 edition for the inpaiting task. The winners used a 3D U-Net network with MAE and SSIM losses. Although the quantitative metrics are better than the remaining solutions, qualitatively the region inpainted of the second place winner (who used a 2D diffusion model) look more realistic. This is justified by the metrics used for evaluation, as they penalize wrong heavier contrast than wrong smooth transitions. Also, even though the second place model produce visually realistic inpainted regions, this might be morphological incorrect. It was also noticed the lack of continuity between slices of the proposed 2D diffusion model, which supports the need for 3D based solutions. Ferreira et al. [7] also proposed a solution for the inpaint task based on the WDM, which got second place in 2024 edition. The use of the mask as additional condition and a repainting based strategy for inference allowed realistic inpaiting. However, 5000 steps were required to achieve these results, what makes this solution very slow.

One of the main challenges in working with generative models is their high computational cost during training, as well as the speed of inference. There is also a growing need for evaluation metrics that go beyond traditional benchmarks and better capture how humans perceive quality. Together, these issues present significant hurdles for researchers and developers in the field. To minimize the problem of slow sampling, Improved Denoising Diffusion Probabilistic Models (IDDPM) [16] and Denoising Diffusion Implicit Models (DDIM) [19] have been explored. Pan et al. [17] explored the use of IDDPM for MRI to CT translation. Their method uses a Swin-Vnet and patch-based inference to allow the use of less computational resources. Each patch has shape of 64x64x4, which allow the use of weaker GPUs. Clipping of the CT scans was performed [-1024, 1650] with linear normalization to [-1, 1]. MRI intensities were independently normalized between [-1, 1]. A timestep respacing of 50 was used, instead of the full 1000 steps. However, in contrast to the original implementation of IDDPM, a linear noise scheduler was used as well as MAE loss instead of MSE.

Due to the high sensitivity and complexity of the data and the results that DDPMs and GANs were having, DDPMs were chosen for both tasks. However, DDPMs are known by their Markov chain of diffusion steps which make the inference process slow. Therefore, a method based on the IDDPM is proposed. Due to the nature of the dataset which comes from distinct institutions as well as the need for faster processing methods, normalization methods and a reduced number of steps were used to ensure both quality and speed of inference. We propose the use of only 25 steps and a large window size which allow realistic and fast synthetic generation.

3 Methods

A cluster node with 6 NVIDIA RTX 6000, 48 GB of VRAM, 1024 GB of RAM, and AMD EPYC 7402 24-Core Processor was used for training and testing. Only one GPU was required for each training. The developed solutions are capable of running on a GPU with as little as 2 GB of VRAM.

3.1 Model Architecture and Experimental Settings

We use a hybrid ResNet – Swin-Unet architecture [4,9]. The top stage (first encoder / last decoder) is pure ResNet. The other three stages are a ResNet followed by a Swin Transformer blocks, with skip connections at each stage, with base channels = 64, and stage multipliers = [1,2,3,4], and time embeddings in all blocks. The base loss function used is presented in Eq. 1, explained with more detail in the next subsections.

$$L = L_{\text{MSE}} + L_{\text{VLB}} + L_{\text{SSIM}} + L_{\text{MAE}}. \tag{1}$$

where MSE and MAE are the mean squared and mean absolute errors, respectively, VLB is the variational lower bound loss and SSIM the structural similarity index measure. AdamW with betas=(0.9, 0.999), weight decay of 1e-5 and lr of 2e-5, linear noise schedule with early stop based on MAE, and sliding windows of shape 128x128x32 were used.

3.2 Task 8 - MRI Synthesis for BraTS

The dataset is composed of 1251 training cases from the BraTS 2023 Glioma dataset [1] and 238 training cases from the BraTS 2023 MET dataset [15]. The modalities T1, T1-Gd, T2 and FLAIR and the respective segmentations are available for each case. In the testing phase, the realism is evaluated using SSIM in tumor and healthy brain regions. To assess downstream utility, the generated modality is used in a automatic pre-trained brain tumour segmentation tool which later compares with the ground truth segmentation and computes the combined Dice and Hausdorff scores for three tumor substructures.

10% of the dataset is randomly selected for local validation with the remaining 90% used for training. To further standardize the data for training the IDDPM model, percentile clipping of 0.1% and 99.9% followed by z-score normalization was applied to reduce the effect of multi-institution multi-parametric data. Due to instability of training, linear normalization to [-1:1] was also applied to ensure more normalized values. Normalization was applied individually to each modality. For the z-score, two methods were tested, i.e., with individual mean and std and with global mean and std per modality. We applied randomized spatial and intensity augmentations (probability 0.5): random affine (rotations ±3°, scale ±3%, shear ±0.05), grid elastic (5×5×5, limit 0.01), 3rd-degree bias field (coeff 0 – 0.05); intensity-only: shift ±0.1, scale ±10%, gamma 0.9 – 1.1, Gaussian blur (σ per axis 0.1 – 0.4) and additive Gaussian noise (σ=0.01). Spatial transforms were applied to images and labels; intensity transforms to the image only.

The loss function is based on the original $L_{MSE} + \lambda L_{vlb}$ [16]. Since SSIM will be used for evaluation of the generated scans, L_{SSIM} is also added to ensure good performance on the evaluation metrics. L_{MAE} is also used to reduce the blurring effect created by the MSE metric. To make the IDDPM conditional, four channels are concatenated with the input of the network used to learn the denoised version of the input. The four modalities are concatenated in the same order, with the missing modality replaced by a volume composed by only "1" values, allowing the network to learn what modality is missing.

As shown in the paper [16], 25 sampling steps are enough to produce reasonable results. However, they trained the network for 1000 steps and them used the same model to infer only on 25 steps. In contrast, we optimized the network to learn these specific 25 steps. By using L_{vlb} and training on those specific sampling steps, it is possible to converge the training faster and optimize the results. In contrast, if 1000 steps were used to training, we would need much more epochs without much improvement, as our goal is to use only this specific 25 steps. Regular resized sampling and DDIM sampling methods were used and compared.

The output is then linearly normalized between 0 and 1. To avoid very small values in the background and in order to better match the pre-trained model used for the segmentation test, the output models are post-processed by thresholding. A threshold of 0.01 is used, i.e., values smaller than 0.01 are set to 0 (background value). In case of using global z-score statistics, the output is de-normalized using the pre-computed mean and std and then normalized between 0 and 1.

3.3 Task 9 - MR Image Inpainting for BraTS

The BraTS 2023 Glioma [1,2,14] dataset is also used for this task. 1251 training cases are available for training, and 219 for validation in the online platform. For this task, only the the modality T1n with the respective unhealthy mask and a random healthy mask are available for training, as explained in [10]. For the testing phase, only the masked T1n scan and the mask are available. The inpainted region (only the healthy part) is evaluated using the SSIM, Peak-Signal-to-Noise-Ratio (PSNR) and MSE.

Similarly to Task 8 (Sect. 3.2), 10% of the dataset is randomly selected for local validation with the remaining 90% used for training. To further standardize the data for training the IDDPM model, percentile clipping of 0.1% and 99.9% followed by z-score normalization is applied on the cases without the region of the mask (both healthy and unhealthy) to ensure reproducibility on the validation and test sets. Linear normalization to [-1:1] is also applied to ensure more normalized values. A solution without this last steps is also tested. For each case, a random mask and a random healthy region are selected for training. Random affine perturbations (rotations $\pm\pi/60 \approx \pm 3°$, scale $\pm 3\%$, shear ± 0.05), coarse grid elastic-like distortions (5,5,5) with distort limit (0.01,0.01,0.01), random axis flips and random 90° rotations are applied on the fly.

The loss function is based on the original $L_{MSE} + \lambda L_{vlb}$ [16]. L_{SSIM} is added to ensure good performance on the evaluation metrics. L_{MAE} of only the region inpainted is used to reduce the blurring effect created by the MSE metric and optimize this specific region. SSIM on the inpainted regions was also evaluated but discarded due to instability caused by the small size of some regions. 25 steps are used to optimize the IDDPM training. Regular resized sampling and DDIM sampling methods are used and compared.

4 Results

4.1 Task 8

The local validation results are presented in Table 1. The DSC is computed using the Docker container available on the BraSyn tutorial GitHub page[1], and the SSIM using the script also available on the GitHub page. The SSIM results presented are computed over the entire volume, and not divided by healthy and tumour regions as it will be during the testing phase. The experiments are divided by the use of individual or global statistics for z-score normalization, and if post-processing was applied (thresholding). Figure 1 presents a comparison between synthetic (left) and real (right) cases for each modality on the left side of the figure. On the right, a violin plot illustrates the SSIM comparison between Exp. 1 and Exp. 2. Table 2 presents the results on the test set computed by the organizers using global statistics with regular sampling and post processed.

Table 1. Performance comparison of Task 8 on the local validation set using DSC and SSIM metrics.

Name	Statistics	Post Processed	Sampling	DSC	SSIM
Real	—	—	—	0.9034	—
Exp. 1	Individual	No	25	0.6801	0.7698
			ddim25	0.6579	0.7703
		Yes	25	0.8455	**0.7709**
			ddim25	0.8469	0.7708
Exp. 2	Global	No	25	0.8107	0.7707
			ddim25	0.8077	0.7707
		Yes	25	**0.8591**	**0.7709**
			ddim25	0.8577	**0.7709**

[1] https://github.com/WinstonHuTiger/BraSyn_tutorial.

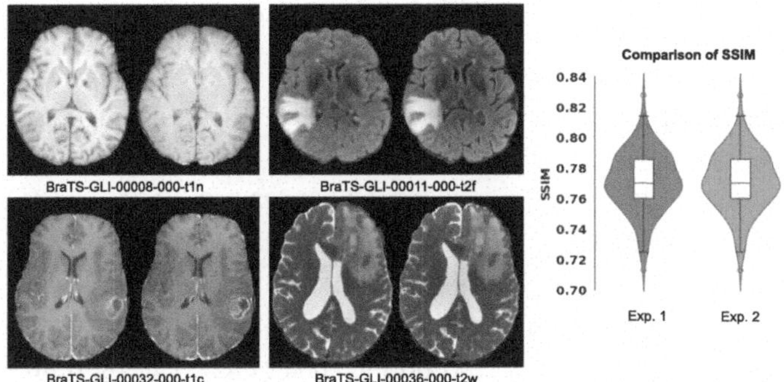

Fig. 1. Results of Task 8. Left: Visual comparison of a sample from each modality alongside the ground truth. Right: Violin plots comparing SSIM.

Table 2. Performance of Task 8 on the test set.

Group	Dice_ET	Dice_TC	Dice_WT	NSD_ET	NSD_TC	NSD_WT	SSIM
GLI	0.82 ± 0.21	0.85 ± 0.24	0.92 ± 0.09	0.57 ± 0.26	0.51 ± 0.27	0.52 ± 0.19	0.95 ± 0.05
MEN	0.80 ± 0.31	0.81 ± 0.30	0.83 ± 0.28	0.59 ± 0.32	0.59 ± 0.32	0.57 ± 0.26	0.95 ± 0.02
ALL	0.80 ± 0.26	0.83 ± 0.27	0.88 ± 0.20	0.56 ± 0.28	0.53 ± 0.29	0.52 ± 0.22	0.95 ± 0.04

4.2 Task 9

As mentioned before, instability is the main reason why normalization from z-score to [-1:1] was performed. However, for this task, we will also present the results of the model trained without it. Table 3 presents the results obtained on the online platform using the validation set (not the local validation set). "Inpaint" refers to the replacement of the known region at each denoising step. However, this was discarded due to the bad results as it increases the inference instability. Therefore, it is not considered in our final solution. Figure 2 shows a comparison of MSE, SSIM, and PSNR using violin plots at the top of the image. At the bottom, the inpainting results for BraTS-GLI-00027-000-t1n are presented, generated by Exp. 1 and Exp. 2. Table 4 contains the results of the testing phase provided by the organizers, using z-scoring followed by linear normalization and regular sampling.

5 Discussion and Conclusions

In Sect. 4.1 is presented the results for Task 8. The low DSC observed in the experiments without any post-processing (Table 1) is related to the way the pre-trained segmentation network, based on nnUNet, operates. When background noise is present and the background value is not set to 0, nnUNet performs more sliding window inferences. This behavior increases the number of False Positives (FP), thereby reducing the overall DSC.

Table 3. Performance comparison of Task 9 on the online validation set using MSE, PSNR, and SSIM metrics.

Name	Norm [-1:1]	Sampling	MSE	PSNR	SSIM
Real	—	—	—	—	—
Exp. 1	No	25	0.007 ±0.005	23.042 ±4.15	0.841 ±0.105
		ddim25	0.007 ±0.005	23.332 ±4.305	0.842 ±0.106
		inpaint25	0.064 ±0.056	15.018 ±6.676	0.686 ±0.184
		inpaint ddim25	0.059 ±0.052	15.37 ±6.632	0.693 ±0.181
Exp. 2	Yes	25	**0.005** ±0.004	24.527 ±4.718	**0.868** ±0.089
		ddim25	0.005 ±0.004	**24.529** ±4.872	0.867 ±0.0901

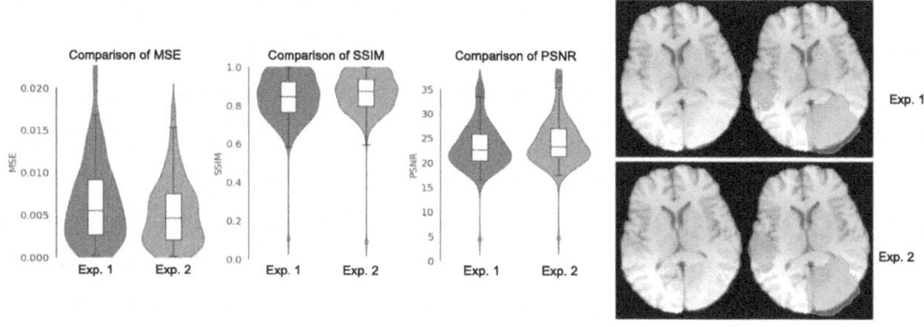

Fig. 2. Results of Task 9. Top: Violin plots comparing MSE, SSIM, and PSNR. Bottom: Visual comparison of sample BraTS-GLI-00027-000-t1n output.

The use of global statistics improves the DSC in 1.61% (comparing the resized sampling method) and 0.3368% the SSIM (considering the DDIM sampling method). Such small improvements are not sufficient to conclude that using global statistics is better than using individual ones. However, their use is justified by the ability to convert back to real intensities. While this may not be necessary during the testing phase, it could be important for other tasks. The training process showed no signs of overfitting, and the validation metrics continued to improve. This suggests that the model's performance could potentially improve further with extended training.

This solution presents a significant improvement in relation to [7] solution as only 25 steps are needed (per patch). Considering that all images have roughly

Table 4. Performance of Task 9 on the test set.

Task	RMSE	PSNR	SSIM
Local inpainting	0.053 ±0.027	26.77 ±5.21	0.918 ±0.089

the same size, each new generation takes around 1 min and 40 s (in our machine), making our solution more than 12 times faster.

In relation to Task 9 (Sect. 4.2), since we use mixed precision for faster processing and lower computational footprint as well as the L_{vlb} and patches, the training was very unstable. Therefore, the model training in the first experiment was stopped upon encountering the first NaN value. This issue was later mitigated by applying normalization between -1 and 1. However, it was not entirely resolved, as some iterations still had to be skipped due to the occurrence of NaN values. Nevertheless, this normalization enabled more stable training.

It can be seen that the use of z-score normalization per case followed by linear normalization to -1 and 1 produces the best results, when resized 25 steps and regular sampling are used. These results represent an improvement over the 2024 edition validation set, where MSE $= 0.007 \pm 0.005$, PSNR $= 23.257 \pm 4.213$, and SSIM $= 0.843 \pm 0.098$ were obtained. A considerable speed-up is achieved with this solution, as each case takes approximately 3 min to inpaint. In contrast, the solution proposed in [7] requires 30 min per case, making our approach roughly 10 times faster. The test results demonstrate performance improvements, as evidenced by a reduction in RMSE from 0.07 to 0.05, an increase in PSNR from 22.8 to 26.8, and a slight increase in SSIM from 0.91 to 0.92.

Training on 1000 steps and inference on 25 steps was also tested. However, such solution was very unstable, producing NaN values, mainly due to the hight values of noise variances predicted by the model, as well as the use of mixed precision. Therefore, no results are presented. The IDDPM gets specialized on the time-steps which is trained on, making it less flexible to more aggressive inference steps (such as T=25). For instance, the model specialized for 25 steps predicted variance values roughly between -2 and 2, whereas the model trained with T=1000 steps produced variances reaching into the dozens or even hundreds. Sampling with DDIM was possible, but produced very bad results. When T=1000 was used no NaN were produced, but the inference was 40 times slower. Therefore, we also discarded this option.

The main drawback of our solutions for both tasks is the use of patches for inference, which leads to artifacts at the edges of the individual patches. In Task 9, the lack of surrounding tissue for each patch worsens the generation due to the lack of context in larger regions to be inpainted. As a future solution, we propose the use of a denoising autoencoder to eliminate the grid effect, and larger patches or a network capable of capturing more distant features for inference.

Acknowledgments. André Ferreira was supported by FCT - Fundação para a Ciência e Tecnologia, I.P. by project reference 2022.11928.BD and DOI identifier https://doi.org/10.54499/2022.11928.BD. This work has been supported by FCT – Fundação para a Ciência e Tecnologia within the R&D Unit Project Scope UID/00319/Centro ALGORITMI (ALGORITMI/UM), and by KITE (Plattform für KI-Translation Essen) from the REACT-EU initiative (EFRE-0801977, https://kite.ikim.nrw/).

Disclosure of Interests. The authors have no competing interests to declare that are relevant to the content of this article.

References

1. Baid, U., et al.: The RSNA-ASNR-MICCAI brats 2021 benchmark on brain tumor segmentation and radiogenomic classification. arXiv preprint arXiv:2107.02314 (2021)
2. Bakas, S., et al.: Advancing the cancer genome atlas glioma MRI collections with expert segmentation labels and radiomic features. Sci. Data **4**(1), 1–13 (2017)
3. Baltruschat, I.M., Janbakhshi, P., Lenga, M.: Brasyn 2023 challenge: missing mri synthesis and the effect of different learning objectives. In: International Challenge on Cross-Modality Domain Adaptation for Medical Image Segmentation, pp. 58–68. Springer (2023)
4. Cao, H., et al.: Swin-unet: Unet-like pure transformer for medical image segmentation. In: European conference on computer vision, pp. 205–218. Springer (2022)
5. Cao, Y., et al.: A comprehensive survey of ai-generated content (AIGC): a history of generative AI from GAN to CHATGPT. arXiv preprint arXiv:2303.04226 (2023)
6. Ferreira, A., Li, J., Pomykala, K.L., Kleesiek, J., Alves, V., Egger, J.: Gan-based generation of realistic 3D volumetric data: a systematic review and taxonomy. Med. Image Anal. **93**, 103100 (2024)
7. Ferreira, A., Luijten, G., Puladi, B., Kleesiek, J., Alves, V., Egger, J.: Brain Tumour removing and missing modality generation using 3D WDM. arXiv preprint arXiv:2411.04630 (2024)
8. Friedrich, P., Wolleb, J., Bieder, F., Durrer, A., Cattin, P.C.: Wdm: 3D wavelet diffusion models for high-resolution medical image synthesis. In: MICCAI workshop on deep generative models, pp. 11–21. Springer (2024)
9. He, K., Zhang, X., Ren, S., Sun, J.: Deep residual learning for image recognition. In: Proceedings of the IEEE Conference on Computer Vision and Pattern Recognition, pp. 770–778 (2016)
10. Kofler, F., et al.: The brain tumor segmentation (brats) challenge: local synthesis of healthy brain tissue via inpainting. arXiv preprint arXiv:2305.08992 (2023)
11. LaBella, D., et al.: Analysis of the brats 2023 intracranial meningioma segmentation challenge. arXiv preprint arXiv:2405.09787 (2024)
12. Li, H.B., et al.: The brain tumor segmentation (brats) challenge 2023: Brain MR image synthesis for tumor segmentation (brasyn). ArXiv pp. arXiv–2305 (2024)
13. Mendes, J.M., Barbar, A., Refaie, M.: Synthetic data generation: a privacy-preserving approach to accelerate rare disease research. Front. Digital Health **7**, 1563991 (2025)
14. Menze, B.H., et al.: The multimodal brain tumor image segmentation benchmark (brats). IEEE Trans. Med. Imaging **34**(10), 1993–2024 (2014)
15. Moawad, A.W., et al.: The brain tumor segmentation-metastases (brats-mets) challenge 2023: brain metastasis segmentation on pre-treatment MRI. ArXiv pp. arXiv–2306 (2024)
16. Nichol, A.Q., Dhariwal, P.: Improved denoising diffusion probabilistic models. In: International Conference on Machine Learning, pp. 8162–8171. PMLR (2021)
17. Pan, S., et al.: Synthetic CT generation from MRI using 3D transformer-based denoising diffusion model. Med. Phys. **51**(4), 2538–2548 (2024)
18. Ricker, J., Damm, S., Holz, T., Fischer, A.: Towards the detection of diffusion model deepfakes. arXiv preprint arXiv:2210.14571 (2022)
19. Song, J., Meng, C., Ermon, S.: Denoising diffusion implicit models. arXiv preprint arXiv:2010.02502 (2020)

Local Brain Tumour Inpainting Using Diffusion Transformers

Alexander Koch[1(✉)], Orhun Utku Aydin[1], Adam Hilbert[1], and Dietmar Frey[1,2]

[1] CLAIM – Charité Lab for AI in Medicine, Charité – Universitätsmedizin Berlin, corporate member of Freie Universität Berlin and Humboldt-Universität zu Berlin, Charitéplatz 1, 101117 Berlin, Germany
{alexander.koch,orhun-utku.aydin,adam.hilbert,dietmar.frey}@charite.de
[2] Department of Neurosurgery, Charité – Universitätsmedizin Berlin, corporate member of Freie Universität Berlin and Humboldt-Universität zu Berlin, Charitéplatz 1, 101117 Berlin, Germany

Abstract. Image inpainting of brain tumour MRI volumes has the potential to correct image artefacts, enable novel data augmentation methods and increase compatibility with automated image preprocessing methods. However, achieving 3D anatomical consistency and radiological fidelity remains a significant challenge, especially in the absence of large, annotated datasets. The BraTS 2025 dataset included T1-weighted brain MRI data from 1251 patients for training and 251 for validation. In our solution, we train an unconditional 3D diffusion transformer model to generate synthetic brain MRI data, operating directly on the high-dimensional pixel space ($240 \times 240 \times 155$). To ensure computationally efficient training, we utilise several architectural choices (Hourglass Transformer, efficient attention variants). The models are trained with affine data augmentations, a sigmoid noise schedule and Min-SNR loss weighting. Importantly, our solution does not use any inpainting-specific training. During inference, in the validation set, our models achieve a mean squared error (MSE) of 0.013, peak-signal-to-noise ratio (PSNR) of 20.23 and a structural similarity index measure (SSIM) of 0.775. Qualitatively, the inpainted regions are anatomically consistent with the surrounding tissue. In conclusion, our solution shows the feasibility of using a fully 3D diffusion model to address the task of healthy tissue inpainting, without inpainting-specific training.

Keywords: Diffusion · Transformer · Deep Learning · Neuroscience

1 Introduction

Synthetic image generation has been explored for various medical use cases, including image inpainting, where a selected region of a radiological scan gets replaced with synthetic content while preserving specified anatomical, pathological, or clinical properties. Image inpainting has been successfully addressed in

S. Bakas et al. (Eds.): MICCAI 2025, LNCS 16377, pp. 133–145, 2026.
https://doi.org/10.1007/978-3-032-16370-7_12

the 2D natural-image domain with use cases such as object removal or scratch filling. However, inpainting medical image volumes requires 3D anatomical consistency and fidelity to the radiological properties of the imaging modality, a substantial requirement to fulfil while annotated datasets remain scarce.

Previous research has highlighted several use cases for medical image inpainting. First, healthy tissue inpainting can enable models trained on normal populations to operate on pathological scans [21]. For instance, healthy versions of pathological images would ensure compatibility with existing brain tissue segmentation tools [12]. Second, the inpainting capabilities can be used to remove motion or other artefacts, improving downstream AI model performance (e.g. skullstripping or segmentation models). Third, inpainting-based data augmentation methods can increase model robustness. Furthermore, He et al. recently proposed inverse-supervised learning [14], where healthy-tissue replacement is used for broad-spectrum head disorder detection. Healthy tissue inpainting using generative models has the potential to improve such existing approaches and foster the development of new methodologies.

Our contributions:

1. Full-scale unconditional diffusion model on $240 \times 240 \times 155$ working directly on pixel space, no autoencoder or other dimensionality-reduction required
2. Hourglass-like transformer architecture with additional tricks
3. General synthesis method with no inpainting-specific training, thus applicable beyond the inpainting task

2 Methods

2.1 Data

Our solution uses single-channel T1-weighted brain MRI data from the BraTS 2025 Local Inpainting Challenge [3–6,17,21,25]. The dataset consists of 1251 training, 219 validation cases, and a held-out test set. The image spacing was $1\,\text{mm}^3$, and the image dimensions were $240 \times 240 \times 155$ voxels. The dataset provides healthy and unhealthy mask regions that allow differentiation between tumour and normal tissue. However, these masks were not used in our solution. We use the unprocessed T1-weighted brain MRI data and perform min-max scaling to $[-1, 1]$ range. We pad the data to be of size $240 \times 240 \times 160$. No additional data was used.

2.2 Background

Diffusion Transformer. The Diffusion Transformer architecture was introduced in [28]. It is a class of diffusion models, entirely based on transformers, specifically vision transformers [9]. Of particular importance is the conditioning introduced in the paper, which is applied to layer normalisation. These are referred to as adaLN-Zero blocks, because they each are initialised with zero. They modulate the layer normalisation before attention blocks and MLP blocks with the timestep signal obtained from the timestep embedding.

Hourglass Diffusion Transformer. The Hourglass Transformer architecture introduced by [27]. Similar to the U-Net architecture, the input is processed in a hierarchical manner with lower-resolution feature maps. However, instead of traditional downsampling and upsampling, simple linear layers are used, which effectively shorten or lengthen the sequence length. The sequence is successively shortened in the encoder stage, followed by the middle blocks and then lengthened again in the decoder stage. As in the U-Net, skip connections are employed. A combination of both the Diffusion Transformer and the Hourglass Transformer is the Hourglass Diffusion Transformer introduced by [8]. The architecture achieves subquadratic scaling of compute with resolution and can thus process high-resolution images in pixel space.

2.3 Our Approach

For our approach, we refrain from using any additional data and discard any mask data. We hypothesise that using an unconditional diffusion model provides the best generalisation as it cannot overfit on the masks and has to learn to model entire brains from scratch. Thus, such a model needs to learn the overall structure of a brain with each of its intricacies.

For this, we train an unconditional pixel-space three-dimensional diffusion model. We refrain from using a variational autoencoder to provide latent features, as this involves a two-stage training process. This would require us to train two separate models, ensuring that both generalise. However, using standard models like U-Net, ADM, or U-ViT does not work because running these on pixel-space easily runs out of memory.

Instead, we opt for the Diffusion Transformer (DiT) as a fast, energy-efficient and trainable alternative. The DiT was recently introduced and is already widely studied and used in state-of-the-art. This comes with a caveat: diffusion transformers are known to have limited to no inductive bias [1]. Thus, when training on a small dataset, the model will likely not converge, especially if the data is three-dimensional. Furthermore, using the classical DiT, we are restricted to large patch sizes, as the model scales quadratically with image size.

Recent work studying the generalisation of diffusion transformers has shown a discrepancy in performance compared to the U-Net, which is the lack of local inductive bias [1]. When trained with enough data, the attention map will attend to neighbouring tokens, close to the token at hand. This effect only happens when trained with sufficient data. We can enforce this behaviour without more data by using localised window attention. The simplest approach to implement this is the shifted window attention, as introduced by the Swin Transformer [22]. Replacing the attention with local attention also allows us to train with smaller patch sizes (patch size 4 instead of 16).

Compared to training a standard DiT of patch size $16 \times 16 \times 16$, the local attention DiT produces smooth images. However, we need a lot of capacity, and global structures are missing. To improve this, we use an Hourglass Transformer, which further reduces the computational overhead, scaling sub-quadratically with the sequence length. In Fig. 1 we show an abstraction of the architecture

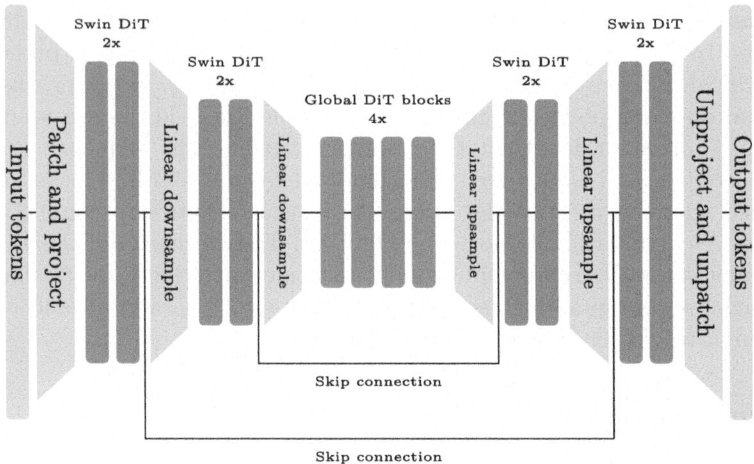

Fig. 1. Architecture visualization.

used. We use two layers of downsampling with two local attention blocks per stage. Each block provides a skip connection. For the middle blocks, we use global attention. For the patch size, we use $6 \times 6 \times 4$. The window size per local attention block is kept constant at four.

2.4 Diffusion Setup

A Gaussian diffusion process begins with the data x and gradually destroys the signal with noise over continuous time $t \in U(0, 1)$:

$$z_t = \alpha_t x + \sigma_t \varepsilon, \text{ where } \varepsilon \in \mathcal{N}(0, I) \tag{1}$$

We use a variance-preserving schedule, i.e. $\alpha_t^2 = 1 - \sigma_t^2$, where $\lambda_t = \log \text{SNR} = \log \alpha_t^2 / \sigma_t^2$ is the log signal-to-noise ratio. A neural network is trained to predict the original image from the noisy data for any timestep: $\hat{x} = \hat{x}_\theta(zt, t)$. To train the neural network, the weighted mean squared error loss is minimised.

$$L(x) = \mathbb{E}_{t \sim U(0,1)} w(\lambda_t) \|x - \hat{x}\|^2 \tag{2}$$

Here $w(\lambda_t)$ is the loss weighting, based on the log signal-to-noise ratio. Instead of predicting the start, we can also predict the noise or the velocity $v_t = \alpha_t \varepsilon_t - \sigma_t x$. We choose to predict the velocity as this has been shown to train more reliably, especially for larger resolutions [15].

The denoising process can be written as follows:

$$q(z_s \mid z_t, x) = \mathcal{N}(\mu_{t \to s}, \sigma_{t \to s}^2 I) \tag{3}$$

where $\mu_{t \to s} = \frac{\alpha_{ts} \sigma_s^2}{\sigma_t^2} z_t + \frac{\alpha_s \sigma_{ts}^2}{\sigma_t^2} x$ and $\sigma_{t \to s}^2 = \frac{\sigma_{ts}^2 \sigma_s^2}{\sigma_t^2}$, $\alpha_{ts} = \alpha_t / \alpha_s$ and $\sigma_{ts}^2 = \sigma_t^2 - \alpha_{ts}^2 \sigma_s^2$ and $t > s$. During sampling, when predicting the start, we clip the values between $[-1, 1]$ to keep the data within the bounds. When performing in-painting, we rescale the data afterwards to obtain the original minimum and maximum values of the data.

2.5 Inpainting

To perform inpainting with an unconditional diffusion model, we require a mask m and a ground truth image x. For the known part of the masked region, we can simply forward sample to obtain the noisy signal for timestep t. For the unknown part of the masked region, we simply perform denoising of the previous timestep. One step of inpainting thus looks as follows:

$$z_s^{\text{known}} = \alpha_s x + \sigma_s \varepsilon \tag{4}$$

$$z_s^{\text{unknown}} = q(z_s \mid z_t, x) \tag{5}$$

$$z_s = m z_s^{\text{known}} + (1 - m) z_s^{\text{unknown}} \tag{6}$$

2.6 Augmentation

For data augmentation, we draw random affine transformations that are applied to the brain scan. These consist of centred scaling, random rotations and voxel shifts. The parametrisation is as follows:

$$\begin{aligned}
\text{translations} &= \{(t_x, t_y, t_z) \mid t_x, t_y, t_z \in U(-3, 3)\} \\
\text{rotations} &= \left\{(r_x, r_y, r_z) \mid r_x \in U\left(0, \frac{\pi}{4}\right), r_y \in U\left(0, \frac{\pi}{4}\right), r_z \in U(0, 2\pi)\right\} \\
\text{scales} &= \{(s_x, s_y, s_z) \mid s_x, s_y, s_z \in U(0.8, 1.2)\}
\end{aligned}$$

We translate three voxels randomly, rotate each axis by 45 degrees, except in the axial plane, where we allow full 360-degree rotations. For the scales, we limit the reduction to 2% points higher or lower than the current scale on each axis. Given each augmentation, we obtain a 4x4 matrix and a transformed image per sample in the batch. Augmentations have a chance to occur per sample in the batch by 50 per cent. Every other time, we provide the identity matrix. This matrix is given as conditioning to our diffusion model. For this, we simply flatten the matrix and pass it through a simple MLP layer, consisting of two linear layers with a SiLU in between. The timestep embedding and matrix embedding are then simply added to obtain the final conditioning vector. During sampling, we set the matrix conditioning to be the identity matrix.

2.7 Bag of Tricks

In this section, we provide a collection of refinements used in our diffusion transformer architecture.

VDM Low-Discrepancy Sampler. We use the low-discrepancy sampler from Variational Diffusion Models (VDM) [19], which lowers the variance of the Monte Carlo estimator of the continuous-time loss, improving the optimisation efficiency. When processing a minibatch of k examples x_i, $i \in \{1, \ldots, k\}$, we require k timesteps t^i sampled from a uniform distribution. Instead of sampling these timesteps independently, we sample a single uniform random number $u_0 \sim U(0, 1)$ and then set $t^i = \text{mod}(u_0 + \frac{i}{k}, 1)$. Each t^i now has the correct uniform marginal distribution, but the minibatch of timesteps covers the space in $[0, 1]$ more equally than when sampling independently. This reduces the variance during training.

Sigmoid Schedule. For diffusion training, we use a sigmoid schedule as defined in [16]:

$$v_{\text{start}} = \sigma(\text{start}/\tau) \tag{7}$$

$$v_{\text{end}} = \sigma(\text{end}/\tau) \tag{8}$$

$$\gamma(t) = -\frac{\sigma(\frac{t(\text{end}-\text{start})+\text{start}}{\tau}) + v_{\text{end}}}{(v_{\text{end}} - v_{\text{start}})} \tag{9}$$

where $\sigma(t)$ is the sigmoid function, start $= -3$, end $= 3$ and $\tau = 1$. In our formulation $\alpha_t = \sqrt{\gamma(t)}$. Thus, we can reformulate the logarithmic signal-to-noise ratio as follows

$$\log \text{SNR}(t) = \log \frac{\alpha_t^2}{\sigma_t^2} = \log \frac{\alpha_t^2}{1 - \alpha_t^2} = \log \gamma(t) - \log(1 - \gamma(t)) \tag{10}$$

Min-SNR. We use the soft version of Min-SNR [8,13]. Min-SNR is a loss weighting scheme for diffusion models, which has been shown to improve diffusion model training [13,20]. Recall the original definition of MinSNR:

$$w_t = \min\{\text{SNR}(t), \gamma\} \tag{11}$$

Here, instead of a hard cut-off at the threshold, the soft version provides a smooth transition. The soft-weighted version can be written as

$$w_t = \frac{\alpha^2}{\sigma^2 + \gamma^{-1}} \tag{12}$$

For our model, we set γ to five as used in the original paper.

LASER Attention. To improve the gradients of attention, we utilise LASER attention [10]. The authors use the log-sum-exp trick to boost the gradient signal. Attention is applied in exponential value space. Given query, key, value as $Q, K, V \in \mathbb{R}^{N \times d}$ with output $O \in \mathbb{R}^{N \times d}$

$$m_j = \max_{i \in \{1,\ldots,N\}} V_{ij},\ j \in \{1,\ldots,d\} \tag{13}$$

$$\hat{V_{ij}} = V_{ij} - m_j \tag{14}$$

$$O = \log(\text{softmax}(QK^\top)\exp(\hat{V})\text{diag}(\exp(m))) \tag{15}$$

$$O_{ij} = (\log(\text{softmax}(QK^\top)\exp(\hat{V})))_{ij} + m_j \tag{16}$$

RMSNorm. Root Mean Square Layer Normalisation (RMSNorm) [32] is a normalisation layer used to stabilise training and improve model convergence. Compared to the commonly used Layer normalisation [2], it is simpler and computationally more efficient. It has been used recently as a drop-in replacement for Layer normalisation and has been found to be the best performing normalisation variant [26]. A simplification to RMSNorm is introduced by [30], where the authors discover that the learned scaling can be disabled without performance degradation. Thus, we use SimpleRMSNorm in our model.

Cosine Similarity Attention. Cosine similarity has been successfully used in recent papers [18,22]. Here, the queries and keys of attention are normed using L2-normalisation.

Shifted Window Attention. As in [8], we add local attention to all levels, except the middle block on the lowest resolution. Here, instead, we use global attention. As for the choice of the local attention, we use shifted windows as introduced by the Swin Transformer [22,23]. Self-attention is computed in partitions of non-overlapping windows instead of the full sequence length. To facilitate connections between the windows, the windows are shifted every second layer. Additionally, a relative positional bias is injected into the self-attention. This reduces the computational complexity and introduces a local inductive bias, similar to using convolutions with a small kernel size. We fix the window size to four for all layers.

Feed-Forward Activation. Instead of commonly used vision transformer MLPs, consisting of two linear layers, with a ReLU in between, we use SwiGLUs [31]. Here, the data itself affects its own modulation. We find that these always provide a performance increase over a classical MLP layer.

Tied Weight Embedding. When training language models [29] recommend tying the weights of the input embedding and the output embedding together. They show that the tied embedding evolves similarly to the output embedding. This method results in performance improvements regarding perplexity and is commonly used in LLMs. We apply the same technique, but instead of text, we are embedding image patches. This reduces the parameter count.

2.8 Training Setup

We use the Adam-atan2 [11] variant. This version of Adam eliminates the epsilon hyperparameter. We set $\beta_1 = 0.9$, $\beta_2 = 0.95$, use bfloat16 precision training, a batch size of four, a learning rate of 5×10^{-4} and a weight decay of $\lambda = 10^{-5}$. The weight decay is decoupled from the learning rate following [24]. We use a learning rate warmup of 10,000 steps and train for a total budget of 300,000 steps. We implement all our models in JAX [7].

3 Results

In Fig. 2, we show two unconditional samples from our model using the identity matrix as conditioning, using 2048 sampling steps. The model generates realistic brains that are structurally sound. In Fig. 3, we show an example of performing inpainting using the same model on the validation set. For inpainting, we sample our model using 256 sampling steps. In our experiments, we found that sampling shorter or too long degrades the performance of the metrics. Given the mask and the voided image, we apply our inpainting algorithm and let the model sample the missing regions. The inpainted regions appear consistent with the surrounding tissue. In Table 1, we show the results of the distance metrics on the training, validation and test set. We measure the distances to the original images and the predicted inpainted ones. Due to time constraints, we were only able to evaluate our training scores for 380 samples. When comparing the training and the validation scores, our model performs better on the training set, achieving lower MSE, PSNR and SSIM scores than on the validation set.

Table 1. Results of the inpainting on the training, validation and test set. We estimate the results on the training set using 380 samples. We provide the mean and the standard deviation per value.

	MSE	RMSE	PSNR	SSIM
Training	0.009 ± 0.007	0.089 ± 0.035	21.63 ± 3.779	0.7989 ± 0.129
Validation	0.013 ± 0.01	N/A	20.229 ± 4.006	0.775 ± 0.133
Test	N/A	0.094 ± 0.043	21.469 ± 4.416	0.837 ± 0.135

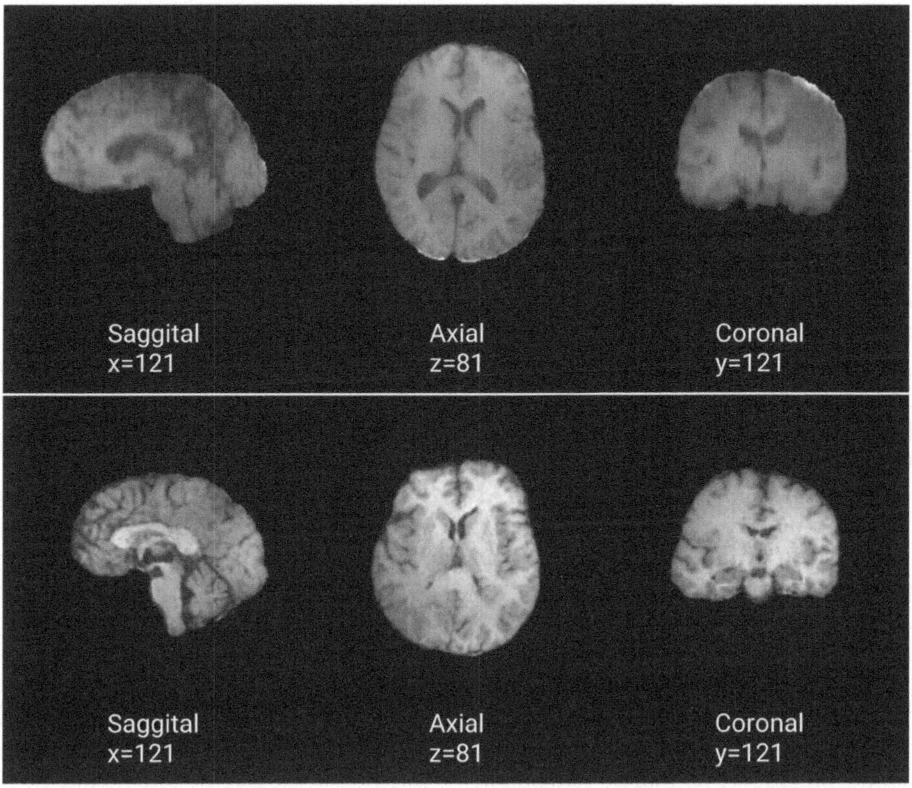

Saggital
x=121

Axial
z=81

Coronal
y=121

Saggital
x=121

Axial
z=81

Coronal
y=121

Fig. 2. Two unconditional samples from the model, sampled using 2048 steps.

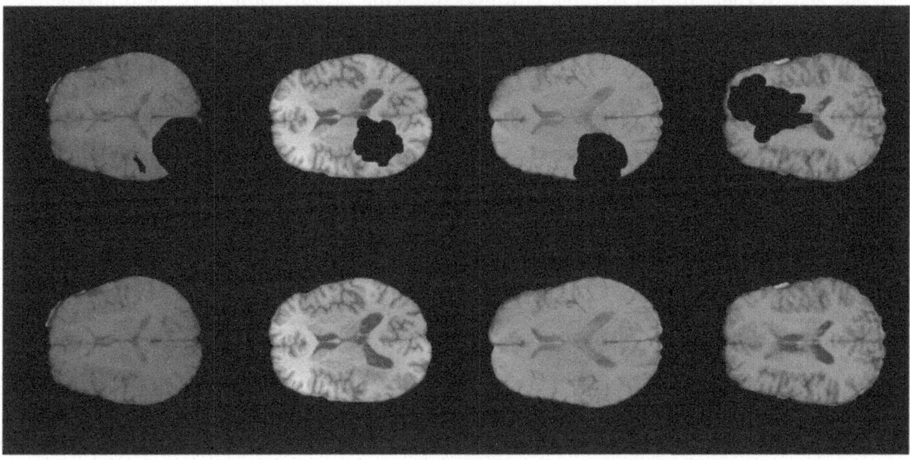

Fig. 3. Inpainting results of full 3D images on the validation set. Here, we show axial slices at z-index 80. The top row shows the voided image and the bottom row the inpainted result. We use 256 sampling steps.

4 Discussion

We demonstrate the feasibility of using a fully 3D diffusion model to address the task of healthy tissue inpainting, without inpainting-specific training. The mask agnostic training of our solution may allow generalisation beyond the mask configurations seen during training and thus reduce overfitting. Moreover, since we omit masks during training, our approach should generalise better in under-represented (i.e. according to regions of interest in training masks) brain regions and is generally applicable for healthy inpainting of any pathology in the brain. When trained to convergence, the proposed model could further be exploited for generic pathology detection beyond inpainting since it models the full brain. Executing step-wise inpainting throughout the whole brain and comparison to the ground truth pathological scan can highlight suspicious areas. This ability of our approach greatly increases potential clinical utility beyond inpainting. One limitation of this approach is that it sacrifices fully controllable generation, especially with respect to healthy and pathological inpainting. We hypothesise that our model can perform better if trained for longer and with a higher batch size using distributed training on multiple GPUs. Especially given the amount of possible augmentations using our method, we believe that our method should generalise with longer training. Due to time constraints, we only trained our model for 300,000 steps. Future works should use the resulting edited images as synthetic data augmentation and evaluate on downstream tasks such as segmentation and classification. Furthermore, the anatomical consistency of inpainted regions should be visually evaluated to establish a ground truth for evaluation beyond pixel-level similarity measures.

Acknowledgments. Computation has been performed on the HPC for Research cluster of the Berlin Institute of Health. Data used in this publication were obtained as part of the Challenge project through Synapse ID syn64153430. The authors acknowledge the financial support by the Federal Ministry of Research, Technology and Space of Germany in the grant program "Forschungsnetzwerk Anonymisierung für eine sichere Datennutzung" (Project number 16KISA042K).

Disclosure of Interests. The authors have no competing interests to declare that are relevant to the content of this article.

References

1. An, J., Wang, D., Guo, P., Luo, J., Schwing, A.G.: On inductive biases that enable generalization of diffusion transformers. CoRR **abs/2410.21273** (2024). https://doi.org/10.48550/ARXIV.2410.21273
2. Ba, L.J., Kiros, J.R., Hinton, G.E.: Layer normalization. CoRR **abs/1607.06450** (2016). http://arxiv.org/abs/1607.06450
3. Baid, U., et al.: The RSNA-ASNR-MICCAI brats 2021 benchmark on brain tumor segmentation and radiogenomic classification. CoRR **abs/2107.02314** (2021). https://arxiv.org/abs/2107.02314

4. Bakas, S., et al.: Advancing the cancer genome atlas glioma MRI collections with expert segmentation labels and radiomic features. Sci. Data **4**(1), 170117 (2017). https://doi.org/10.1038/sdata.2017.117
5. Bakas, S., et al.: Segmentation labels and radiomic features for the pre-operative scans of the TCGA-GBM collection. Cancer Imaging Archive (2017). https://doi.org/10.7937/K9/TCIA.2017.KLXWJJ1Q
6. Bakas, S., et al.: Segmentation labels and radiomic features for the pre-operative scans of the TCGA-LGG collection. Cancer Imaging Archive (2017). https://doi.org/10.7937/K9/TCIA.2017.GJQ7R0EF
7. Bradbury, J., et al.: JAX: composable transformations of Python+NumPy programs (2018). http://github.com/jax-ml/jax
8. Crowson, K., et al.: Scalable high-resolution pixel-space image synthesis with hourglass diffusion transformers. In: Forty-first International Conference on Machine Learning, ICML 2024, Vienna, Austria, July 21-27, 2024. OpenReview.net (2024). https://openreview.net/forum?id=WRIn2HmtBS
9. Dosovitskiy, A., et al.: An image is worth 16x16 words: transformers for image recognition at scale. In: 9th International Conference on Learning Representations, ICLR 2021, Virtual Event, Austria, May 3-7, 2021. OpenReview.net (2021). https://openreview.net/forum?id=YicbFdNTTy
10. Duvvuri, S.S., Dhillon, I.S.: LASER: attention with exponential transformation. CoRR **abs/2411.03493** (2024). https://doi.org/10.48550/ARXIV.2411.03493
11. Everett, K.E., et al.: Scaling exponents across parameterizations and optimizers. In: Forty-first International Conference on Machine Learning, ICML 2024, Vienna, Austria, July 21-27, 2024. OpenReview.net (2024). https://openreview.net/forum?id=0ksNeD1SJT
12. Fischl, B.: Freesurfer. Neuroimage **62**(2), 774–781 (2012)
13. Hang, T., et al.: Efficient diffusion training via Min-SNR weighting strategy. In: IEEE/CVF International Conference on Computer Vision, ICCV 2023, Paris, France, October 1-6, 2023, pp. 7407–7417. IEEE (2023). https://doi.org/10.1109/ICCV51070.2023.00684
14. He, Y., et al.: Disorder-free data are all you need—inverse supervised learning for broad-spectrum head disorder detection. NEJM AI **1**(4), AIoa2300137 (2024). https://doi.org/10.1056/AIoa2300137
15. Hoogeboom, E., Heek, J., Salimans, T.: simple diffusion: End-to-end diffusion for high resolution images. In: Proceedings of the 40th International Conference on Machine Learning, pp. 13213–13232. PMLR (2023). https://proceedings.mlr.press/v202/hoogeboom23a.html, iSSN: 2640-3498
16. Jabri, A., Fleet, D.J., Chen, T.: Scalable adaptive computation for iterative generation. In: Krause, A., Brunskill, E., Cho, K., Engelhardt, B., Sabato, S., Scarlett, J. (eds.) International Conference on Machine Learning, ICML 2023, 23-29 July 2023, Honolulu, Hawaii, USA. Proceedings of Machine Learning Research, vol. 202, pp. 14569–14589. PMLR (2023). https://proceedings.mlr.press/v202/jabri23a.html
17. Karargyris, A., et al.: Federated benchmarking of medical artificial intelligence with MEDPERF. Nat. Mach. Intell. **5**(7), 799–810 (2023). https://doi.org/10.1038/s42256-023-00652-2
18. Karras, T., Aittala, M., Lehtinen, J., Hellsten, J., Aila, T., Laine, S.: Analyzing and improving the training dynamics of diffusion models. In: IEEE/CVF Conference on Computer Vision and Pattern Recognition, CVPR 2024, Seattle, WA, USA, June 16-22, 2024, pp. 24174–24184. IEEE (2024). https://doi.org/10.1109/CVPR52733.2024.02282

19. Kingma, D.P., Salimans, T., Poole, B., Ho, J.: Variational diffusion models. CoRR **abs/2107.00630** (2021). https://arxiv.org/abs/2107.00630
20. Koch, A., et al.: Cross-modality image synthesis from TOF-MRA to CTA using diffusion-based models. Med. Image Anal. **105**, 103722 (2025)
21. Kofler, F., et al.: The brain tumor segmentation (brats) challenge 2023: local synthesis of healthy brain tissue via inpainting. CoRR **abs/2305.08992** (2023). https://doi.org/10.48550/ARXIV.2305.08992
22. Liu, Z., et al.: Swin transformer V2: scaling up capacity and resolution. In: IEEE/CVF Conference on Computer Vision and Pattern Recognition, CVPR 2022, New Orleans, LA, USA, June 18-24, 2022, pp. 11999–12009. IEEE (2022). https://doi.org/10.1109/CVPR52688.2022.01170
23. Liu, Z., et al.: Swin transformer: hierarchical vision transformer using shifted windows. In: 2021 IEEE/CVF International Conference on Computer Vision, ICCV 2021, Montreal, QC, Canada, October 10-17, 2021, pp. 9992–10002. IEEE (2021). https://doi.org/10.1109/ICCV48922.2021.00986
24. Loshchilov, I., Hutter, F.: Decoupled weight decay regularization. In: 7th International Conference on Learning Representations, ICLR 2019, New Orleans, LA, USA, May 6-9, 2019. OpenReview.net (2019). https://openreview.net/forum?id=Bkg6RiCqY7
25. Menze, B.H., et al.: The multimodal brain tumor image segmentation benchmark (brats). IEEE Trans. Med. Imaging **34**(10), 1993–2024 (2015). https://doi.org/10.1109/TMI.2014.2377694
26. Narang, S., et al.: Do transformer modifications transfer across implementations and applications? In: Moens, M., Huang, X., Specia, L., Yih, S.W. (eds.) Proceedings of the 2021 Conference on Empirical Methods in Natural Language Processing, EMNLP 2021, Virtual Event / Punta Cana, Dominican Republic, 7-11 November, 2021, pp. 5758–5773. Association for Computational Linguistics (2021). https://doi.org/10.18653/V1/2021.EMNLP-MAIN.465
27. Nawrot, P., et al.: Hierarchical transformers are more efficient language models. In: Carpuat, M., de Marneffe, M., Ruíz, I.V.M. (eds.) Findings of the Association for Computational Linguistics: NAACL 2022, Seattle, WA, United States, July 10-15, 2022, pp. 1559–1571. Association for Computational Linguistics (2022). https://doi.org/10.18653/V1/2022.FINDINGS-NAACL.117
28. Peebles, W., Xie, S.: Scalable diffusion models with transformers. In: IEEE/CVF International Conference on Computer Vision, ICCV 2023, Paris, France, October 1-6, 2023, pp. 4172–4182. IEEE (2023). https://doi.org/10.1109/ICCV51070.2023.00387
29. Press, O., Wolf, L.: Using the output embedding to improve language models. In: Lapata, M., Blunsom, P., Koller, A. (eds.) Proceedings of the 15th Conference of the European Chapter of the Association for Computational Linguistics, EACL 2017, Valencia, Spain, April 3-7, 2017, Volume 2: Short Papers, pp. 157–163. Association for Computational Linguistics (2017). https://doi.org/10.18653/V1/E17-2025
30. Qin, Z., et al.: Scaling TransNormer to 175 billion parameters. CoRR **abs/2307.14995** (2023). https://doi.org/10.48550/ARXIV.2307.14995

31. Shazeer, N.: GLU variants improve transformer. CoRR **abs/2002.05202** (2020). https://arxiv.org/abs/2002.05202
32. Zhang, B., Sennrich, R.: Root mean square layer normalization. In: Wallach, H.M., Larochelle, H., Beygelzimer, A., d'Alché-Buc, F., Fox, E.B., Garnett, R. (eds.) Advances in Neural Information Processing Systems 32: Annual Conference on Neural Information Processing Systems 2019, NeurIPS 2019, December 8-14, 2019, Vancouver, BC, Canada. pp. 12360–12371 (2019). https://proceedings.neurips.cc/paper/2019/hash/1e8a19426224ca89e83cef47f1e7f53b-Abstract.html

Post-processing Methods for Improving Accuracy in MRI Inpainting

Nishad Kulkarni[1], Krithika Iyer[1], Austin Tapp[1], Abhijeet Parida[1,2], Daniel Capellán-Martín[1,2], Zhifan Jiang[1], María J. Ledesma-Carbayo[2], Syed Muhammad Anwar[1,3], and Marius George Linguraru[1,3](✉)

[1] Sheikh Zayed Institute for Pediatric Surgical Innovation, Children's National Hospital, Washington, DC, USA
mlingura@childrensnational.org

[2] Universidad Politécnica de Madrid and CIBER-BBN, ISCIII, Madrid, Spain

[3] School of Medicine and Health Sciences, George Washington University, Washington, DC, USA

Abstract. Magnetic Resonance Imaging (MRI) is the primary imaging modality used in the diagnosis, assessment, and treatment planning for brain pathologies. However, most automated MRI analysis tools, such as segmentation and registration pipelines, are optimized for healthy anatomies and often fail when confronted with large lesions such as tumors. To overcome this, image inpainting techniques aim to locally synthesize healthy brain tissues in tumor regions, enabling the reliable application of general-purpose tools. In this work, we systematically evaluate state-of-the-art inpainting models and observe a saturation in their standalone performance. In response, we introduce a methodology combining model ensembling with efficient post-processing strategies such as median filtering, histogram matching, and pixel averaging. Further anatomical refinement is achieved via a lightweight U-Net enhancement stage. Comprehensive evaluation demonstrates that our proposed pipeline improves the anatomical plausibility and visual fidelity of inpainted regions, yielding higher accuracy and more robust outcomes than individual baseline models. By combining established models with targeted post-processing, we achieve improved and more accessible inpainting outcomes, supporting broader clinical deployment and sustainable, resource-conscious research. Our 2025 BraTS inpainting docker is available at hub.docker.com/layers/aparida12/brats2025/inpt.

Keywords: Brain tumor · Inpainting · MRI · Post-processing · Ensemble

1 Introduction

Magnetic Resonance Imaging (MRI) and automated analysis are critical for monitoring brain pathologies [1]. However, existing segmentation and registration

N. Kulkarni, K. Iyer and A. Tapp—Equal contribution.

S. Bakas et al. (Eds.): MICCAI 2025, LNCS 16377, pp. 146–157, 2026.
https://doi.org/10.1007/978-3-032-16370-7_13

tools, designed for healthy anatomies, perform poorly in the presence of large lesions such as glioma, limiting their clinical utility [1]. To address these limitations, recent efforts have explored the use of image inpainting to locally synthesize healthy-appearing brain tissue in regions affected by tumors. Inpainting, a well-established task in computer vision, involves reconstructing missing or corrupted parts of an image using contextual information [1,13]. While traditionally applied to 2D natural images, in the context of neuroimaging, inpainting offers the potential to restore anatomical plausibility in 3D MR volumes, enabling the application of standard processing pipelines even in the presence of pathology [23,29].

The Brain Tumor Segmentation (BraTS) challenge has historically focused on benchmarking algorithms for tumor segmentation in MRI scans of glioma patients [17,18]. In 2023, the challenge introduced a new task focused on 3D inpainting of T1-weighted MRIs, where tumor regions were masked out and participants were asked to synthesize realistic, healthy tissue in their place. This task has both clinical and research relevance: in-painted images can improve image registration, facilitate whole-brain parcellation, and support studies of tumor – brain interactions by enabling analysis of the underlying brain anatomy in the absence of visible lesions [23]. Building on this foundation, the BraTS 2025 inpainting challenge continues to advance the field by encouraging the development of robust, generalizable algorithms for localized 3D brain tissue synthesis.

As the field advances, however, critical questions emerge regarding the direction and efficiency of model development for medical image inpainting. In recent years, deep learning models have reached a plateau, with leading algorithms showing only marginal differences in performance metrics [16,26]. Moreover, even with architectural advances, issues like anatomical implausibility, blurred inpainted regions, and imperfect integration with surrounding tissue persist in many models [16,21]. This diminishing return prompts reflection: does the field benefit from continually training larger, more complex models, or should efforts shift toward more intelligent utilization of existing resources and data? Medical imaging inherently suffers from data scarcity compared to natural image domains, making continued escalation in model complexity impractical and often counterproductive. Overly complex models not only demand significant computational resources but also risk overfitting, reduced interpretability, and high environmental cost factors that collectively limit real-world clinical translation, especially in resource-constrained clinical sites [5,10].

A notable limitation of existing inpainting approaches lies in underutilizing abundant healthy brain scans [7,15]. Current models often struggle with generating high-fidelity, realistic tissue, occasionally resulting in inpainted images that are blurry or anatomically implausible [24]. In contrast, adopting general purpose yet robust architectures such as denoising autoencoders trained on large, healthy image patches offers a promising, generalizable route for enhancing image quality [6,24]. These models facilitate the restoration of anatomical consistency without needing large, complex networks by focusing on domain-specific feature extraction from healthy regions. Additionally, traditional image processing techniques provide straightforward, computationally efficient post-processing strategies, including median filtering, pixel averaging (ensemble methods), and sharpening [25]. Combined with lightweight learning-based models, these tools have the potential to consistently outperform many computationally intensive approaches, eliminating the need for repeated, large-scale model training [3,11]. Such solutions could dramatically lower GPU and memory requirements, reduce total energy consumption, and lend themselves to be readily deployable on-site—characteristics that address practical and sustainability considerations for clinical implementation [22]. Additionally, recent studies have demonstrated how intuitively designed methodologies demonstrate robust, generalizable pipelines across diverse clinical environments, as shown in recent efforts leveraging ensemble models for brain tumor segmentation and adaptation in under-resourced settings [2,8,9,20]. Thus, streamlined, ensembled methodologies pave the way for building equity in model deployment [27]. Inequality in access to high-end computational infrastructure is a persistent barrier; therefore, optimizing and reusing established tools democratizes advanced neuroimaging workflows, enabling broader access and more consistent standards of care.

2 Methods

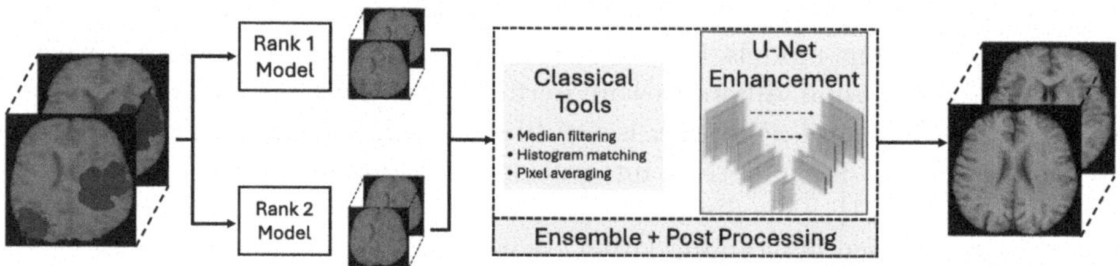

Fig. 1. Overview of the proposed post-processing pipeline for MRI inpainting. Inpainted outputs from the top two models from the BraTS 2024 inpainting challenge are first aggregated using classical tools like pixel-level averaging. The ensemble result is then refined by post-processing, a basic U-Net trained on synthetically blurred healthy brain regions, or a mix of both. This multi-stage pipeline improves anatomical fidelity and reconstruction sharpness while maintaining computational efficiency.

2.1 Dataset

The BraTS local inpainting dataset (2025) [12] is derived from the BraTS glioma segmentation dataset, which contains multi-modal scans (T1, T1ce, T2, and FLAIR) [19]. However, the local inpainting challenge exclusively utilizes the T1-weighted MRI scans for both training and validation. The training set comprises 1251 cases, with each case including the T1 scan, the mask segmenting healthy and unhealthy regions, the full mask, and a voided T1 scan where the lesion region is removed. The validation set consists of 219 cases, each providing only the voided T1 scan and the mask segmenting healthy and unhealthy regions. This structure enables focused development and evaluation of inpainting algorithms on the T1 modality, distinct from segmentation challenges that use all four modalities.

2.2 Proposed Pipeline

Our pipeline integrates multiple stages to generate high-quality, healthy brain tissue inpaintings from masked MRI scans, as illustrated in Fig. 1. Pre-trained models, specifically the top-performing U-Net by Zhang et al. [28] and the 3D Wavelet Diffusion model by Ferreira et al. [4], produce inpainted predictions. These outputs then undergo post-processing steps, including classical pixel averaging filters and a dedicated U-Net-based enhancement module trained to denoise and refine anatomical details. The enhanced outputs from these combined procedures form the final synthesized healthy brain tissue volumes. In the following sections, we describe each component of this pipeline in detail.

State-of-the-Art (SOTA) Inpainting Model Details.

U-Net Based Healthy 3D Brain Tissue Inpainting, J.Zhang et al. [28] As part of our model ensemble, we incorporate the U-Net-based brain tissue inpainting method developed by Zhang et al. Last year, this model was the top performer in the BraTS Local Synthesis of Tissue via Inpainting challenge, establishing it as the SOTA approach for healthy 3D brain tissue synthesis within masked regions of T1-weighted MRI volumes. This strong benchmark performance makes it a highly robust and justifiable choice for inclusion in our pipeline.

In our approach, we leverage the published implementation and utilize the pre-trained weights, ensuring faithful reproducibility with the original SOTA methodology. The architecture is a sophisticated 3D U-Net with three levels of downsampling and upsampling, skip connections, and a ReLU-activated bridge; regularization techniques include instance normalization and dropout (0.2). The loss function combines mean absolute error within the healthy mask regions and structural similarity index over the entire volume. For our ensemble, masked T1 images are input to the pre-trained U-Net model, with the output inpainted regions seamlessly integrated back into the original image context.

Conditional Wavelet Diffusion Model, A. Ferreira et al. [4]. We incorporate the 3D Wavelet Diffusion Model (WDM) developed by Ferreira et al. as part of our brain tumor inpainting ensemble. This approach achieved second place in the BraTS 2024 Local Synthesis of Tissue via Inpainting challenge, demonstrating competitive performance and complementing the SOTA U-Net model.

The model leverages conditional diffusion processes applied in the wavelet domain, allowing full-resolution 3D brain MRI volumes to be processed without patching or downsampling. This preserves high spatial fidelity during inpainting synthesis while maintaining manageable GPU memory usage. Unlike conventional voxel-space diffusion models, the wavelet transform disentangles spatial frequency components, improving the learning efficiency and reconstruction quality of fine details. The conditional input includes masked MRI images paired with binary masks denoting regions for inpainting. The model was trained to iteratively denoise wavelet coefficients conditioned on these inputs, reconstructing healthy tissue in the tumor-masked regions.

Inference operates by feeding masked MRI data through the trained wavelet diffusion network to generate consistent, high-fidelity tissue inpaintings and synthesized modalities. The outputs are inverse wavelet transformed back into image space and seamlessly integrated into the original volumes for downstream analysis. By incorporating the pre-trained 3D Wavelet Diffusion Model, our ensemble benefits from an advanced generative approach optimized for high-resolution, volumetric brain MRI synthesis with efficient memory usage and strong inpainting accuracy. Together with the U-Net model, this provides complementary strengths in reproducing realistic healthy brain tissue across diverse pathological scenarios.

Post-processing

1. Pixel Averaging: Median/Geometric Approach: After obtaining inpainted outputs from leading SOTA models, classical image processing techniques are employed to enhance visual consistency and reduce instability across the synthesized regions. Specifically, pixel-level aggregation strategies such as voxel-wise average, median, and geometric mean filters are applied to ensemble multiple model predictions. These techniques operate at the voxel level, aggregating pixel intensities across aligned predictions to produce a representative consensus output. Averaging provides a smooth blend of input predictions, minimizing high-frequency disagreement, while the geometric mean is more robust to multiplicative outliers. Notably, when only two predictions are available, average and median aggregations yield mathematically equivalent results. However, the pipeline is designed to accommodate richer ensemble configurations, enabling maximum intensity projection, variance-based adaptive fusion, or hybrid aggregation strategies in future expansions. Collectively, these pixel-level operations offer a robust and interpretable post-processing mechanism that harmonizes multi-model predictions and reduces synthesis variability across diverse MR volumes.

2. Post-averaging Smoothing: We employ two classical denoising strategies to refine the ensembled output. First, we apply a 3D median filter with a $3 \times 3 \times 3$ kernel, which effectively removes localized outlier voxels while preserving edge structure and anatomical boundaries. This median filter is highly effective when ensembling three or more predictions, such as the top three ranked challenge submissions or hybrid combinations (e.g., two predictions from the first-place model and one from the second-place model). In such cases, the median serves as an outlier-resistant estimator that preserves sharp transitions while rejecting spurious values introduced by any single model and makes it especially beneficial in areas where individual model outputs may hallucinate inconsistent textures or misaligned anatomical boundaries. Second, we apply Gaussian smoothing with a small standard deviation ($\sigma = 0.5$), which gently suppresses high-frequency noise and improves voxel-wise consistency without overly blurring tissue interfaces.

3. Histogram Matching: Following smoothing, we perform histogram matching using the output of the Rank 1 model as the reference. This step aligns the intensity distribution of the ensembled prediction with that of the most reliable single-model output. By correcting for model-specific intensity shifts and ensuring consistency with the original intensity range, histogram matching enhances perceptual realism and improves cross-sample comparability, especially in downstream analyses where intensity drift may affect quantitative accuracy.

4. Deep Learning Enhancement. As a learned post-processing step, a U-Net model was trained using a synthetic inpainting dataset designed to enable supervised learning of image refinement. To construct this dataset, we started with the original inpainting training dataset and applied random Gaussian blurring to the healthy brain regions defined by the provided healthy masks. This localized degradation mimics the smooth, low-detail appearance of BraTS inpainting methods. The resulting blurred images serve as inputs to the U-Net, while the original, high-resolution MR scans provide the ground truth targets. The network minimizes mean squared error during this task in an attempt to improve ensemble scores. The U-Net effectively minimizes anatomical error, delineates structural boundaries, and optimizes residual smoothing artifacts by leveraging the ground truth healthy tissue appearance. This context-aware enhancement approach complements classical pixel-wise filtering by addressing limitations that ensemble averaging alone cannot resolve. As a result, the U-Net serves as a robust and flexible final-stage enhancement module, significantly improving the perceptual quality and clinical realism of inpainted brain MR volumes.

3 Experiments

3.1 Metrics

To assess image inpainting quality, we use three main metrics. Structural similarity (SSIM) measures how closely the synthetic image matches the real one in structure, contrast, and luminance; values closer to 1 reflect higher perceptual similarity. Peak signal-to-noise ratio (PSNR) quantifies the ratio between signal and noise based on pixel errors, with higher decibel values indicating better reconstruction quality. Mean squared error (MSE) calculates the average squared difference between predicted and ground truth images, where lower values mean closer pixel-wise agreement.

We optimized the thresholds and chose the best model with the ranking approach proposed by the BraTS team LaBella *et al.* [14]. The evaluation is done in a hidden test set, computing lesion-wise metrics in all regions and comparing ranks of all the submissions rather than the metrics. To replicate this procedure, we built an internal ranking metric that produces a single score, where a smaller value means better performance on MSE, SSIM, and PSNR. The code is available on GitHub[1].

The ranking metric approach is robust to outlier predictions, allowing us to optimize for a single value while aligning with the contest evaluation pipeline.

3.2 Models for Comparison

We compare five setups: (1) output from Zhang's U-Net [28], (2) output from Ferreira's 3D Wavelet Diffusion [4], (3) an ensemble of Zhang's and Ferreira's models via geometric or pixel-level averaging, (4) the same ensemble further refined with classical filters such as median or Gaussian, and (5) the filtered ensemble with an additional U-Net-based denoising stage for enhanced image quality. Filter implementation followed a straightforward scheme: model outputs from Zhang and Ferreira were combined voxelwise using equal 50/50 weighting, either via geometric averaging (primary setting) or alternative strategies (mean, median, max, min). The refined outputs were subsequently matched to their corresponding references using histogram matching to preserve intensity distributions. For the U-Net model, training was conducted for 1000 epochs with 250 iterations per epoch, including 50 validation iterations. We optimized with SGD (momentum $= 0.99$, Nesterov), weight decay $= 3 \times 10^{-5}$, an initial learning rate of 1×10^{-2}, and polynomial decay. Batch size and patch size were 2 and $96 \times 160 \times 160$, respectively. Simple augmentations of rotations ($\pm 30°$ per axis or anisotropy-aware), uniform scaling [0.7, 1.4], Gaussian noise ($p = 0.1$), Gaussian blur ($\sigma \in [0.5, 1.0]$, $p = 0.2$), brightness scaling ($\times[0.75, 1.25]$, $p = 0.15$), contrast adjustment ($p = 0.15$), simulated low resolution (zoom $\in [0.5, 1.0]$, $p = 0.25$), and gamma corrections ($p = 0.1/0.3$), with mirroring and oversampling of foreground regions were used (0.33). The refinement U-Net minimized mean squared error without deep supervision or additional augmentation. Training used a 5-fold cross-validation split, and results were reported as the equal-weight (50/50) ensemble of model probabilities across folds. This design enables us to assess the impact of model combination and each post-processing step against the state of the art (Fig. 2).

4 Results

Table 1 presents the quantitative results for our validation-phase experiments using the BraTS 2025 inpainting benchmark. The table summarizes how various post-processing strategies affect the perceptual and quantitative quality of inpainted brain MR volumes. All reported mean $\pm$ standard deviation values are

[1] https://github.com/Pediatric-Accelerated-Intelligence-Lab/BraTS-Unofficial-Ranker.

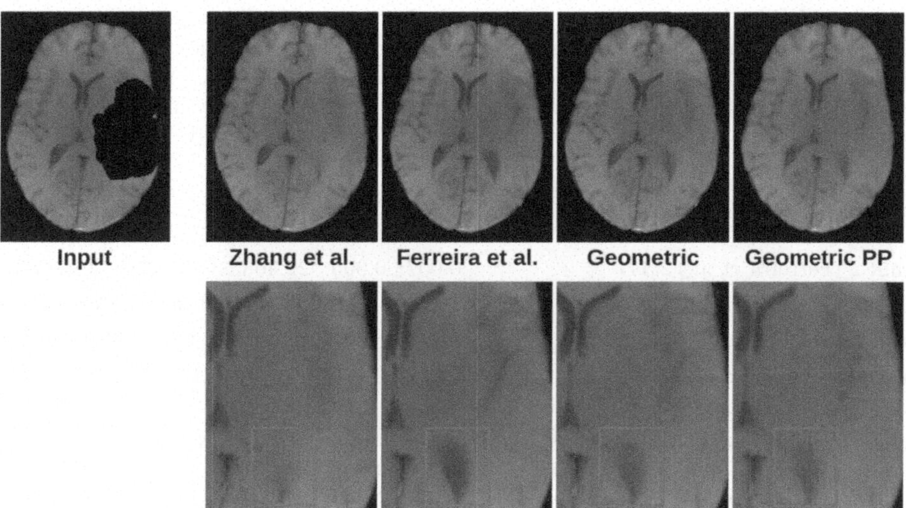

Fig. 2. Qualitative Results Comparison of inpainted brain MR images from different methods visualized in ITK-SNAP. From left to right: Rank 1 (Zhang et al.), Rank 2 (Ferreira et al.), median ensemble, and geometric mean ensemble. All views are centered at the same voxel coordinate (164, 110, 78), but demonstrate differing image intensity values under the cursor: 931.1 (Rank 1), 664.2 (Rank 2), 797.6 (Geometric), and 796.4 (Geometric with median filter postprocessing). Notably, the bottom-left ventricle appears more faded and ill-defined in the Rank 1 output, while it is clearly delineated in the Rank 2 image. The ventricle is slightly more apparent in both the median and geometric ensemble outputs than in Rank 1, indicating partial recovery of anatomical detail through pixel-wise fusion strategies. These variations highlight differences in tissue reconstruction fidelity between individual models and ensemble-based approaches.

provided directly by the BraTS validation server, where the standard deviation reflects variation across individual validation cases rather than variation across cross-validation folds. Results on the testing set are included in Table XY.

The baseline Rank 1 and Rank 2 models (Ferreira et al. [4] and Zhang et al. [28], respectively) yield identical values for MSE (0.007±0.005) and nearly identical SSIM (0.841±0.103 vs. 0.842±0.099), but differ in PSNR: 23.257±4.213 for Rank 1 and 22.463±3.776 for Rank 2. Simple ensembling of these models yields strong improvements across all metrics, with MSE reduced to 0.006±0.004, PSNR increased to 23.652±4.092, and SSIM elevated to 0.854±0.094. Importantly, this approach also lowers the standard deviations for all metrics, suggesting more stable and consistent performance. Adding classical post-processing filters preserves the MSE and maintains low variance, but leads to slightly reduced PSNR (23.385±3.908) and SSIM (0.851±0.095) relative to ensembling alone (Table 2).

In contrast, the U-Net-enhanced ensemble results in performance that, while still stable, shows a decline in mean values: MSE increases to 0.007±0.004, PSNR

Table 1. Validation Set Quantitative results on the BraTS 2025 inpainting validation set. Performance is evaluated using Structural Similarity Index (SSIM, ↑), Peak Signal-to-Noise Ratio (PSNR, ↑), and Mean Squared Error (MSE, ↓). Metrics reflect perceptual similarity, reconstruction quality, and pixel-level fidelity, respectively. The best performing configuration for each metric is highlighted in **bold**.

Model	Ranking Metric (↓)	MSE(↓)	PSNR(↑)	SSIM(↑)
Rank 1 (Zhang et al.)	1.970	0.007±0.005	23.257±4.213	0.841±0.103
Rank 2 (Ferreira et al.)	2.441	0.007±0.005	22.463±3.776	0.842±0.099
Ensemble (R1 + R2)	**1.223**	**0.006±0.004**	**23.652±4.092**	**0.854±0.094**
Ensemble + Filters	**1.223**	**0.006±0.004**	23.385±3.908	0.851±0.095
Ensemble + U-Net	2.366	0.007±**0.004**	22.740±**3.670**	0.843±0.096

Table 2. Test Set Quantitative results on the BraTS 2025 inpainting testing set. Performance is evaluated using Structural Similarity Index (SSIM, ↑), Peak Signal-to-Noise Ratio (PSNR, ↑), and Mean Squared Error (MSE, ↓). Metrics reflect perceptual similarity, reconstruction quality, and pixel-level fidelity, respectively.

Model	MSE(↓)	PSNR(↑)	SSIM(↑)
Ensemble + Filters	0.007±0.004	23.955±4.989	0.867±0.1312

drops to 22.740±3.670, and SSIM falls to 0.843±0.096. According to the overall ranking metric, the best configuration is the ensemble with classical filters (1.223), followed by Rank 1 (1.970), then the U-Net-enhanced ensemble (2.366). These results suggest that while the U-Net refiner introduces plausible structural detail and reduced variability, it may require further training to outperform simpler, well-tuned classical strategies.

5 Discussion

Motivated by the observed saturation in performance among state-of-the-art inpainting models, we proposed a modular pipeline that combines predictions from previous winners' methods with classical image processing filters and a U-Net-based enhancement module trained on synthetically degraded healthy tissue. The synthetically degraded tissue uses a simple method that applies a Gaussian blur to healthy brain regions, and using these artificially degraded scans as inputs, we generated a rich supervised training dataset for the enhancement model without additional manual annotations. This allowed the U-Net to learn a targeted correction function aimed at restoring anatomical similarity in artifact-prone outputs from existing inpainting models.

Our results indicate that simple model ensembling leads to clear performance improvements across SSIM, PSNR, and MSE while reducing variability compared to individual model outputs. Adding classical post-processing filters preserves these gains with minimal overhead, and ranks best overall across quantitative metrics. Our metrics reflect a third place ranking in the BraTS 2025 inpainting challenge with a strategy that emphasizes using an ensemble of existing models and lightweight post-processing rather than creating and training increasingly complex architectures. For the 2025 validation set, the 2024 baseline Rank-1 (Ferreira et al. [4]) and Rank-2 (Zhang et al. [28]) systems yield identical MSE (0.007 ± 0.005) and near-identical SSIM (0.841 ± 0.103 vs. 0.842 ± 0.099), but differ in PSNR (23.257 ± 4.213 vs. 22.463 ± 3.776). A simple ensemble of these models produces consistent improvements across all metrics (MSE 0.006 ± 0.004, PSNR 23.652 ± 4.092, SSIM 0.854 ± 0.094) and meaningfully reduces standard deviations, indicating more stable performance across slices/cases. Adding classical filters preserves the ensemble's MSE and low variance but slightly lowers means (PSNR 23.385 ± 3.908, SSIM 0.851 ± 0.095). The U-Net-based refinement showed slight reductions in mean SSIM and PSNR, along with an increase in MSE. These results suggest that while conceptually promising and effective at maintaining low standard deviation, the U-Net enhancement model in its current training configuration may require additional fine-tuning or regularization to outperform traditional averaging and filtering approaches.

Importantly, the components of our postprocessing pipeline are computationally lightweight, reproducible, and deployable in resource-constrained settings. This efficiency not only reduces the burden on GPU memory and energy consumption but also makes high-fidelity inpainting more accessible across diverse research and clinical environments. By strategically leveraging existing models, healthy data cohorts, and simple yet effective post-processing methods, our approach offers a sustainable and modular path forward for medical image inpainting and supports bridging the gap between benchmark performance and real-world applicability.

6 Conclusion

Our work shows that strong brain tissue inpainting performance can be achieved without resorting to ever larger or more complex models. By ensembling established, high-performing models and applying lightweight classical post-processing tools alongside a U-Net-based enhancement module trained on healthy scans, we obtain high-fidelity results in a resource-efficient manner. These approaches do not require extensive GPU resources and are simple to implement, demonstrating that carefully selected and combined methods, rather than sheer model scale, can provide reliable, clinically useful brain image synthesis. This strategy supports scalable and accessible solutions for medical image inpainting in both research and clinical practice.

References

1. Bonato, B., Nanni, L., Bertoldo, A.: Advancing precision: a comprehensive review of MRI segmentation datasets from brats challenges (2012–2025). Sens. (Basel, Switzerland) **25**(6), 1838 (2025)
2. Capellán-Martín, D., et al.: Model ensemble for brain tumor segmentation in magnetic resonance imaging. In: International Challenge on Cross-Modality Domain Adaptation for Medical Image Segmentation, pp. 221–232. Springer (2023)
3. Dede, A., et al.: Intelligent systems with applications (2018)
4. Ferreira, A., Luijten, G., Puladi, B., Kleesiek, J., Alves, V., Egger, J.: Brain tumour removing and missing modality generation using 3D WDM. arXiv preprint arXiv:2411.04630 (2024)
5. Guizard, N., Nakamura, K., Coupé, P., Fonov, V.S., Arnold, D.L., Collins, D.L.: Non-local means inpainting of MS lesions in longitudinal image processing. Front. Neurosci. **9**, 456 (2015)
6. He, K., Chen, X., Xie, S., Li, Y., Dollár, P., Girshick, R.: Masked autoencoders are scalable vision learners. In: Proceedings of the IEEE/CVF Conference on Computer Vision and Pattern Recognition, pp. 16000–16009 (2022)
7. Iglesias, J.E., et al.: Synthsr: a public ai tool to turn heterogeneous clinical brain scans into high-resolution t1-weighted images for 3D morphometry. Sci. Adv. **9**(5), eadd3607 (2023)
8. Jiang, Z., et al.: Enhancing generalizability in brain tumor segmentation: model ensemble with adaptive post-processing. In: 2024 IEEE International Symposium on Biomedical Imaging (ISBI), pp. 1–4. IEEE (2024)
9. Jiang, Z., et al.: Magnetic resonance imaging feature-based subtyping and model ensemble for enhanced brain tumor segmentation. arXiv preprint arXiv:2412.04094 (2024)
10. Kamraoui, R.A., Mansencal, B., Manjon, J.V., Coupé, P.: Longitudinal detection of new MS lesions using deep learning. Front. Neuro. **1**, 948235 (2022)
11. Kaur, A., Dong, G.: A complete review on image denoising techniques for medical images. Neural Process. Lett. **55**(6), 7807–7850 (2023)
12. Kofler, F., et al.: The brain tumor segmentation (brats) challenge: local synthesis of healthy brain tissue via inpainting. arXiv preprint arXiv:2305.08992 (2023)
13. Kofler, F., et al.: Brats orchestrator: Democratizing and disseminating state-of-the-art brain tumor image analysis. arXiv preprint arXiv:2506.13807 (2025)
14. LaBella, D., et al.: Analysis of the BraTS 2023 intracranial meningioma segmentation challenge. J. Mach. Learn. Biomed. Imaging **3**, 38–58 (2025)
15. Liu, X., Xing, F., Yang, C., Kuo, C.C.J., El Fakhri, G., Woo, J.: Symmetric-constrained irregular structure inpainting for brain MRI registration with tumor pathology. In: International MICCAI Brainlesion Workshop, pp. 80–91. Springer (2020)
16. Liu, X., Xiang, C., Lan, L., Li, C., Xiao, H., Liu, Z.: Lesion region inpainting: an approach for pseudo-healthy image synthesis in intracranial infection imaging. Front. Microbiol. **15**, 1453870 (2024)
17. Maleki, N., et al.: Analysis of the MICCAI brain tumor segmentation–metastases (brats-mets) 2025 lighthouse challenge: Brain metastasis segmentation on pre-and post-treatment MRI. arXiv preprint arXiv:2504.12527 (2025)
18. Menze, B.H., et al.: The multimodal brain tumor image segmentation benchmark (brats). IEEE Trans. Med. Imaging **34**(10), 1993–2024 (2014)

19. Menze, B.H., et al.: The multimodal brain tumor image segmentation benchmark (brats). IEEE Trans. Med. Imaging **34**(10), 1993–2024 (2015)
20. Parida, A., et al.: Adult glioma segmentation in sub-Saharan Africa using transfer learning on stratified finetuning data. arXiv preprint arXiv:2412.04111 (2024)
21. Pollak, C., Kügler, D., Bauer, T., Rüber, T., Reuter, M.: Fastsurfer-lit: lesion inpainting tool for whole-brain MRI segmentation with tumors, cavities, and abnormalities. Imaging neuroscience **3**, imag_a_00446 (2025)
22. Prajwal, R., et al.: A study on energy consumption in ai-driven medical image segmentation. J. Imaging **11**(6), 174 (2025)
23. Santos, J.C., Tomás Pereira Alexandre, H., Seoane Santos, M., Henriques Abreu, P.: The role of deep learning in medical image inpainting: a systematic review. ACM Trans. Comput. Healthcare **6**(3), 1–24 (2025)
24. Sumathi, G., Devi, M.U.: High-resolution image inpainting using a probabilistic framework for diverse images with large arbitrary masks. Front. Artif. Intell. **8**, 1614608 (2025)
25. Susan, J., Subashini, P.: Deep learning inpainting model on digital and medical images-a review. Int. Arab J. Inf. Technol. **20**(6), 919–936 (2023)
26. Torrado-Carvajal, A., et al.: Inpainting as a technique for estimation of missing voxels in brain imaging. Ann. Biomed. Eng. **49**(1), 345–353 (2021)
27. Ueda, D., et al.: Fairness of artificial intelligence in healthcare: review and recommendations. Jpn. J. Radiol. **42**(1), 3–15 (2024)
28. Zhang, J., Weng, Y., Chen, K.: U-net based healthy 3D brain tissue inpainting. arXiv preprint arXiv:2507.18126 (2025)
29. Zhu, R., Zhang, X., Pang, H., Xu, C., Ye, C.: Advancing brain tumor inpainting with generative models. arXiv preprint arXiv:2402.01509 (2024)

Context-Aware Healthy Brain Inpainting: A Multi-stage DDIM Approach for the BraTS 2025 Challenge

Yaxuan Dai(✉), Yuan Bi, Nassir Navab, and Zhongliang Jiang

Chair for Computer Aided Medical Procedures (CAMP), TU Munich, Munich, Germany
yaxuan.dai@tum.de

Abstract. This work presents our solution to the BraTS Inpainting 2025 Challenge, which focuses on the reconstruction of healthy brain tissue in magnetic resonance images (MRI) where certain regions are missing or corrupted. The objective is to synthesize realistic and structurally coherent content in voided regions using only partial anatomical context. To address this, we propose a conditional denoising diffusion probabilistic model (DDPM) trained exclusively on healthy tissue. During training, we leverage all voided slices from the dataset while computing supervision only on voxels marked as healthy, ignoring regions labeled as pathological to ensure that the model learns a prior over healthy brain anatomy. For inference, we adopt a multi-stage denoising process based on DDIM (Denoising Diffusion Implicit Models), enhanced by fusion of unmasked context into each denoising stage. This strategy encourages gradual refinement and consistency with the surrounding brain structure, enabling the model to generate high-fidelity inpainting results. We evaluate our method on the challenge validation set using standard image reconstruction metrics including RMSE, PSNR, and SSIM, computed only within healthy regions. Experimental results demonstrate that our approach achieves high reconstruction accuracy and produces visually plausible results across various cases. Our findings highlight the potential of 2D conditional diffusion models, when equipped with contextual fusion, to tackle complex medical inpainting tasks in 3D volumes.

Keywords: Medical Image Inpainting · BraTS Inpainting Challenge · Diffusion Denoising · DDIM · Context Fusion

1 Introduction

Medical imaging plays a pivotal role in clinical diagnosis, surgical planning, and treatment evaluation. However, due to various factors such as imaging artifacts, occlusions, lesion resection, or privacy-preserving procedures, medical images often contain regions of missing or corrupted information. In this context, image inpainting—the process of restoring missing content based on surrounding context—has garnered increasing attention within the medical image analysis

S. Bakas et al. (Eds.): MICCAI 2025, LNCS 16377, pp. 158–167, 2026.
https://doi.org/10.1007/978-3-032-16370-7_14

community. This task is especially critical in brain magnetic resonance imaging (MRI), where accurately reconstructing missing or abnormal regions with plausible healthy tissue can aid clinicians in understanding anatomical structure and enhance the quality of downstream tasks such as segmentation, registration, and analysis.

Traditional inpainting approaches, such as interpolation based on image priors, patch-matching methods like PatchMatch [4], and energy-based reconstruction models [6], struggle to cope with the structural complexity and rich semantic information inherent in medical images. In recent years, deep learning-based methods, particularly those utilizing Generative Adversarial Networks (GANs) and diffusion models, have demonstrated substantial improvements in inpainting performance. Notable examples include Contextual Attention GAN [13], Partial Convolution [9], and more recently, generation models based on Denoising Diffusion Probabilistic Models (DDPM) [7] and DDIM-based inference [11], which have proven effective in producing structurally coherent and perceptually realistic results [5].

The BraTS Inpainting 2025 Challenge focuses on the automatic reconstruction of healthy brain tissue in voided regions of MRI scans. Participants are required to synthesize anatomically consistent and detail-rich completions of the missing areas, based solely on partial image context. This task presents significant challenges in generative modeling and emphasizes the need for generalization and stability in complex medical structures. The challenge also provides a unified benchmark for data, evaluation, and reproducibility, facilitating further progress in the practical application of medical image inpainting.

In this work, we propose a diffusion-based solution based on tailored for this challenge based on the multi-stage denoising scheme [5]. Our method learns the distribution of healthy brain anatomy by training a conditional diffusion model exclusively on non-pathological tissue. During inference, we employ a multi-stage DDIM denoising strategy, incorporating the visible context from unmasked regions at each stage to progressively guide and refine the reconstruction. This stage-wise fusion mechanism enables the model to generate anatomically consistent and semantically meaningful content within the voided regions.

The remainder of this report is organized as follows: Sect. 2 describes the task setting and evaluation metrics. Section 3 details our model architecture, training pipeline, and inference strategy. Section 4 presents experimental results and visual analyses. Section 5 concludes the report with a discussion of our findings and future directions.

2 Task

The BraTS Inpainting 2025 challenge [1–3, 8, 10, 12] focuses on the task of reconstructing healthy brain tissue in MRI scans from voided or masked regions. The training dataset consists of five aligned volumetric inputs per case: the original t1n image, its corresponding voided version (voided-t1n), and three binary masks that indicate the voided region, healthy tissue, and unhealthy tissue (typically tumor or lesion areas), respectively. During inference (validation and test), only the voided-t1n image and its associated voided region mask are provided, and the goal is to inpaint these regions with plausible healthy content.

The training set comprises a total of 1252 subjects, while the validation set contains 219 subjects. The model operates on axial slices extracted from the 3D volumes. Each slice of 2D image is resampled from 240×240 to 256×256, and normalized to [-1, 1] during preprocess. We applied no augmentation to the training data.

Performance is quantitatively evaluated using three widely adopted image quality metrics: Root Mean Squared Error (RMSE), Peak Signal-to-Noise Ratio (PSNR), and Structural Similarity Index Measure (SSIM). All metrics are computed only over the inpainted healthy regions (as defined by the healthy mask in the ground truth), in accordance with the challenge's focus on realistic and anatomically consistent tissue reconstruction. RMSE measures pixel-level intensity deviation from ground truth, PSNR reflects the overall fidelity of the reconstructed image, and SSIM evaluates structural similarity and perceptual quality (Fig. 1).

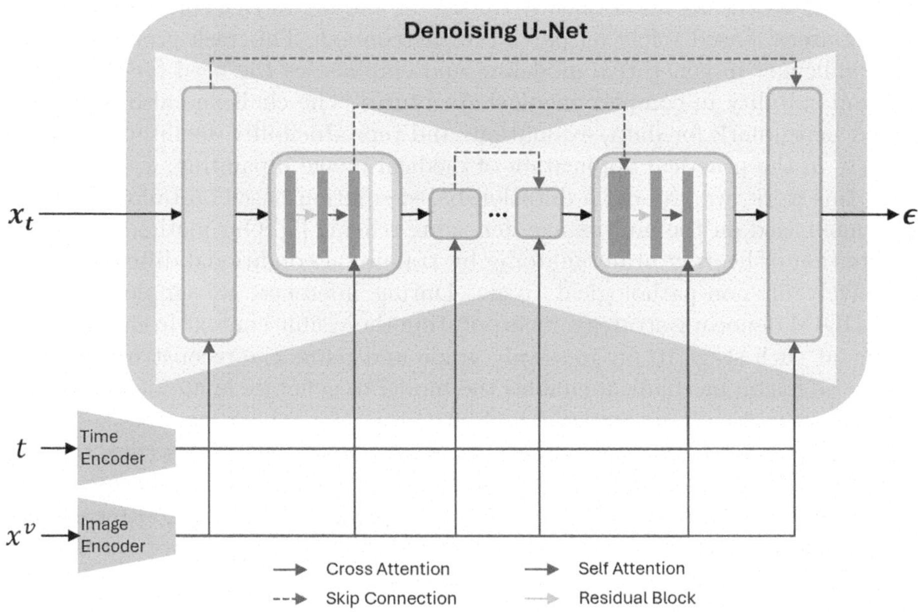

Fig. 1. Model Structure.

3 Method

In this section, we present the overall methodology of our proposed approach, including the model architecture, training strategy, and inference procedure.

Our solution is based on a 2D conditional diffusion model designed to reconstruct healthy brain tissue in 3D MRI volumes. During training, we leverage all provided voided slices from the dataset and employ conditional generation to learn the underlying distribution of healthy tissue. At inference time, we propose a progressive context fusion strategy to enhance the structural consistency and semantic plausibility of the reconstructed regions.

3.1 Model Architecture

We operate on 2D image slices extracted along the axial direction of the 3D volume, treating each slice independently. Our model adopts a UNet-based conditional denoising architecture integrated into a Gaussian diffusion framework.

The UNet backbone consists of two residual blocks at each resolution level, and multi-scale self-attention layers are applied at feature resolutions of 32, 16, and 8. Each attention layer employs two heads with 64 channels each. The network is conditioned on two inputs: the current diffusion timestep t (encoded as a time embedding), the voided input image x^v with its learned embedding extracted using a CLIP image encoder. These conditioning signals are fused into the intermediate layers of the UNet through a cross-attention mechanism.

For the forward diffusion process, we use a Gaussian noising schedule with T=1000 steps and adopt a cosine beta schedule. During reverse sampling, the model performs denoising using the DDIM formulation.

3.2 Training Procedure

During training, we use all available voided slices from the dataset to improve the model's robustness to various occlusion patterns. For each training pair, the process follows these steps:

Given an original image x_0 and its corresponding voided version, we randomly sample a timestep $t \in [1, T]$ and apply the forward diffusion process $q(x_t \mid x_0)$ to generate a noisy input x_t based on Gaussian noise ϵ^*.

The model then receives the noised image x_t, with current timestep t and the voided image x^v as condition inputs, predicts the noise component $\hat{\epsilon}_\theta$ for the current timestep.

To ensure that the model focuses on reconstructing only the healthy brain tissue, we compute the training loss solely over the healthy regions. Specifically, we exclude pixels within annotated lesion areas (where the unhealthy mask is `True`) and define the loss as:

$$\mathcal{L}_{\texttt{healthy}} = \frac{1}{|\mathcal{H}|} \sum_{i \in \mathcal{H}} \left\| \epsilon_{(i)} - \epsilon^*_{(i)} \right\|^2,$$

where $\mathcal{H}$ denotes the set of pixels out of the unhealthy region. This selective loss formulation allows the model to learn the structural distribution of normal tissue while ignoring abnormal areas during optimization (Fig. 2).

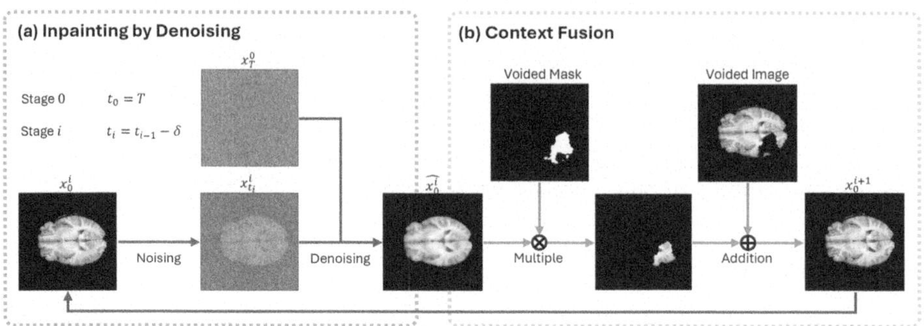

Fig. 2. Main inference pipeline consisting of two components: (a) Multi-stage inpainting by denoising, where noise levels t_i decrease by fixed increments δ at each stage. In our setup, we perform $s = 20$ stages of denoising with a total of $T = 1000$ noising steps, resulting in $\delta = T/s = 50$. (b) Context fusion, which updates the denoised output by inpainting the voided region of the denoised image $\hat{x_0^i}$ into the voided image x^v. The fused image then serves as the input image x_0^{i+1} to the next stage.

3.3 Inference Procedure

At inference time, the objective is to reconstruct healthy tissue within the voided region, starting from random Gaussian noise. We employ a multi-stage DDIM denoising process augmented with a context-aware fusion mechanism, guiding the model toward anatomically plausible reconstructions. The stage number s of DDIM denoising stage is set to 20, offering a balance between reconstruction quality and computational efficiency.

We begin by sampling a noisy image from the standard Gaussian distribution as the denoising input $x^0_{t_0=T}$ of stage 0. At each stage i, a forward diffusion process $q(x^i_{t_i}|x^i_0)$ is applied with its noising timestep t_i reduce by $\delta = T/s$ steps from timestep t_{i-1} of previous stage. Then a denoised image $\hat{x_0^i}$ is generated by the denoising diffusion model, conditioned on timestep t_i and the voided image x^v.

After every denoising inference, we inpaint the voided region of the denoised image $\hat{x_0^i}$ into the voided image x^v to prevent contextual information from being lost. This fusion strategy ensures that the reconstruction remains consistent with the available surrounding tissue across all denoising stages.

After completing all DDIM stages, the model outputs a fully reconstructed image in which the previously missing regions are filled with coherent and anatomically realistic brain tissue, guided by both learned priors and visible context. This progressive fusion substantially improves the fidelity and realism of inpainted regions by anchoring generation to actual anatomical structures throughout the denoising trajectory.

4 Results

4.1 Experimental Settings

We conducted our experiments using a consistent training and inference configuration across all evaluations. During training, the model was optimized using the Adam optimizer with a learning rate of 1×10^{-3}, first and second momentum terms $(\beta_1, \beta_2) = (0.9, 0.999)$, and no weight decay. To ensure numerical stability during training, we applied gradient clipping with a norm threshold of 1.0. The input slices were resized to 256×256, and gradient accumulation was used to achieve an effective batch size of 64.

For inference, we adopt a DDIM-based denoising procedure with a fixed number of stages $s = 25$. We empirically evaluated different configurations—10, 25, and 50 stages. While 50 stages yielded slightly better results, the 25-stage schedule offered comparable quality with nearly double the speed. We also compared two denoising strategies: multi-stage single-step DDIM versus single-stage multi-step DDIM. The multi-stage approach consistently outperformed the single-stage variant.

Table 1. Quantitative results on the validation set, averaged over all 219 cases.

Model	SSIM ↑	PSNR ↑	MSE ↓
Pix2Pix3D	0.7739 ± 0.1300	19.12 ± 3.22	0.0151 ± 0.0098
Ours ($s = 10$)	0.7207 ± 0.1532	17.70 ± 3.02	0.0205 ± 0.0128

4.2 Quantitative Results

Table 1 reports the average performance of our method on the validation set using three standard metrics: Root Mean Squared Error (RMSE), Peak Signal-to-Noise Ratio (PSNR), and Structural Similarity Index Measure (SSIM). All evaluations were restricted to the healthy brain tissue regions, aligning with the challenge requirements. Our model achieved low RMSE and high PSNR/SSIM values, demonstrating its ability to accurately reconstruct structurally plausible and perceptually consistent content within the voided regions. For the test set results, we refer the reader to Table xy.

4.3 Qualitative Results

Figure 3 presents the visual comparison of inpainting results along different anatomical axes, specifically slices from both the axial (z-axis) and sagittal (x-axis) planes. The reconstructed regions exhibit coherent texture and anatomical correctness, with minimal artifacts and smooth blending into surrounding brain tissue.

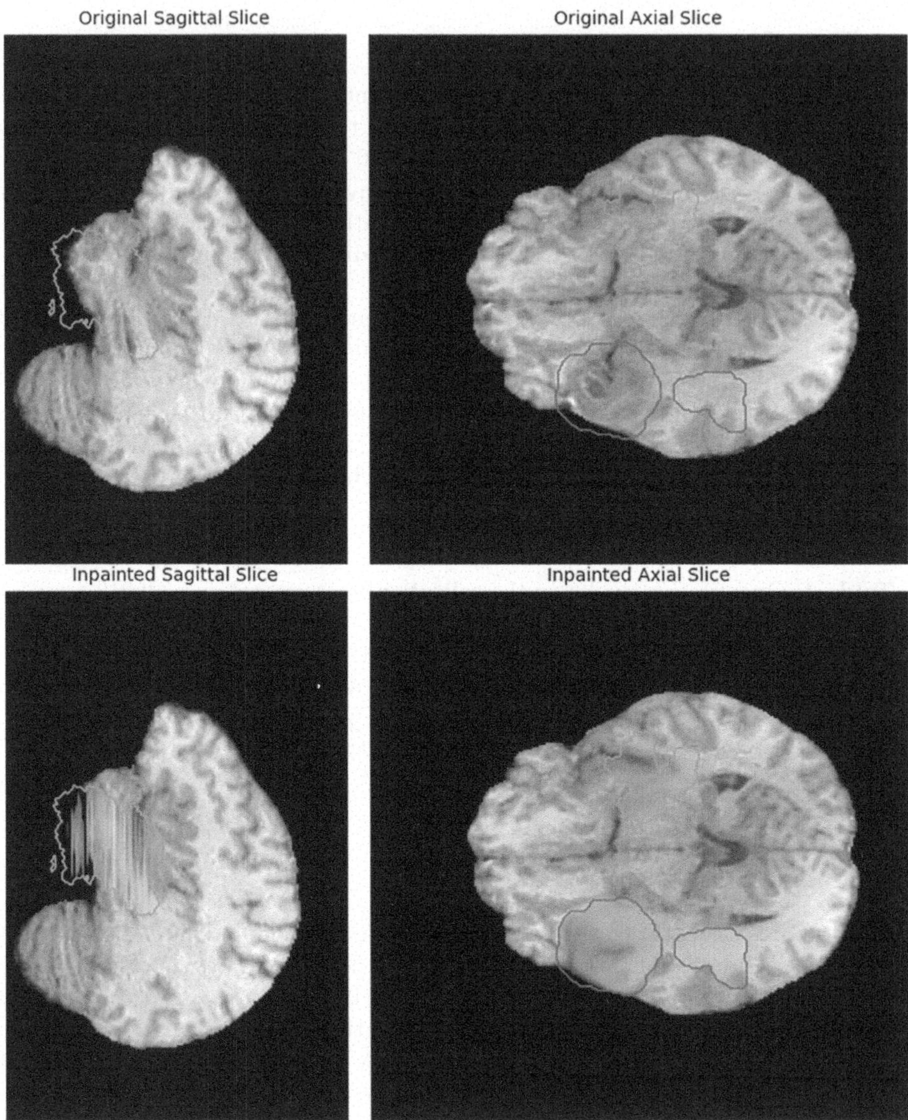

Fig. 3. Examples of inpainting results shown in both sagittal and axial views. The original images (top row) and the corresponding inpainted outputs (bottom row) are overlaid with contours of healthy (green) and unhealthy (red) regions. Since our inpainting model operates on 2D axial slices, the reconstructions exhibit strong structural and contextual consistency within each axial plane. However, due to the absence of inter-slice modeling, the sagittal view reveals weaker continuity across adjacent slices, highlighting a common limitation of purely 2D approaches when applied to 3D volumetric data. (Color figure online)

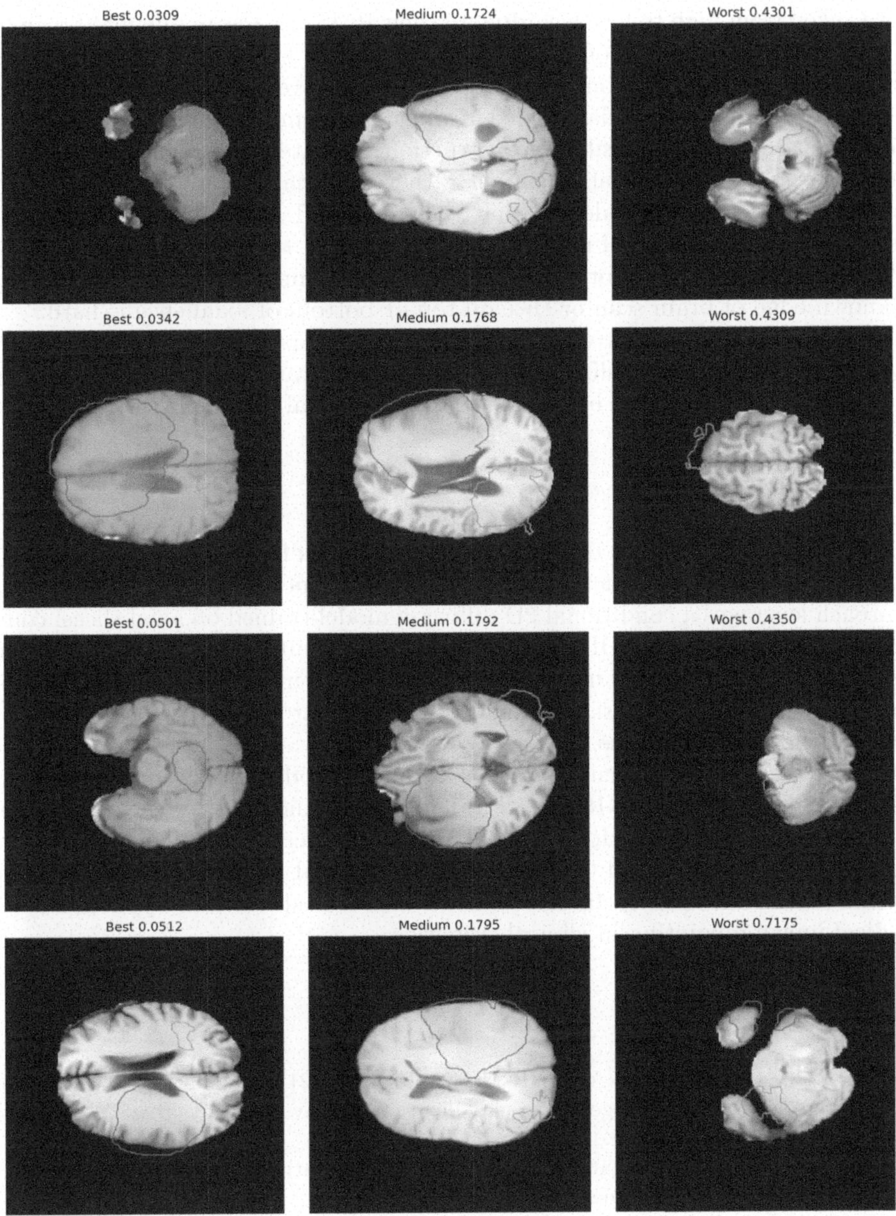

Fig. 4. Representative inpainting results, sorted from best (left) to worst (right) based on RMSE within the healthy regions. For each case, we visualize the inpainted image overlaid with contours of healthy (green) and unhealthy (red) areas. Samples with healthy region pixel counts less than 100 are excluded. The RMSE value for the healthy region of each axial slice is also provided. (Color figure online)

To further examine model behavior across different cases, we visualize samples ranked from high to low according to their RMSE scores in inpainted regions in Fig. 4. High-scoring reconstructions preserve fine structural details and are nearly indistinguishable from ground truth, while lower-scoring cases often correspond to large or irregular voided regions with limited context, which pose greater challenges for plausible reconstruction. Despite this, the model still produces anatomically reasonable content rather than hallucinated or structurally incorrect patterns. We could see that the unpainted region have blurry tissue structure, might because of using MSE loss and tend to prevent from large mistakes. Small voided region or region with roughly symmetrical refer is easy, while unknown edge of brain scan or slice on top or bottom of axial slice is hard.

Overall, both quantitative metrics and visual inspections confirm the effectiveness of our proposed diffusion-based inpainting framework in reconstructing healthy brain regions with high fidelity and structural plausibility.

5 Conclusion

In this work, we proposed a diffusion-based framework for medical image inpainting, targeting the reconstruction of healthy brain tissue in 3D MRI volumes. Our approach leverages a conditional 2D diffusion model trained on axial slices, combined with a multi-stage DDIM denoising strategy and a context-aware fusion mechanism. By reinserting unmasked regions during inference, the model maintains strong structural consistency and generates anatomically plausible content across diverse void patterns.

Experimental results demonstrate that our method achieves superior performance across RMSE, PSNR, and SSIM metrics, indicating its effectiveness in restoring missing tissue with high fidelity and visual realism. Moving forward, we plan to extend our method to fully three-dimensional architectures and explore multimodal integration to further enhance the robustness and applicability of medical image inpainting in clinical scenarios.

References

1. Baid, U., et al.: The RSNA-ASNR-MICCAI brats 2021 benchmark on brain tumor segmentation and radiogenomic classification. arXiv preprint arXiv:2107.02314 (2021)
2. Bakas, S., et al.: Segmentation labels for the pre-operative scans of the TCGA-LGG collection. Cancer Imaging Archive (2017)
3. Bakas, S., et al.: Advancing the cancer genome atlas glioma MRI collections with expert segmentation labels and radiomic features. Sci. Data **4**(1), 1–13 (2017)
4. Barnes, C., Shechtman, E., Finkelstein, A., Goldman, D.B.: Patchmatch: a randomized correspondence algorithm for structural image editing. ACM Trans. Graph. **28**(3), 24 (2009)
5. Bi, Y., et al.: Synomaly noise and multi-stage diffusion: a novel approach for unsupervised anomaly detection in medical images. Med. Image Anal. 103737 (2025)

6. Guan, Y., Tu, Z., Wang, S., Liu, Q., Wang, Y., Liang, D.: MRI reconstruction using deep energy-based model. arXiv preprint arXiv:2109.03237 (2021)
7. Ho, J., Jain, A., Abbeel, P.: Denoising diffusion probabilistic models. Adv. Neural. Inf. Process. Syst. **33**, 6840–6851 (2020)
8. Kofler, F., et al.: The brain tumor segmentation (brats) challenge: local synthesis of healthy brain tissue via inpainting (2024). https://arxiv.org/abs/2305.08992
9. Liu, G., Reda, F.A., Shih, K.J., Wang, T.C., Tao, A., Catanzaro, B.: Image inpainting for irregular holes using partial convolutions. In: Proceedings of the European Conference on Computer Vision (ECCV), pp. 85–100 (2018)
10. Menze, B.H., et al.: The multimodal brain tumor image segmentation benchmark (brats). IEEE Trans. Med. Imaging **34**(10), 1993–2024 (2014)
11. Song, J., Meng, C., Ermon, S.: Denoising diffusion implicit models. arXiv preprint arXiv:2010.02502 (2020)
12. Spyridon, B., et al.: Segmentation labels and radiomic features for the pre-operative scans of the TCGA-GBM collection. Cancer Imaging Archive (2017)
13. Yu, J., Lin, Z., Yang, J., Shen, X., Lu, X., Huang, T.S.: Generative image inpainting with contextual attention. In: Proceedings of the IEEE Conference on Computer Vision and Pattern Recognition, pp. 5505–5514 (2018)

PSegGAN: Pseudo-Segmentation-Guided GANs for Brain Tissue Inpainting

Juhyung Ha[1], Jong Sung Park[2], Jiyeong Oh[1], and David Crandall[1](✉)

[1] Computer Science, Indiana University, Bloomington, IN 47408, USA
djcran@iu.edu
[2] Intelligent Systems Engineering, Indiana University, Bloomington, IN 47408, USA

Abstract. Brain inpainting presents unique challenges compared to natural image inpainting, including increased problem complexity arising from the volumetric nature of 3D MRI and the need to ensure anatomical plausibility in addition to visual realism. To address these challenges, we propose a Pseudo-Segmentation-Guided GAN (PSegGAN) for tumor-to-healthy brain inpainting. Our framework consists of three cooperating networks: (i) a generator that reconstructs masked brain volumes conditioned on both healthy and tumor masks, (ii) a discriminator that enforces perceptual realism by distinguishing reconstructed from inpainted regions, and (iii) a segmentator that provides structural guidance through a perceptual masked loss derived from whole-brain segmentation. We evaluate our method on the BraTS 2025 Inpainting Challenge dataset. While our results show that the proposed model does not surpass the state-of-the-art in standard voxel-wise metrics such as MSE, PSNR and SSIM, qualitative assessment demonstrates that it produces more realistic and anatomically plausible reconstructions. Our findings suggest that incorporating structural priors can enhance anatomical plausibility in medical image synthesis and may offer additional insights for supporting medical image analysis. We share our code in https://github.com/juhha/BraTS-inpainting-2025-PSegGAN.

Keywords: Brain Inpainting · GAN · MRI

1 Introduction

Image inpainting refers to the task of reconstructing missing or corrupted regions of an image while ensuring perceptual consistency with surrounding structures. In natural image domains, inpainting has been widely studied for applications such as photo restoration [4,12], object removal [5,36,37], and image editing [28], with generative models demonstrating the ability to synthesize plausible textures and structures. In the medical imaging field, inpainting has attracted increasing attention for tasks such as artifact correction, missing slice completion, and lesion filling. While many studies focus on 2D inpainting of radiological scans [3,30,34], extending this problem to the volumetric domain remains challenging due to the

S. Bakas et al. (Eds.): MICCAI 2025, LNCS 16377, pp. 168–180, 2026.
https://doi.org/10.1007/978-3-032-16370-7_15

high dimensionality and the need to preserve anatomical fidelity across three dimensions [13,22].

To advance research in this area, the Brain Tumor Segmentation (BraTS) initiative introduced the tumor inpainting challenge in 2023 [24] as part of its long-standing benchmark series. This task targeted the synthesis of healthy-appearing tissue in regions affected by tumors. The objective is to enable downstream algorithms that typically assume healthy brain morphology, such as registration, parcellation, and morphometric analysis, by providing a tumor-free counterpart of the patient's MRI. This could potentially facilitate a deeper understanding of the tumor's mass effect and provide a consistent baseline for post-treatment analysis. The challenge was repeated in 2024 [26] and 2025 [1].

Top-performing methods in the BraTS inpainting challenges have centered around two main architectures: Generative Adversarial Networks (GANs) [39] and Denoising Diffusion Probabilistic Models (DDPMs) [10,11]. GAN-based approaches leverage a generator to synthesize the missing region and a discriminator to distinguish between real and synthetic images, often employing advanced perceptual and style losses to enhance realism. More recently, diffusion models have shown much success by learning to reverse a gradual noising process, allowing them to generate highly realistic and diverse image content. While these methods excel at creating texturally convincing inpainting results, ensuring long-range anatomical plausibility remains a significant open challenge.

To address this limitation, we propose Pseudo-Segmentation-Guided GANs (PSegGAN) for brain tissue inpainting for tumor-to-healthy inpainting. Our method is designed to not only restore realistic appearance but also enforce anatomical plausibility in the inpainted regions. Specifically, we employ three networks: (i) a generator that synthesizes healthy and tumorous brain regions from the mask, (ii) a discriminator that encourages perceptual similarity between reconstructed and inpainted regions, and (iii) a segmentator that provides anatomical guidance via a perceptual masked loss in feature space. For anatomical guidance via segmentator, we incorporate pseudo-anatomical segmentation maps obtained from SynthSeg [6] for structural priors.

2 Related Work

2.1 Image Inpainting

Inpainting has been a long-standing research problem in computer vision, with early techniques based on partial differential equations (PDEs) and exemplar-based patch matching [5,8]. Classic approaches [5] demonstrated diffusion-based filling of missing regions, while Exemplar-Based Image Inpainting [8] introduced patch-based methods that propagated texture information into occluded areas. In recent years with the advent of deep learning, the field has been dominated by two powerful generative modeling paradigms, Generative Adversarial Networks (GANs) [7,21,39] and Denoising Diffusion Probabilistic Models (DDPMs) [9,17,29], which have become the standards for state-of-the-art inpainting.

In medical imaging, inpainting has been explored for tasks such as lesion filling, artifact correction, and missing slice completion. Many studies have focused on 2D applications, including GAN-based lesion filling in brain MRI [2], chest X-ray inpainting for pathology localization [41], and CT inpainting guided by edge and organ boundary awareness [33]. Extending to the volumetric domain remains more challenging due to high dimensionality and the requirement to preserve anatomical fidelity across three dimensions. Approaches such as 3D CNN-based inpainting of MR volumes [22] and 3D diffusion-based synthesis for MRI and CT [23] have begun addressing these difficulties. Overall, both GANs and DDPMs also dominate in the medical domain.

2.2 Generative Adversarial Networks (GANs)

Generative Adversarial Networks (GANs) [15] introduced a framework in which a generator synthesizes data and a discriminator distinguishes real from synthetic. In image generation, important models include conditional GANs such as Pix2Pix [19] and cycle-consistent GANs [40], which have been widely applied in medical imaging, including modality translation, super-resolution, and lesion synthesis. For inpainting, GAN-based methods have proven effective at producing realistic local structures, with extensions incorporating style-based losses to improve visual fidelity [32,38].

In medical image inpainting, GANs have been applied to lesion inpainting and artifact correction in both 2D and 3D settings. For example, ipA-MedGAN [3] demonstrated arbitrary-shape inpainting in brain MRI, while GANs have also been used to fill lesions in neurodegenerative disorders to facilitate morphometric analysis. Within the BraTS inpainting challenges, top-performing teams have adopted 3D U-Net GAN variants [24], using adversarial and perceptual losses to synthesize healthy tissue in tumor regions. These results illustrate the continuing importance of GANs in producing sharp, realistic reconstructions, though they often struggle with long-range anatomical consistency.

2.3 Denoising Diffusion Models

Denoising Diffusion Probabilistic Models (DDPMs) [17] are a class of generative models that have recently achieved state-of-the-art results in image synthesis [9, 29]. The core idea involves a two-stage process: a forward "diffusion" process that systematically adds Gaussian noise to an image until it becomes pure noise, and a learned reverse "denoising" process. The model, typically a U-Net, is trained to predict the noise added at each step, allowing it to reverse the process and generate a clean image from a random noise input.

Compared to GANs, diffusion models often produce more diverse and higher-fidelity outputs and have a more stable training process. However, this comes at the cost of significantly increased computational complexity during inference, as the denoising process requires many iterative steps. This runtime challenge is exacerbated in 3D medical imaging due to the cubic growth in data size as resolution increases, although various acceleration techniques are being actively investigated [14,31]. For inpainting, diffusion models are conditioned on the unmasked portion of the image to guide the reverse process, generating content for the missing region that is coherent with its surroundings [27]. This approach has proven extremely powerful, with diffusion-based solutions securing top ranks in the BraTS Inpainting challenges [24,26].

2.4 Semantic Segmentation as Anatomical Guidance

One of the core ideas of our work involves structure-guided learning to inpaint anatomically plausible brain tissues. To build the explicit structural priors for guided learning, we used semantic segmentation maps, which assign an anatomical label to every voxel, providing an ideal source for such guidance. SynthSeg [6], in particular, has demonstrated robustness across varying contrasts, resolutions, and pathologies by training with synthetic data, making it highly suitable for tasks requiring generalizability. In our framework, we leverage SynthSeg to generate pseudo-anatomical segmentations. By incorporating anatomical information through a segmentator network and a perceptual masked loss, we encourage our generator to produce inpainted outputs that are not only visually realistic but also structurally consistent with brain anatomy.

3 Method

In this section, we detail our proposed inpainting method including the data processing, the model architecture, our strategy for generating synthetic brain tissue segmentation labels, the end-to-end training and inference pipelines, and the official evaluation metrics used to assess performance.

3.1 Data Processing

Our data processing is designed to prepare the medical imaging data for both the training and inference stages of our framework. The pipeline begins with three primary inputs for each subject: a T1 brain MRI, a manually annotated tumor mask, and a synthetically generated healthy tissue mask. The tumor mask is derived directly from the ground truth annotations provided in the dataset, while the healthy mask is generated by randomly sampling spherical regions within the brain parenchyma, avoiding areas overlapping with the tumor.

From these initial inputs, we derive two additional data products that serve as the primary inputs to our network: a masked T1 image and a pseudo-anatomy segmentation map. The masked T1 image is created by first combining the tumor and healthy masks into a single comprehensive mask, which is then used to zero-out the corresponding voxels in the original T1 image. Then it is channel-wise concatenated with healthy and tumor mask, making the final input a 3-channel masked T1 image. The pseudo-anatomy segmentation is generated by processing the original, non-masked T1 image with SynthSeg [6].

In training, we use a patch-based sampling strategy to manage computational cost and batch-processing. First, we perform random 3D cropping of 128^3 voxel patches from each subject's brain volume. To ensure that these patches primarily contain meaningful information, we employ a weighted index sampling strategy that assigns zero weight to background voxels, effectively focusing the cropping on foreground brain tissue. Following the cropping, the intensity values of each patch are rescaled from their original range to a normalized range of [-1, 1].

In inference, we first crop out background regions consisting of zero-valued voxels to reduce unnecessary computation. To instruct the model to inpaint the tumor region as healthy tissue, we prepare the 3-channel input by using the given tumor mask in place of the "healthy mask" channel, and an all-zero mask for the "tumor mask" channel. This configuration signals to the generator that the region defined by the original tumor mask should be filled in with content that mimics healthy anatomical structures.

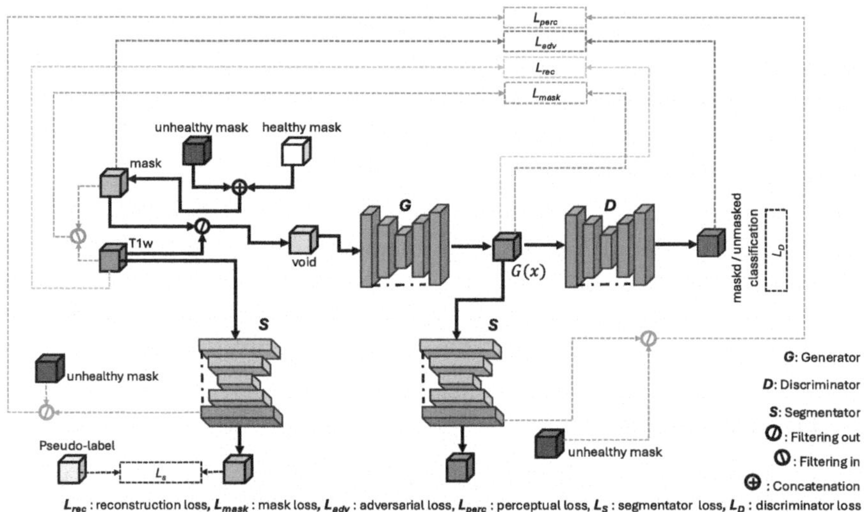

Fig. 1. Overall model architecture. There are three models including Generator (G), Discriminator (D), and Segmentator (S). Each model has its own training loss. However, every model contributes in training to the Generator model, so that it can produce both realistic and more anatomically plausible output. Details about model training and loss formulation are in Sect. 3.3.

3.2 Model Architecture

Our proposed framework (Figure 1) is composed of three distinct deep neural networks: a Generator (G), a Discriminator (D), and a Segmentator (S). Each network plays a specialized role in ensuring the final inpainted output is both realistic and anatomically correct.

Generator (G). The generator is the core synthesis engine of our framework, tasked with producing a complete T1 brain image by inpainting the masked region. It takes the 3-channel volume—comprising the masked T1 image, the healthy mask, and the tumor mask—as input. Its objective is twofold: to accurately reconstruct the unmasked regions to be nearly identical to the original image, and to inpaint the masked regions with plausible, high-fidelity brain tissue. We employ a U-Net architecture for the generator, as its encoder-decoder structure with skip connections is highly effective at preserving multi-scale spatial context, which is crucial for generating coherent anatomical structures.

Discriminator (D). Unlike conventional GANs that distinguish between entire real and fake images with a binary label, our discriminator is designed to enforce regional consistency within the generator's output. It operates on the synthesized T1 image and learns to discriminate between voxels from the reconstructed (originally unmasked) regions and those from the inpainted (originally masked) regions. The intuition is that the well-reconstructed regions, which are generated with full contextual information, can serve as a benchmark for realism. By training the generator to fool this discriminator, we minimize the perceptual difference between the inpainted and reconstructed areas. The discriminator is implemented with a U-Net architecture that performs voxel-wise classification, providing a localized adversarial loss signal that pushes the generator to produce more seamless and realistic inpainting.

Segmentator (S). The segmentator provides anatomical guidance during training. It is a 3D segmentation network trained to predict pseudo-anatomical labels produced by SynthSeg [6]. To encourage the generator to produce anatomically meaningful outputs, the segmentator introduces a perceptual loss in the feature space. Specifically, features extracted from the ground-truth T1 image are compared with those from the reconstructed T1 image, but only within the non-tumor regions. Minimizing this loss encourages the generator to synthesize tissue that the segmentator "perceives" as anatomically correct, thereby reinforcing the structural plausibility of the inpainted brain regions.

3.3 Training Pipeline with Loss Formulation

Our training process involves a multi-step optimization of the generator (G), discriminator (D), and segmentator (S) networks. Each component is updated sequentially in the following order: (1) discriminator, (2) segmentator, and (3) generator. This design ensures stable adversarial training while leveraging anatomical guidance from the segmentator.

Training the Discriminator. At each iteration, the generator first produces an inpainted image $\hat{I} = G(x)$. The discriminator is then trained to classify voxels from the reconstructed (unmasked) regions as "real" (label 1) and voxels from the inpainted (masked) regions as "fake" (label 0). The discriminator loss is defined by the binary cross-entropy (BCE) function,

$$\mathcal{L}_D = -\frac{1}{N}\sum_{i=1}^{N}\Big[\mathbb{E}\big[\log D\big(G(x_i)\odot(1-M_i)\big)\big]+\mathbb{E}\big[\log\big(1-D(G(x_i)\odot M_i)\big)\big]\Big], \quad (1)$$

where N is the number of voxels, x_i is the voxel itself, D is discriminator, G is generator, and M is the mask including both healthy and tumor. In this loss, the discriminator learns to classify inpainted masked region as "fake" and reconstructed but unmasked region as "real."

Training the Segmentator. The segmentator is trained as a stand-alone anatomical feature extractor. We feed the ground-truth T1 image into the segmentator and optimize it against pseudo-labels generated by SynthSeg [6]. We exclude the tumorous (unhealthy) region in the loss calculation, ensuring the segmentator learns only from valid, healthy anatomical examples. The segmentation loss is a voxel-wise cross-entropy,

$$\mathcal{L}_S = -\frac{1}{|M_i^H|}\sum_{i\in H_i^H}\sum_{c=1}^{C} y_{i,c}\log(S(x_{i,c})), \quad (2)$$

where M_i^H is the healthy mask, C is the number of unique segmentation classes, S is the segmentation model, and $y_{i,c}$ is the pseudo-annotation used as ground-truth label.

Training the Generator. Finally, the generator is updated while keeping both discriminator and segmentator frozen. The generator is trained with a combination of four complementary losses including reconstruction (L_{rec}), mask (L_{mask}), adversarial (L_{adv}), and perceptual loss (L_{perc}),

$$\mathcal{L}_G = \lambda_1 L_{\text{rec}} + \lambda_2 L_{\text{mask}} + \lambda_3 L_{\text{adv}} + \lambda_4 L_{\text{perc}}, \quad (3)$$

with weighting coefficients $\lambda_1 = \lambda_2 = 1$ and $\lambda_3 = \lambda_4 = 0.1$. The individual losses are,

$$\mathcal{L}_{\text{rec}} = \frac{1}{N}\|\hat{I} - I\|_1, \quad (4)$$

$$\mathcal{L}_{\text{mask}} = \frac{1}{|M|}\|\hat{I}_{\text{M}} - I_{\text{M}}\|_1, \quad (5)$$

$$\mathcal{L}_{adv} = -\frac{1}{|M^H|}\sum_{i\in M_i^H}\mathbb{E}\big[\log D\big(G(x_i)\big)\big], \quad (6)$$

$$\mathcal{L}_{\text{perc}} = \frac{1}{|M^H|}\sum_{i\in M^H}|S(I_i) - S(\hat{I}_i)|, \quad (7)$$

Table 1. Image Quality Assessment (IQA) results using mean squared error (MSE), peak signal-to-noise ratio (PSNR), and structural similarity index (SSIM). Our IQA results show underperformance compared to the previously top-performing team [24, 26].

	MSE $\downarrow$ (10^{-3})	PSNR $\uparrow$	SSIM $\uparrow$
Ying Weng et al. [24,26]	6.50 ± 4.66	23.4 ± 4.26	0.841 ± 0.103
Ours	8.99 ± 6.25	21.8 ± 3.99	0.808 ± 0.117

where N is the total number of voxels, I and $\hat{I}$ are ground-truth and reconstructed images, and I_{M} and $\hat{I_{\text{M}}}$ are the masked regions from ground-truth and reconstructed images.

This multi-loss formulation enables the generator to simultaneously capture low-level intensity fidelity (L_{rec}), enforce accurate inpainting of missing regions (L_{mask}), improve perceptual realism (L_{adv}), and ensure anatomical plausibility through structural guidance (L_{perc}).

3.4 Inference Pipeline

At inference time, the objective is to generate a tumor-to-healthy reconstruction of the brain given a T1 scan and its corresponding mask. To construct the generator input, we reassign the mask as the "healthy" mask channel, while setting the tumor mask channel to all zeros. In this way, the generator treats the mask as a healthy region to be inpainted. Furthermore, we crop out the voxels with zero intensity to reduce computational overhead. Finally, the generator takes 3-channel input and produces a completed T1 image in which the masked region is replaced with anatomically plausible healthy tissue.

4 Results

4.1 Dataset

We evaluated our method using the dataset provided by the BraTS 2025 Inpainting Challenge [1]. This challenge offers a large, multi-institutional collection of brain MRI scans specifically created to help develop algorithms capable of synthesizing healthy-appearing brain tissue in regions affected by pathology. The dataset is divided into three parts: a development set of 1,251 cases, a validation set of 219 cases, and a hidden test set maintained by the challenge organizers for final benchmarking. Each case in the development set includes three elements: (i) a T1 brain MRI, (ii) a randomly generated healthy mask, and (iii) a tumor mask derived from expert annotations. For the validation and test sets, only masked T1 brain images and the corresponding masks are provided.

4.2 Model Performance

In this section, we present both quantitative and qualitative evaluations of our method, compared against the top-ranked solution (Ying Weng et al. [24,26]) from the previous BraTS Inpainting Challenge.

Quantitative Analysis. Table 1 summarizes the performance of our method on the validation set using standard image quality assessment (IQA) metrics: mean squared error (MSE), peak signal-to-noise ratio (PSNR), and structural similarity index (SSIM). Our approach achieved a MSE of 8.99, PSNR of 21.8, and SSIM of 0.808. These values correspond to relative differences of −2.49 in MSE, −1.6 in PSNR, and −0.033 in SSIM compared to the prior best-performing method. While our model underperforms in terms of these standard quantitative measures, the results remain competitive in qualitative terms, as we now discuss.

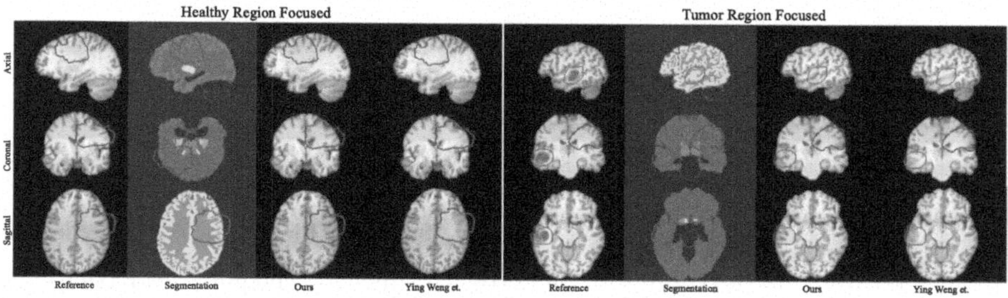

Fig. 2. Sample results from the development set. Ground-truth and pseudo-segmentation provide reference information corresponding to reconstructed samples. Blue and Red boundaries indicate healthy and tumor regions, respectively. The Blue boundary shows the inpainting quality compared to real brain tissue, whereas the Red boundary shows the generation quality of healthy tissue compared to the tumor region. (Color figure online)

Qualitative Analysis. Visual inspection of Figs. 2 and 3 suggest that our method generates more realistic and anatomically plausible reconstructions. Figure 2 is obtained from the development set, where ground-truth T1 and pseudo-segmentation are available as reference. Blue and Red boundaries in the figure represent the healthy and tumor mask, respectively. Blue boundaries show the model performance compared to the ground-truth, whereas Red boundaries indicate how the different models inpaint tumor regions into healthy tissue. Figure 3 is obtained from the validation set, where no references are available for comparison. In both figures, the inpainted tissue produced by our framework demonstrates improved structural coherence and sharper local details, which are less reflected in the quantitative analysis.

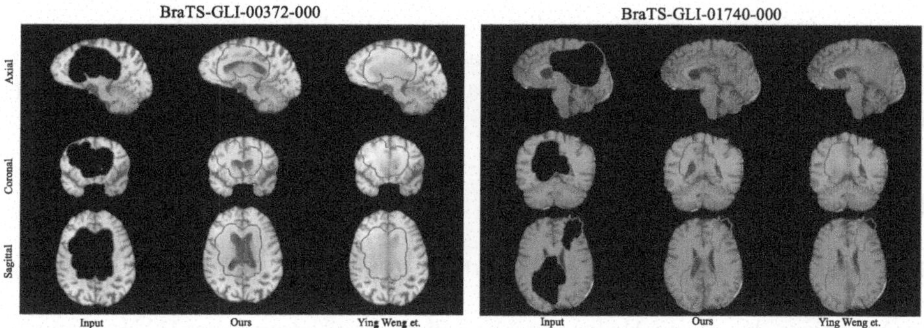

Fig. 3. Sample results from the validation set. The ground-truth information for this sample is explicitly held-out from the development and not publicly provided. Thus, the inpainted regions indicate the final model performance in the competition.

This observation is consistent with prior findings in the field of image quality assessment, which have shown that conventional pixel-wise metrics may correlate poorly with human perception of image realism [18,20,25,35]. Traditional measures rely heavily on low-level differences and often assume additive Gaussian noise, making them less sensitive to high-level perceptual and anatomical consistency.

5 Discussion

While traditional image quality assessment (IQA) metrics such as MSE, PSNR, and SSIM provide useful benchmarks, our findings highlight a gap between voxel-wise measures and human perception of medical image realism. In particular, voxel-level discrepancies may fail to capture high-level perceptual quality or medically relevant structural consistency. Although our method underperforms the previous winning solution on IQA scores, qualitative analysis indicates that it generates more visually realistic and anatomically plausible inpainting results. This underscores the importance of incorporating perceptual or clinically motivated metrics alongside traditional quantitative measures [16].

6 Conclusion

In this paper, we introduced an pseudo-segmentation-guided 3D GAN framework for the challenging task of tumor-to-healthy inpainting in brain MRI. Our approach integrates three key components: a generator that synthesizes realistic reconstructions conditioned on masked inputs, a discriminator that enforces perceptual similarity between reconstructed and inpainted regions, and a segmentator that provides anatomical guidance through a perceptual masked loss. Together, these components help generate inpainted brain tissue that is both visually convincing and structurally coherent. We demonstrated that our approach, while not achieving state-of-the-art results on traditional pixel-wise metrics, produces outputs that are qualitatively superior in terms of anatomical plausibility and visual realism.

References

1. Aboian, M., et al.: MICCAI 2025 lighthouse challenge: brain tumor segmentation cluster of challenges (brats) (2024)
2. Armanious, K., et al.: Medgan: medical image translation using GANs. Comput. Med. Imaging Graph. **79**, 101684 (2020)
3. Armanious, K., Kumar, V., Abdulatif, S., Hepp, T., Gatidis, S., Yang, B.: IPA-MEDGAN: Inpainting of arbitrary regions in medical imaging. In: 2020 IEEE International Conference on Image Processing (ICIP), pp. 3005–3009. IEEE (2020)
4. Barcelos, C.A.Z., Batista, M.A.: Image restoration using digital inpainting and noise removal. Image Vis. Comput. **25**(1), 61–69 (2007)
5. Bertalmio, M., Sapiro, G., Caselles, V., Ballester, C.: Image inpainting. In: Proceedings of the 27th Annual Conference on Computer Graphics and Interactive Techniques, pp. 417–424 (2000)
6. Billot, B., et al.: Synthseg: segmentation of brain MRI scans of any contrast and resolution without retraining. Med. Image Anal. **86**, 102789 (2023)
7. Brock, A., Donahue, J., Simonyan, K.: Large scale GAN training for high fidelity natural image synthesis. arXiv preprint arXiv:1809.11096 (2019)
8. Criminisi, A., Pérez, P., Toyama, K.: Region filling and object removal by exemplar-based image inpainting. IEEE Trans. Image Process. **13**(9), 1200–1212 (2004)
9. Dhariwal, P., Nichol, A.Q.: Diffusion models beat GANs on image synthesis. arXiv preprint arXiv:2105.05233 (2021)
10. Durrer, A., Bieder, F., Friedrich, P., Menze, B., Cattin, P.C., Kofler, F.: fastwdm3d: Fast and accurate 3D healthy tissue inpainting. arXiv preprint arXiv:2507.13146 (2025)
11. Durrer, A., et al.: Denoising diffusion models for 3D healthy brain tissue inpainting. In: MICCAI Workshop on Deep Generative Models, pp. 87–97. Springer (2024)
12. Elharrouss, O., Almaadeed, N., Al-Maadeed, S., Akbari, Y.: Image inpainting: a review. Neural Process. Lett. **51**(2), 2007–2028 (2020)
13. Friedrich, P., Frisch, Y., Cattin, P.C.: Deep generative models for 3D medical image synthesis. In: Generative Machine Learning Models in Medical Image Computing, pp. 255–278. Springer (2024)
14. Geng, Z., Deng, M., Bai, X., Kolter, J.Z., He, K.: Mean flows for one-step generative modeling. arXiv preprint arXiv:2505.13447 (2025)
15. Goodfellow, I.J., et al.: Generative adversarial nets. In: Advances in Neural Information Processing Systems (NeurIPS), pp. 2672–2680 (2014)
16. Ha, J., Park, J.S., Crandall, D., Garyfallidis, E., Zhang, X.: Multi-resolution guided 3D gans for medical image translation. In: Proceedings of the IEEE/CVF Winter Conference on Applications of Computer Vision (WACV) (2025)
17. Ho, J., Jain, A., Abbeel, P.: Denoising diffusion probabilistic models. arXiv preprint arXiv:2006.11239 (2020)
18. Huynh-Thu, Q., Ghanbari, M.: Scope of validity of PSNR in image/video quality assessment. Electron. Lett. **44**(13), 800–801 (2008)

19. Isola, P., Zhu, J.Y., Zhou, T., Efros, A.A.: Image-to-image translation with conditional adversarial networks. In: Proceedings of the IEEE Conference on Computer Vision and Pattern Recognition (CVPR) (2017)
20. Johnson, J., Alahi, A., Fei-Fei, L.: Perceptual losses for real-time style transfer and super-resolution. In: European Conference on Computer Vision (ECCV), pp. 694–711 (2016)
21. Kang, M., Lee, J., Choo, J.: Gigagan: Scaling up GANs for text-to-image synthesis. arXiv preprint arXiv:2303.05511 (2023)
22. Kang, S.K., et al.: Deep learning-based 3D inpainting of brain MR images. Sci. Rep. **11**(1), 1673 (2021)
23. Khader, F., et al.: Medical diffusion: denoising diffusion probabilistic models for 3D medical image generation. Sci. Rep. **12**, 8130 (2022)
24. Kofler, F., et al.: The brain tumor segmentation (brats) challenge: local synthesis of healthy brain tissue via inpainting. arXiv preprint arXiv:2305.08992 (2023)
25. Kundu, D., Evans, B.: Full-reference visual quality assessment for synthetic images: a subjective study. In: Proceeding IEEE International Conference on Image Processing (2015)
26. Li, H.B., et alet al.: The brain tumor segmentation (brats) challenge 2023: brain MR image synthesis for tumor segmentation (brasyn). ArXiv pp. arXiv–2305 (2024)
27. Lugmayr, A., Danelljan, M., Romero, A., Yu, F., Timofte, R., Van Gool, L.: Repaint: inpainting using denoising diffusion probabilistic models. In: Proceedings of the IEEE Conference on Computer Vision and Pattern Recognition (CVPR), pp. 11461–11471 (2022)
28. Qureshi, M.A., Deriche, M., Beghdadi, A., Amin, A.: A critical survey of state-of-the-art image inpainting quality assessment metrics. J. Vis. Commun. Image Represent. **49**, 177–191 (2017)
29. Rombach, R., Blattmann, A., Lorenz, D., Esser, P., Ommer, B.: High-resolution image synthesis with latent diffusion models. In: Proceedings of the IEEE/CVF Conference on Computer Vision and Pattern Recognition (CVPR), pp. 10684–10695 (2022)
30. Sogancioglu, E., Hu, S., Belli, D., van Ginneken, B.: Chest x-ray inpainting with deep generative models. arXiv preprint arXiv:1809.01471 (2018)
31. Song, J., Meng, C., Ermon, S.: Denoising diffusion implicit models. In: International Conference on Learning Representations (2021)
32. Suvorov, R., et al.: Resolution-robust large mask inpainting with Fourier convolutions. In: Proceedings of the IEEE/CVF Winter Conference on Applications of Computer Vision (WACV), pp. 2149–2159 (2022)
33. Tran, K.S., Nguyen, Q.T., Jeong, M., Park, S.J.: Multi-task learning for medical image inpainting based on organ boundary awareness. Appl. Sci. **11**(9), 4247 (2021)
34. Tran, M.T., Kim, S.H., Yang, H.J., Lee, G.S.: Multi-task learning for medical image inpainting based on organ boundary awareness. Appl. Sci. **11**(9), 4247 (2021)
35. Wang, Z., Bovik, A.: Mean squared error: love it or leave it? A new look at signal fidelity measures. IEEE Signal Process. Mag. **26**(1), 98–117 (2009)
36. Xiong, W., et al.: Foreground-aware image inpainting. In: Proceedings of the IEEE/CVF Conference on Computer Vision and Pattern Recognition, pp. 5840–5848 (2019)
37. Yang, C., Lu, X., Lin, Z., Shechtman, E., Wang, O., Li, H.: High-resolution image inpainting using multi-scale neural patch synthesis. In: Proceedings of the IEEE Conference on Computer Vision and Pattern Recognition, pp. 6721–6729 (2017)

38. Yu, J., Lin, Z., Yang, J., Shen, X., Lu, X., Huang, T.S.: Generative image inpainting with contextual attention. In: Proceedings of the IEEE Conference on Computer Vision and Pattern Recognition (CVPR), pp. 5505–5514 (2018)
39. Zeineldin, R.A., Mathis-Ullrich, F.: Ensemble learning and 3D pix2pix for comprehensive brain tumor analysis in multimodal MRI. In: International Challenge on Cross-Modality Domain Adaptation for Medical Image Segmentation, pp. 24–34. Springer (2023)
40. Zhu, J.Y., Park, T., Isola, P., Efros, A.A.: Unpaired image-to-image translation using cycle-consistent adversarial networks. In: Proceedings of the IEEE International Conference on Computer Vision (ICCV) (2017)
41. Çallı, E., Sogancioglu, E., van Ginneken, B., van Leeuwen, K.G., Murphy, K.: Deep learning for chest x-ray analysis: a survey. Med. Image Anal. **72**, 102125 (2021)

Challenge 10 – BraTS-Path

Patch-Level Classification of Histopathological Subregions in Glioblastoma

Jia Son[1] and Tae Hoon Roh[2](✉)

[1] Yonsei University Health System, Seoul, Korea
zson202@gmail.com
[2] Department of Neurosurgery, Yonsei University College of Medicine, Seoul, Korea
throh@yuhs.ac

Abstract. Glioblastoma is a highly aggressive primary brain tumor with histopathological heterogeneity. Identifying relevant structures in histology images is crucial for diagnosis and treatment, yet manual interpretation is tedious. To address this, we developed a deep learning model for the classification of histopathological subregions in glioblastoma. In this work, we present one of the top-performing methods in the BraTS-Path 2025 Challenge, a competition aimed at developing computational pathology solutions for glioblastoma. We adapted a Vision Transformer pretrained on a large-scale histology dataset. To achieve a balance between efficiency and performance, we employed parameter-efficient fine-tuning with Low-Rank Adaptation. To address class imbalance and enhance generalization, we used stratified cross-validation, data augmentation, and ensemble inference. The results indicate that our approach performs robustly and can assist histopathological analysis in neuro-oncology. The code is available at http://github.com/oikosohn/brats25-path.

Keywords: BraTS · challenge · brain · tumor · pathology · classification · deep learning · artificial intelligence · low-rank adaptation

1 Introduction

Glioblastoma is the most common primary malignant brain tumor in adults. It is the most aggressive subtype of gliomas. Although the number of long-term survivors has increased in recent years, its prognosis remains substantially worse than that of any other brain tumor [16]. Histopathological analysis plays a critical role in diagnosing glioma and planning appropriate treatment. It provides valuable visual information to support rapid decision making [7]. However, manual interpretation is time-consuming, labor-intensive and requires specialized expertise. Even among professionals, qualified neuro-pathologists are scarce. To support neuro-pathologists, we develop a deep learning model that classifies square patches from whole slide histopathology images (WSI) into specific subregions.

S. Bakas et al. (Eds.): MICCAI 2025, LNCS 16377, pp. 183–192, 2026.
https://doi.org/10.1007/978-3-032-16370-7_16

Early computer vision models based on neural networks were dominated by convolutional neural networks, which proved effective for a variety of visual recognition tasks due to their ability to extract local patterns [8,11,12,15]. Building on its success in natural language processing [17], the Transformer architecture was extended to vision tasks, where images are represented as patch sequences and self-attention mechanisms are employed to capture long-range spatial relationships [2,6,13,19]. Transformer-based vision models have achieved state-of-the-art performance on various computer vision benchmarks. In this work, we leverage a foundation model based on the Vision Transformer (ViT) to classify histopathological image tiles, capturing the inherent heterogeneity of glioblastoma tissue.

2 Data Description

The BraTS-Path 2025 Challenge dataset includes digitized FFPE H&E-stained glioblastoma tissue sections sourced from 11 international medical institutions [1, 3]. It comprises 1,047,801 image patches, which constitute the development set for this study. This set is divided into two splits: Train split 1 (749,269 patches) and Train split 2 (298,532 patches). Each patch is 512×512 pixels and serves as an input instance for classification, with representative examples shown in Fig. 1.

There is a notable class imbalance in the distribution of these patches, as summarized in Table 1. In particular, a substantial disparity exists between majority classes such as Cellular Tumor (CT) or Necrosis (NC) and minority classes like Presence of Lymphocytes (PL) or Dense Macrophages (DM). This class imbalance may affect the model's ability to generalize to underrepresented classes.

Table 1. Class distribution in the BraTS-Path 2025 development set.

Class	# of Train split 1	# of Train split 2	Total
Cellular Tumor (CT)	250,370	85,903	336,273
Dense Macrophages (DM)	4,359	556	4,915
Infiltration into Cortex (IC)	126,773	58,735	185,508
Leptomeningeal Infiltration (LI)	6,419	4,663	11,082
Microvascular Proliferation (MP)	21,349	221	21,570
Necrosis (NC)	259,329	88,821	348,150
Presence of Lymphocytes (PL)	1,998	793	2,791
Pseudopalisading Necrosis (PN)	38,821	2,773	41,594
White Matter (WM)	39,851	56,067	95,918
Grand Total	**749,269**	**298,532**	**1,047,801**

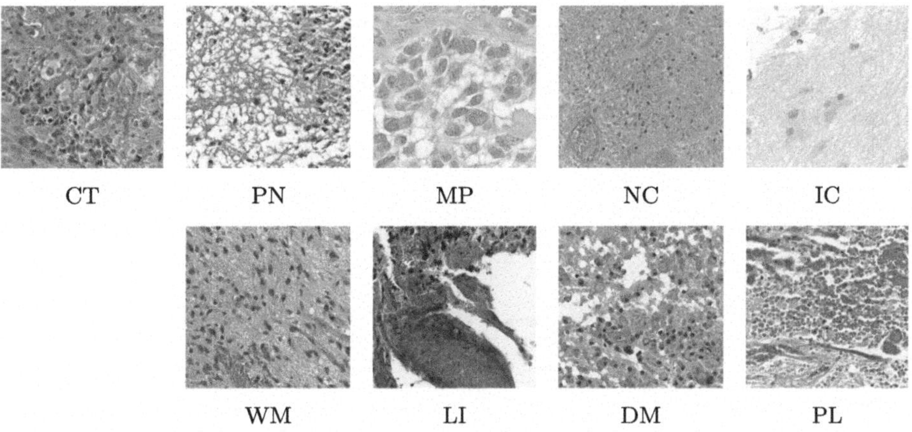

Fig. 1. Representative histopathology examples of glioblastoma subregions from the BraTS-Path 2025 dataset. Images show patches corresponding to CT (Cellular Tumor), PN (Pseudopalisading Necrosis), MP (Microvascular Proliferation), NC (Necrosis), IC (Infiltration into Cortex), WM (White Matter), LI (Leptomeningeal Infiltration), DM (Dense Macrophages), and PL (Presence of Lymphocytes).

3 Method

3.1 Data Preprocessing

The images were resized to 224×224 pixels and stored as NumPy arrays. For input normalization, we applied the RGB channel mean and standard deviation from the ImageNet dataset [5] to align with the ViT backbone. The values were:

$$\begin{aligned} \text{mean} &= [0.485,\ 0.456,\ 0.406] \\ \text{standard deviation} &= [0.229,\ 0.224,\ 0.225] \end{aligned}$$

3.2 Model

To classify histopathological subregions, we adopted **Virchow2**, a pathology-specific foundation model based on a ViT-H backbone, pretrained with self-supervised learning on a large-scale histopathology dataset consisting of 3.1 million WSI tiles from Memorial Sloan Kettering Cancer Center (MSKCC) [18,21]. Virchow2 incorporates pathology-specific modifications to the DINOv2 framework [4,14], including the replacement of the KoLeo regularizer with a kernel density estimator and the use of extended-context translation (ECT) to preserve cell morphology.

To tailor the foundation model to our task, we applied parameter-efficient fine-tuning (PEFT) using Low-Rank Adaptation (LoRA) [9,20]. Specifically, LoRA was applied to the query (`Q`), key (`K`), and value (`V`) projections of the self-attention layers in each Transformer block, as illustrated in Fig. 2. The classifier head is a linear layer that operates on the concatenation of the class token and the mean of the patch tokens. During training, only the LoRA-injected parameters and the classifier head were set to be trainable, while the rest of the backbone was frozen to stabilize fine-tuning and reduce computational cost.

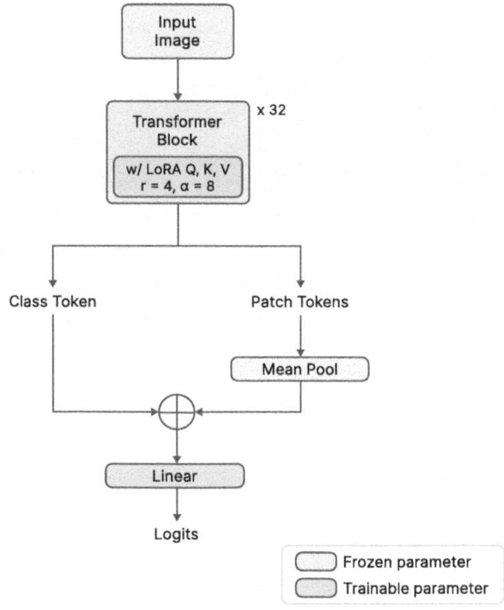

Fig. 2. Simplified architecture of our model. Only the `Q`, `K` and `V` projection layers and the linear classifier are trainable; the backbone is frozen.

3.3 Training

To mitigate class imbalance and enhance generalization to underrepresented classes, we approached the training data strategically. The models were trained on the development set provided by the challenge, which comprises all available labeled data. Stratified k-fold cross-validation was employed in combination with data augmentation to maximize learning from underrepresented classes. Gradient accumulation was used to simulate larger batch sizes, while mixed-precision training accelerated convergence. Model checkpoints and evaluation metrics were recorded at the end of each epoch to monitor performance.

3.4 Inference

Outputs from models trained on each fold were ensembled by averaging the softmax probabilities, and the final class was determined by selecting the one with the highest averaged probability. Test-time augmentation (TTA) with horizontal and vertical flips was also applied to improve robustness.

3.5 Hyperparameters

The hyperparameters that achieved top performance in the BraTS-Path 2025 Challenge are summarized in Table 2. Hyperparameter settings were guided by preliminary experiments and constrained by the available hardware resources.

Training was conducted with a batch size of 32 with gradient accumulation over 4 steps. Data augmentation included random color jittering, horizontal and vertical flips, and rotations by discrete angles. A 4-fold cross-validation strategy was adopted, with each fold trained independently on a separate GPU to enable simultaneous training. The AdamW optimizer was utilized to accelerate convergence, with a learning rate of 5×10^{-5} and weight decay of 1×10^{-2}. Cosine annealing with warm restarts was used for learning rate scheduling. The loss function was cross-entropy, incorporating label smoothing with a rate of 0.1. LoRA was applied with a rank (r) of 4 and an alpha (α) of 8, which resulted in approximately 10% of the model parameters being trainable—double that of linear probing (about 5%)—while preserving computational efficiency. To handle the large number of patches and parameters, mixed precision with brain floating point (bfloat16) was employed, which reduced training time while achieving performance comparable to full-precision training [10].

3.6 Computing Hardware and Software

All experiments and analysis in this study were implemented using Python 3.9.21 and PyTorch 2.7.0 (CUDA 11.8). Both training and inference were conducted using four 24 GB NVIDIA RTX A5000 GPUs.

4 Results

4.1 Metric

Matthews Correlation Coefficient and F1-score are the primary evaluation metrics of the BraTS-Path 2025, and are particularly informative when class distributions are skewed.

Matthews Correlation Coefficient (MCC) summarizes the confusion matrix into a single correlation-like score. It ranges from -1 when predictions are entirely incorrect, to 1 when perfectly accurate, while a value of 0 indicates that predictive capability is no better than random guessing. MCC is defined as:

$$\text{MCC} = \frac{TP \times TN - FP \times FN}{\sqrt{(TP + FP)(TP + FN)(TN + FP)(TN + FN)}}$$

where TP, TN, FP, and FN denote true positives, true negatives, false positives, and false negatives, respectively.

F1-score is the harmonic mean of precision and recall, providing a balanced measure that accounts for both false positives and false negatives. The F1-score is defined as:

$$\text{F1-score} = \frac{2 \times \text{Precision} \times \text{Recall}}{\text{Precision} + \text{Recall}}$$

Table 2. Hyperparameter settings for training and inference.

Phase	Hyperparameter	Value
Training & Inference	Input size	224 × 224
	Input normalization mean/std	ImageNet mean/std
	Automatic mixed precision	bfloat16
	Image augmentation	Yes
Training	Number of epochs	50
	Number of folds	4
	Batch size	32
	Gradient accumulation steps	4
	Loss function	Cross-entropy
	Label smoothing rate	0.1
	Optimizer	AdamW
	Learning rate	5e−5
	Weight decay	1e−2
	Scheduler	CosineAnnealingWarmRestarts
	LoRA r	4
	LoRA α	8
Inference	Batch size	128
	Ensembling	Yes

4.2 Model Evaluation on Development Set

Table 3 summarizes the performance of the model on the development set across four cross-validation folds. By epoch 50, training losses had decreased and evaluation scores had improved; however, convergence remained unstable.

The per-fold confusion matrices shown in Fig. 3 illustrate how the model predicts each class on the internal validation set. Notably, the model shows relatively higher confusion among Cellular Tumor (CT), Pseudopalisading Necrosis (PN), and Microvascular Proliferation (MP). This tendency may be due either to the considerably smaller number of PN and MP images compared to CT, or to the morphological similarities among these classes in challenge dataset.

Table 3. Performance metrics on the internal validation set for each fold at epoch 50.

Fold	Train		Internal Validation	
	MCC	F1-score	MCC	F1-score
Fold 1	0.9975	0.9932	0.9954	0.9886
Fold 2	0.9964	0.9894	0.9948	0.9864
Fold 3	0.9968	0.9911	0.9952	0.9889
Fold 4	0.9925	0.9843	0.9912	0.9806
Mean	0.9958	0.9895	0.9942	0.9861
Std	0.0020	0.0036	0.0019	0.0034

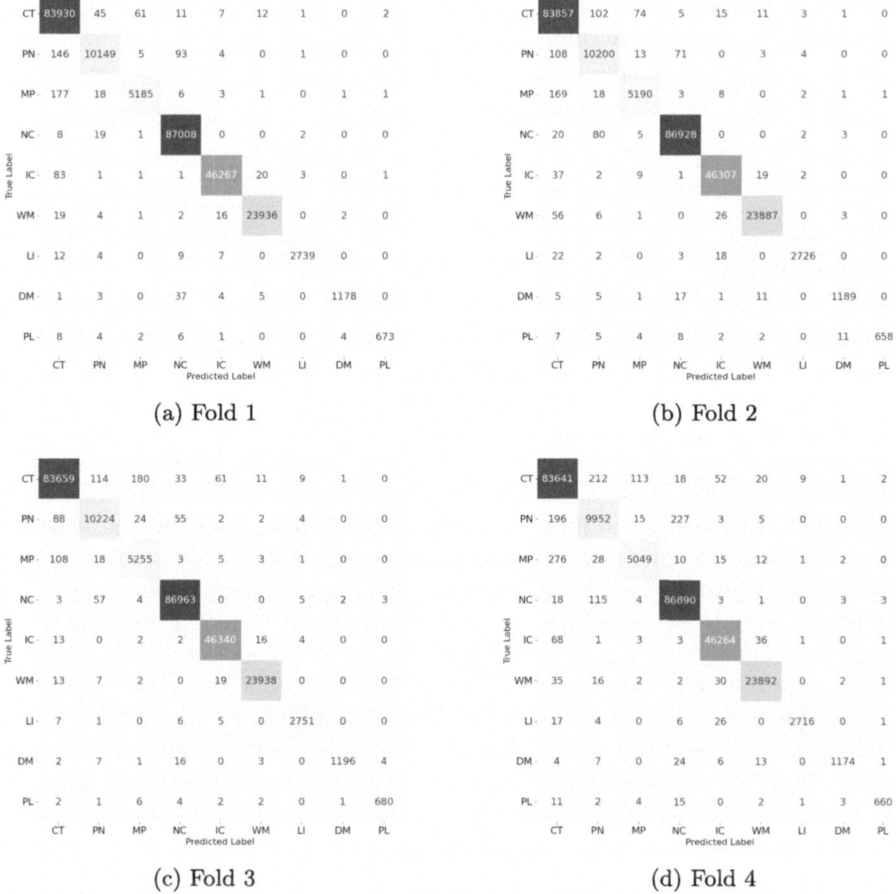

Fig. 3. Confusion matrices on the internal validation set for each fold at epoch 50.

4.3 Model Evaluation on External Validation and Test Sets

The proposed approach achieved a top-three ranking in the BraTS-Path 2025 Challenge, and Table 4 summarizes the metrics obtained on the external validation sets. These results suggest that our approach demonstrates reliable performance. However, the observed performance gaps between the training and external validation may indicate potential generalization challenges, highlighting the need for further analysis of underrepresented classes and unseen data.

Table 4. Performance of the proposed approach on the BraTS-Path 2025 external validation sets.

Metrics	External Validation
MCC	0.7089
F1-Score	0.7717
Accuracy	0.7717
Recall	0.7717
Specificity	0.9746

5 Discussion

In this study, we fine-tuned a foundation model with low-rank adaptation to predict histopathological subregions of glioblastoma. Despite pronounced class imbalance and subtle morphological differences between classes, the model achieved robust performance. Since the internal validation loss was still decreasing at epoch 50, extending the training epochs may lead to further gains.

It is expected that hyperparameter optimization could further improve model performance. Increasing the input image and batch size, lowering the learning rate, and adopting a more advanced learning rate scheduler could promote stable convergence. Adjusting LoRA r and α may also improve performance, although this change would require additional GPU memory. Alternative loss functions may be beneficial. For instance, Focal or Dice loss could better handle class imbalance by re-weighting minority classes. Metric-based losses such as ArcFace or Triplet loss could improve class separability by enlarging the margin.

Additional data-centric approaches may improve model performance. Incorporating blur transformations could make the model more resilient, particularly given the presence of blurry patches in the dataset. Pseudo-labeling on the external validation set could enhance the representation of minority labels and alleviate distributional imbalance. Data generation based on the morphological analysis of glioblastoma may further enhance the ability to distinguish between subregions.

Acknowledgements. The dataset employed in this paper was sourced from "Assessing the Heterogeneous Histologic Landscape of Glioma (BraTS-Path 2025)," a task within the BraTS-Lighthouse 2025 Challenge. It is accessible on Synapse (syn64153430).

This work was supported by the National Research Foundation of Korea (NRF) grant funded by the Korea government (MSIT) (RS-2023-00253964).

References

1. Bakas, S., et al.: BraTS-path challenge: assessing heterogeneous histopathologic brain tumor sub-regions (2024). arXiv preprint
2. Carion, N., Massa, F., Synnaeve, G., Usunier, N., Kirillov, A., Zagoruyko, S.: End-to-end object detection with transformers. In: Vedaldi, A., Bischof, H., Brox, T., Frahm, J.-M. (eds.) ECCV 2020. LNCS, vol. 12346, pp. 213–229. Springer, Cham (2020). https://doi.org/10.1007/978-3-030-58452-8_13
3. Clark, K., et al.: The cancer imaging archive (TCIA): maintaining and operating a public information repository. J. Digit. Imaging **26**(6), 1045–1057 (2013)
4. Darcet, T., Oquab, M., Mairal, J., Bojanowski, P.: Vision transformers need registers. In: The Twelfth International Conference on Learning Representations (2024)
5. Deng, J., Dong, W., Socher, R., Li, L.J., Li, K., Fei-Fei, L.: ImageNet: a large-scale hierarchical image database. In: CVPR (2009)
6. Dosovitskiy, A., et al.: An image is worth 16x16 words: transformers for image recognition at scale. In: ICLR (2021)
7. Fuchs, T.J., Buhmann, J.M.: Computational pathology: challenges and promises for tissue analysis. Comput. Med. Imaging Graph. **35**(7), 515–530 (2011)
8. He, K., Zhang, X., Ren, S., Sun, J.: Deep residual learning for image recognition. In: CVPR (2016)
9. Hu, E.J., et al.: LoRA: low-rank adaptation of large language models. In: ICLR (2022)
10. Kalamkar, D., et al.: A study of bfloat16 for deep learning training 2019 (2019). arXiv preprint
11. Krizhevsky, A., Sutskever, I., Hinton, G.E.: ImageNet classification with deep convolutional neural networks. In: NeurIPS (2012)
12. LeCun, Y., et al.: Backpropagation applied to handwritten zip code recognition. Neural Comput. **1**(4), 541–551 (1989)
13. Liu, Z., et al.: Swin transformer: hierarchical vision transformer using shifted windows. In: ICCV (2021)
14. Oquab, M., et al.: DINOv2: learning robust visual features without supervision. TMLR (2024)
15. Ronneberger, O., Fischer, P., Brox, T.: U-Net: convolutional networks for biomedical image segmentation. In: Navab, N., Hornegger, J., Wells, W.M., Frangi, A.F. (eds.) MICCAI 2015. LNCS, vol. 9351, pp. 234–241. Springer, Cham (2015). https://doi.org/10.1007/978-3-319-24574-4_28
16. Tan, A.C., Ashley, D.M., López, G.Y., Malinzak, M., Friedman, H.S., Khasraw, M.: Management of glioblastoma: state of the art and future directions. Cancer J. Clin. **70**(4), 299–312 (2020)
17. Vaswani, A., et al.: Attention is all you need. In: NeurIPS (2017)
18. Vorontsov, E., et al.: A foundation model for clinical-grade computational pathology and rare cancers detection. Nat. Med. **30**(10), 2924–2935 (2024)

19. Wu, B., et al.: Visual transformers: token-based image representation and processing for computer vision (2020). arXiv preprint
20. Zhu, Y., et al.: MeLo: low-rank adaptation is better than fine-tuning for medical image diagnosis. In: 2024 IEEE International Symposium on Biomedical Imaging (2024)
21. Zimmermann, E., et al.: Virchow2: scaling self-supervised mixed magnification models in pathology (2024). arXiv preprint

Patch-Level Glioblastoma Subregion Classification with a Contrastive Learning-Based Encoder

Juexin Zhang, Qifeng Zhong, Ying Weng(✉), and Ke Chen

University of Nottingham Ningbo China, Ningbo 315100, China
{juexin.zhang,qifeng.zhong,ying.weng,ke.chen2}@nottingham.edu.cn

Abstract. The significant molecular and pathological heterogeneity of glioblastoma, an aggressive brain tumor, complicates diagnosis and patient stratification. While traditional histopathological assessment remains the standard, deep learning offers a promising path toward objective and automated analysis of whole slide images. For the BraTS-Path 2025 Challenge, we developed a method that fine-tunes a pre-trained Vision Transformer (ViT) encoder with a dedicated classification head on the official training dataset. Our model's performance on the online validation set, evaluated via the Synapse platform, yielded a Matthews Correlation Coefficient (MCC) of 0.7064 and an F1-score of 0.7676. On the final test set, the model achieved an MCC of 0.6509 and an F1-score of 0.5330, which secured our team second place in the BraTS-Pathology 2025 Challenge. Our results establish a solid baseline for ViT-based histopathological analysis, and future efforts will focus on bridging the performance gap observed on the unseen validation data.

Keywords: Deep learning · Digital Pathology · BraTS 2025 · Glioblastoma

1 Introduction

Glioblastoma is a highly aggressive primary brain tumor associated with poor patient outcomes, which makes accurate diagnosis and prognostic assessment critical for guiding therapy [12]. One of the main challenges lies in the marked histopathological heterogeneity of these tumors. Such heterogeneity is evident both across patients (inter-tumoral) and within individual tumors (intra-tumoral), and is reflected in differences in cellular morphology, phenotypic profiles, and treatment responses [9], thereby complicating prognostic evaluation.

Glioblastoma is an aggressive primary brain tumor associated with poor patient outcomes, which makes accurate diagnosis and prognostic prediction critical for guiding therapy [12]. The main challenge lies in the marked histopathological heterogeneity of these tumors. This diversity exists both between patients

J. Zhang and Q. Zhong—Contributed equally to this work.

S. Bakas et al. (Eds.): MICCAI 2025, LNCS 16377, pp. 193–202, 2026.
https://doi.org/10.1007/978-3-032-16370-7_17

(inter-tumoral) and within a single tumor (intra-tumoral), manifesting as variations in cellular morphology, phenotypic expression, and therapeutic response [9], which makes the prognosis more complicated.

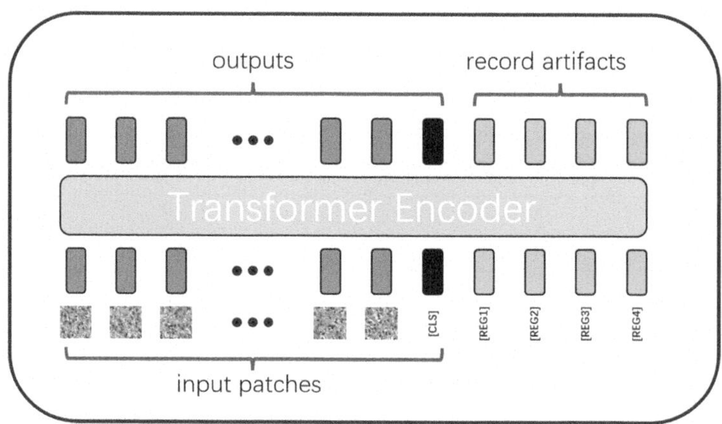

Fig. 1. Virchow2 uses four registers to mitigate local information loss and enhance global contextual information by storing artifact tokens, thereby enabling better feature extraction. Adapted from [2].

The diagnosis of brain tumors has usually relied on pathology, where tissue samples are examined under a microscope to get subtypes of tumors and give treatment plans. In recent years, this traditional workflow has been reshaped by the rise of digital pathology, which replaces glass slides with high-resolution digital images of tissue sections. With the development of computational tools, digital pathology is redefining how brain tumors are studied and classified. The availability of whole-slide imaging also opens the door to artificial intelligence methods, especially deep learning models such as convolutional neural networks, which can detect subtle histological features and support faster, more accurate diagnoses.

Building upon this progress, large-scale foundation models pretrained on histopathology data, such as CTransPath [11] and Virchow [13]. As reported by Neidlinger et al. [7], Virchow excels at extracting fine-grained features and outperforms many alternatives. We use the pretrained Virchow2 as a feature extraction backbone, leveraging its ability to capture discriminative tile-level features. For classification, we attach a head consisting of two linear layers to predict the class of each sub-region patch.

2 Methods

For our study, we selected Virchow2 [13] as the foundational pretrained model, chosen for its state-of-the-art performance in computational pathology. The architecture of Virchow2 is built upon the powerful Vision Transformer (ViT-H/14) [3], a high-capacity model known for its ability to capture complex spatial relationships in image data, as illustrated in Fig. 1. The power of Virchow2 stems from its extensive pretraining on a massive and diverse dataset comprising approximately 3.1 million whole slide images (WSIs) from over 225,000 patients. This dataset provides comprehensive coverage of nearly 200 tissue types and multiple staining modalities, including the widely used hematoxylin and eosin (H&E) as well as various immunohistochemical (IHC) stains. This robust pretraining ensures the model learns a rich hierarchy of generalizable features relevant to histopathology. Virchow2's feature representation capabilities were developed using DINOv2 [8], a sophisticated self-supervised learning framework. This approach enables the model to learn meaningful features directly from unlabeled images without requiring manual annotations.

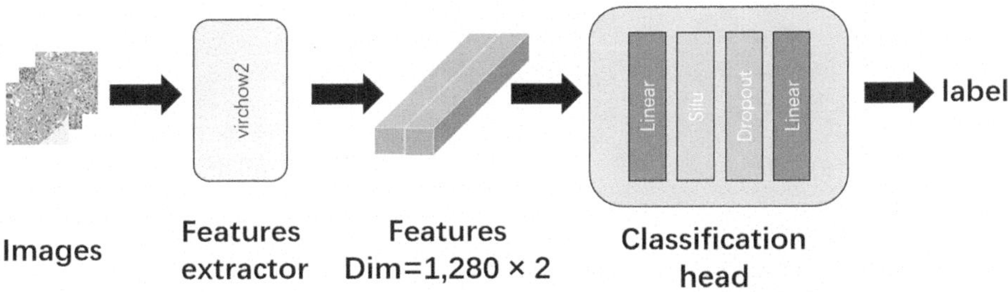

Fig. 2. The network architecture of our model.

To tailor the pretrained Virchow2 for our specific 9-class sub-region classification task, we replace the original classification head with a new one, as depicted in Fig. 2. Our approach is designed to create a highly informative feature representation from each input patch before classification. The process begins by dividing each input patch into 256 non-overlapping tiles. These tiles are processed by the Virchow2 encoder, which generates 256 corresponding feature tokens, each with a dimensionality of 1280. To create a comprehensive feature representation for the entire patch, we combine two distinct signals:

- Global Average Representation: We compute the mean of all 256 tokens to produce a single 1×1280 vector. This provides a global summary of the patch's overall texture, cellularity, and morphology.
- Semantic Class Token: We also retain the original class token (1×1280), which the Vision Transformer learns to use as an aggregate representation of the most critical semantic information in the image.

The averaged feature token and the class token are concatenated and flattened to form a final, rich feature vector of size 2560. This dual-representation strategy ensures our classifier has access to both a holistic summary and the most salient features identified by the transformer. This combined feature vector is then passed to our newly designed classification head, which consists of the following sequential layers:

- A linear layer that projects the 2560-dimensional input to a 256-dimensional space, acting as a feature bottleneck to condense information.
- A SiLU (Sigmoid-weighted Linear Unit) activation function to introduce non-linearity, allowing the model to learn more complex decision boundaries.
- A dropout layer with a rate of 0.5, which randomly deactivates neurons during training to effectively mitigate overfitting.
- A final linear output layer that maps the 256-dimensional features to the 9 target class logits, producing the final predictions.

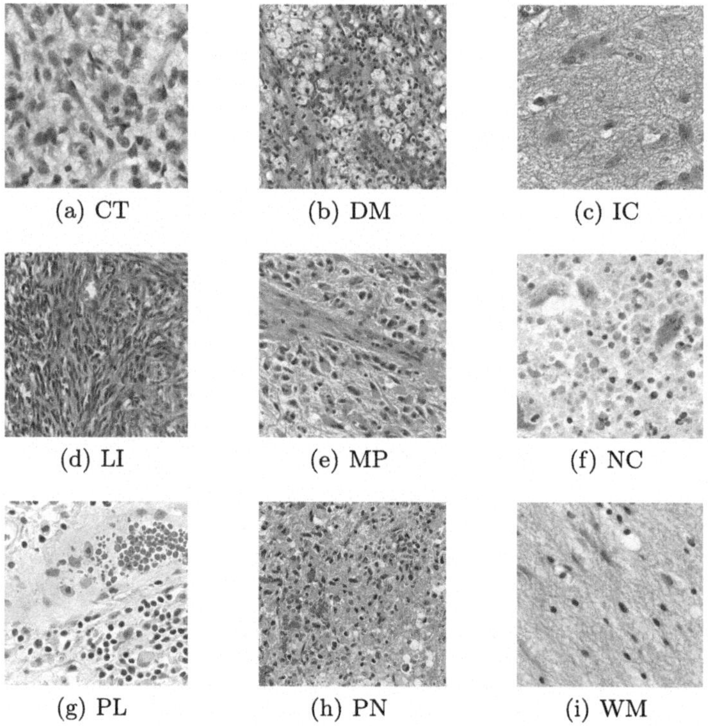

Fig. 3. Illustration of the annotated histologic areas of interest.

3 Experiments

3.1 Dataset

No external unlabeled pathology dataset was used, all operations in this paper were performed on the labeled BraTS-Path dataset [1,4], provided by the official BraTS 2025 challenge [10]. Which consists of H&E-stained Formalin-Fixed,

Paraffin-Embedded (FFPE) tissue sections from the TCGA-GBM and TCGA-LGG collections. The data have been reclassified according to updated World Health Organization (WHO) criteria, focusing on glioblastoma cases. Expert annotations segment the slides into patches representing distinct histological regions. The dataset [1,10] covers nine histological categories:

1. Presence of cellular tumor (CT)
2. Pseudopalisading necrosis (PN)
3. Areas abundant in microvascular proliferation (MP)
4. Geographic necrosis (NC)
5. Infiltration into the cortex (IC)
6. Penetration into white matter (WM)
7. Leptomeningial infiltration (LI)
8. Regions with dense macrophages (DM)
9. Presence of lymphocytes (PL)

Figure 3 provides a qualitative overview of the dataset with representative images from each of the nine classes. The dataset is highly unbalanced, exhibiting a long-tailed class distribution as quantitatively detailed in Fig. 4.

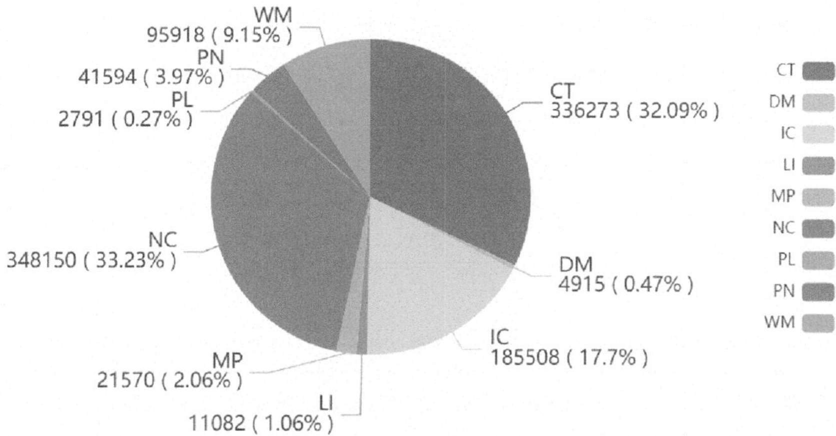

Fig. 4. Class distribution of the dataset, detailing the number and percentage of samples for each category.

3.2 Data Pre-processing

Histopathological patches were input data from nine classes. To ensure uniform input for training and evaluation and ensure the generalization ability of the model, all input images were transformed using a pre-processing pipeline implemented via:

- **Resize:** All images were resized to a fixed size(resolution) of 224×224 pixels, ensuring uniform spatial dimensions of inputs.
- **ToTensor:** Images were converted into PyTorch tensors, scaling pixel values to the $[0, 1]$ range and rearranging the channel order to (C, H, W).
- **Normalization:** Pixel intensities were normalized using ImageNet statistics with mean [0.485, 0.456, 0.406] and standard deviation [0.229, 0.224, 0.225], which facilitates convergence during training process.

3.3 Evaluation Metrics

Let TP, TN, FP, and FN denote true positives, true negatives, false positives, and false negatives. The evaluation metrics used are defined as follows:

$$\text{Accuracy} = \frac{TP + TN}{TP + TN + FP + FN} \tag{1}$$

$$\text{Precision} = \frac{TP}{TP + FP} \tag{2}$$

$$\text{Recall} = \frac{TP}{TP + FN} \tag{3}$$

$$\text{F1-Score} = \frac{2 \cdot \text{Precision} \cdot \text{Recall}}{\text{Precision} + \text{Recall}} \tag{4}$$

$$\text{Specificity} = \frac{TN}{TN + FP} \tag{5}$$

$$\text{MCC} = \frac{TP \cdot TN - FP \cdot FN}{\sqrt{(TP + FP)(TP + FN)(TN + FP)(TN + FN)}} \tag{6}$$

A confusion matrix $C \in \mathbb{R}^{K \times K}$ was also used, where C_{ij} represents the proportion of samples from class i predicted as class j, and K is the number of classes. All metrics were computed on the validation set.

3.4 Experiment Settings

A 5-fold stratified cross-validation [5] scheme was used to evaluate model generalizability. Let $\mathcal{D}_f^{\text{val}}$ denote the validation sets for fold f, and let $\mathcal{M}_f$ be the model trained after fold f. The final performance metrics were obtained by averaging over the 5 validation folds:

$$\text{Metric}_{\text{avg}} = \frac{1}{5} \sum_{f=1}^{5} \text{Metric}(\mathcal{M}_f, \mathcal{D}_f^{\text{val}})$$

For each fold, we utilized the Adam optimizer with an initial learning rate of $1 \times e^{-5}$ and a weight decay of 0.01. To ensure stable convergence, the learning rate schedule included a one-epoch warmup followed by a cosine annealing scheduler, reducing the learning rate to a minimum of $1 \times e^{-6}$. All models were trained on 4 NVIDIA V100 GPUs using a batch size of 256 and FP16 mixed-precision for computational efficiency.

4 Results

4.1 Local Validation

The model's performance was first evaluated on the local validation set using a 5-fold cross-validation methodology. A summary of key performance metrics for each class is provided in Table 1. The results show a wide range of performance across classes. High-performing classes, such as NC, were identified with exceptional reliability, achieving scores above 95% for all metrics. Moderately performing classes like IC and CT scored around 90%, though CT exhibited lower precision (0.86) while IC had a comparatively low recall (0.82). For the remaining classes, while overall accuracy remained high, their recall and F1-scores were significantly lower, a trend particularly pronounced for LI, DM, and PL.

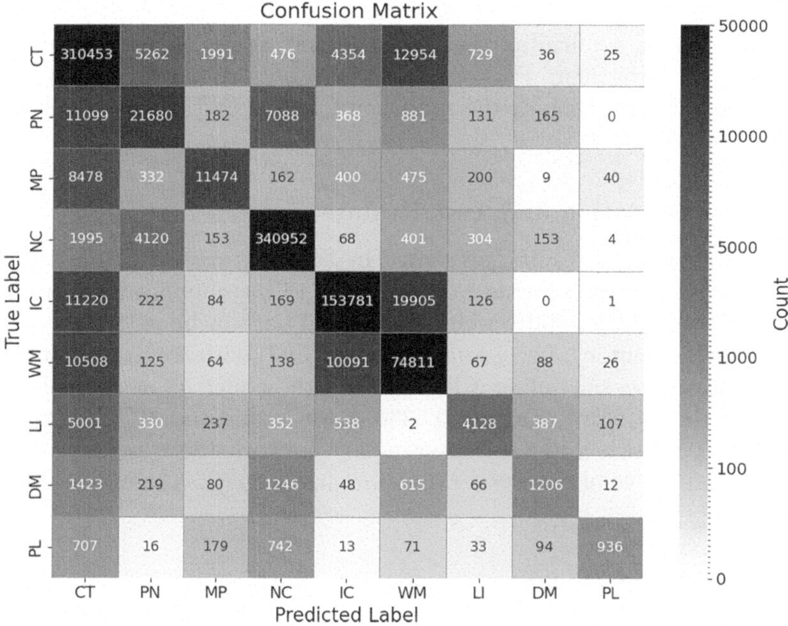

Fig. 5. Aggregated confusion matrix from the 5-fold cross-validation on the local validation set.

Table 1. The class-wise performance on the local validation set. We calculate the micro average of different metrics.

Metric	CT	PN	MP	NC	IC	WM	LI	DM	PL	Average
Accuracy	0.9272	0.9709	0.9875	0.9832	0.9546	0.9462	0.9918	0.9956	0.9980	0.8775
Precision	0.8603	0.6711	0.7944	0.9705	0.9064	0.6794	0.7137	0.5641	0.8132	0.8775
Recall	0.9232	0.5212	0.5319	0.9793	0.8290	0.7799	0.3725	0.2454	0.3354	0.8775
Specificity	0.9291	0.9894	0.9971	0.9852	0.9816	0.9629	0.9984	0.9991	0.9998	0.9847
F1	0.8906	0.5867	0.6372	0.9749	0.8660	0.7262	0.4895	0.3420	0.4749	0.8775
MCC	–	–	–	–	–	–	–	–	–	0.8347

A deeper analysis of these results was conducted using the aggregated confusion matrix from all five folds, visualized in Fig. 5. The matrix reveals that CT, the majority class, is a primary source of confusion. The high concentration of false positives in its column indicates that samples from other classes are frequently misclassified as CT, which directly explains its lower precision. In contrast, NC, despite being the second-largest class, shows highly discriminative performance with minimal confusion.

The most notable trend is the model's difficulty with minority classes. The low recall values for LI, DM, and PL correspond directly to their small sample sizes in the dataset, confirming that the model struggles to learn their features and correctly identify them. Furthermore, the confusion matrix highlights other specific error patterns, such as the tendency for WM and IC to be misclassified as one another.

4.2 Online Validation and Test Resluts

The model's evaluation results, presented in Table 2, reveal a significant performance degradation when moving from the local to the online validation set. The model performed exceptionally well on the local data, achieving uniform scores of 0.8787 across Accuracy, Precision, Recall, and F1, with a corresponding MCC of 0.825. However, on the online validation set, these metrics declined sharply to 0.7677, with the F1-score reaching 0.5330 ± 0.036 and the MCC decreasing to 0.65087 ± 0.006. Such a marked discrepancy between the two validation environments is indicative of poor generalization and suggests a significant degree of overfitting. [6].

Table 2. Online validation and test results.

	Accuracy	Precision	Recall	Specificity	F1	MCC
Validation set	0.76766	0.76766	0.76766	0.97418	0.76766	0.70646
Test set	N/A	N/A	N/A	N/A	0.53301	0.65087

5 Conclusion

In this work, we presented a deep learning approach for the classification of glioblastoma histopathological subtypes by fine-tuning a pre-trained Virchow2 Vision Transformer. Our model demonstrated strong performance on a local validation set, achieving an F1-score of 0.8775 and an MCC of 0.8347, establishing it as a robust baseline for this complex classification task. The analysis revealed high accuracy for well-represented classes like Cellular Tumor (CT) and Necrosis (NC) but highlighted challenges with minority classes, which were often misclassified due to significant data imbalance.

In the BraTS-Pathology 2025 Challenge, our model achieved a second-place finish. It obtained an F1-score of 0.7676 and an MCC of 0.7064 on the Synapse online validation set, which decreased to 0.5330 and 0.6509, respectively, on the final test set. This performance discrepancy suggests that the model overfitted to the validation data, revealing a generalization gap. To address this, our future work will prioritize improving generalization by implementing advanced data augmentation and regularization strategies. Furthermore, we will investigate techniques specifically designed for long-tailed distributions to boost performance on less frequent histological classes.

Acknowledgements. This work was supported by Ningbo Major Science & Technology Project under Grant 2022Z126.

References

1. Bakas, S., et al.: BraTS-path challenge: assessing heterogeneous histopathologic brain tumor sub-regions (2024). https://arxiv.org/abs/2405.10871
2. Darcet, T., Oquab, M., Mairal, J., Bojanowski, P.: Vision transformers need registers (2024). https://arxiv.org/abs/2309.16588
3. Dosovitskiy, A., et al.: An image is worth 16x16 words: transformers for image recognition at scale. CoRR abs/2010.11929 (2020). https://arxiv.org/abs/2010.11929
4. Karargyris, A., et al.: Federated benchmarking of medical artificial intelligence with MedPerf. Nat. Mach. Intell. **5**(7), 799–810 (2023). https://doi.org/10.1038/s42256-023-00652-2
5. Kohavi, R.: A study of cross-validation and bootstrap for accuracy estimation and model selection. In: Proceedings of the 14th International Joint Conference on Artificial Intelligence - Volume 2, IJCAI 1995, pp. 1137–1143. Morgan Kaufmann Publishers Inc., San Francisco, CA, USA (1995)
6. Lin, T.Y., Goyal, P., Girshick, R., He, K., Dollár, P.: Focal loss for dense object detection (2018). https://arxiv.org/abs/1708.02002
7. Neidlinger, P., et al.: A deep learning framework for efficient pathology image analysis (2025). https://arxiv.org/abs/2502.13027
8. Oquab, M., et al.: DINOv2: learning robust visual features without supervision (2024). https://arxiv.org/abs/2304.07193

9. Piana, D., et al.: Phenotyping tumor heterogeneity through proteogenomics: study models and challenges. Int. J. Mol. Sci. **25**(16) (2024). https://doi.org/10.3390/ijms25168830
10. Synapse: Brain tumor pathology dataset (2025). https://www.synapse.org/Synapse:syn64153130/wiki/631458. Accessed 10 July 2024
11. Wang, X., et al.: Transformer-based unsupervised contrastive learning for histopathological image classification. Med. Image Anal. **81**, 102559 (2022). https://doi.org/10.1016/j.media.2022.102559. https://www.sciencedirect.com/science/article/pii/S1361841522002043)
12. Zhang, X., Zhang, W., Cao, W.D., Cheng, G., Zhang, Y.Q.: Glioblastoma multiforme: molecular characterization and current treatment strategy (review). Exp. Ther. Med. **3**(1), 9–14 (2012). https://doi.org/10.3892/etm.2011.367
13. Zimmermann, E., et al.: Virchow2: scaling self-supervised mixed magnification models in pathology (2024). https://arxiv.org/abs/2408.00738

Efficient Classification of Glioblastoma Sub-regions Using MobileNetV2

Ashley Daud, Dimitrios Makris(✉), and Farzana Rahman

Kingston University, London, UK
{K2441726,d.makris,farzana}@kingston.ac.uk

Abstract. Glioblastoma is one of the most aggressive brain tumours, and analysing its histopathology images is essential for accurate diagnosis and prognosis. However, identifying distinct tumour structures in stained tissue sections remains a challenging and time-consuming task for pathologists. In this paper, we present a deep learning approach for multi-class classification of nine distinct tumour sub-regions in H&E-stained histology slides, developed in the context of the BraTS-Path 2025 challenge. We leverage transfer learning with MobileNetV2 as a baseline, then progressively improve it through advanced optimisation techniques. We further validated the model's generalisability using rigorous 5-fold cross-validation. The experimental results demonstrate a substantial improvement over the baseline: the optimised pipeline achieves high overall accuracy (98.54%) and robust class-wise performance (macro-averaged F1-score 95.05%). The optimised model achieves robust and consistent outcomes for each of the 9 tumour classes, as evidenced by per-class receiver operating characteristic curves and confusion matrices.

Keywords: Glioblastoma · Histopathology · Deep Learning · MobileNetV2 · Classification · BraTS-Path 2025

1 Introduction

Glioblastoma is one of the most aggressive brain tumours, and analysing its histopathology images is essential for accurate diagnosis and treatment planning [3]. However, identifying distinct tumour structures in stained tissue sections remains a challenging and time-consuming task for pathologists. Automated deep learning methods offer a promising solution to this problem by providing fast and consistent analysis. BraTS-Path 2025, a recent challenge dataset of glioblastoma pathology images, exemplifies the need for robust algorithms that can classify different tumour sub-regions in whole slide images [2]. The dataset comprises annotated H&E-stained tissue patches from glioblastoma cases, each labelled as one of 9 histological classes or background. These include cellular tumor (CT), pseudopalisading necrosis (PN), microvascular proliferation (MP), geographic necrosis (NC), infiltration into the cortex (IC), white matter (WM),

S. Bakas et al. (Eds.): MICCAI 2025, LNCS 16377, pp. 203–212, 2026.
https://doi.org/10.1007/978-3-032-16370-7_18

leptomeningeal infiltration (LI), dense macrophages (DM), and lymphocytes (PL). These subregions reflect the morphological complexity of glioblastoma and enable fine-grained classification at the patch level. (Fig. 1a).

Yet many state-of-the-art models are complex and computationally intensive, which can be impractical for gigapixel pathology images where each slide may contain thousands of high-resolution patches. Models such as TransUNet and Swin-Unet, which combine convolutional backbones with transformer-based attention mechanisms, have achieved impressive accuracy in histopathology segmentation, but have high computational and memory requirements [5,7]. Earlier approaches in digital pathology used CNNs like ResNet and Inception to classify cancers at patch level, including breast and lung cancer, demonstrating the viability of automated diagnosis [4,6]. More recent efforts have applied U-Net variants for pixel-wise tumour segmentation in whole slide images, achieving accurate delineation of tumour subregions [10]. However, these networks often struggle to scale efficiently for large-scale histopathological workflows. This motivates the need to explore whether more lightweight and computationally efficient architectures can retain high segmentation performance while improving deployment feasibility in real-world clinical settings [8].

We introduce a deep learning approach for multi-class brain tumour pathology image classification using a MobileNetV2 convolutional neural network [12]. MobileNetV2 was chosen for its lightweight architecture and proven feature extraction capabilities, which are advantageous given the large size of pathology images. We leverage transfer learning with MobileNetV2 as a baseline, then progressively improve it through advanced optimisation techniques. Specifically, we froze most of the pre-trained layers initially to establish a baseline performance, and subsequently employed Bayesian hyperparameter optimisation to fine-tune the model and improve its accuracy [13]. We further validated the model's generalisation using rigorous 5-fold cross-validation (Fig. 1b). The following sections detail our methodology, experimental results, discussion of findings, and a conclusion.

2 Method

2.1 Dataset and Preprocessing

We conducted our experiments on the BraTS-Path 2025 histopathology dataset, which contains H&E-stained tissue images of glioblastoma with multi-class labels for different tumour structures. Each image patch is assigned to one of several classes corresponding to distinct tumour histologic features. The dataset was split into training 70%, validation 15%, and test 15% subsets to ensure unbiased evaluation. All images were resized to the input resolution required by MobileNetV2 (224×224 pixels), and pixel values were scaled to a range 0–1.

2.2 Baseline Model Training MobileNetV2

We used a pre-trained MobileNetV2 model for classification [11]. In the baseline configuration, all the convolutional layers of MobileNetV2 were frozen (kept at

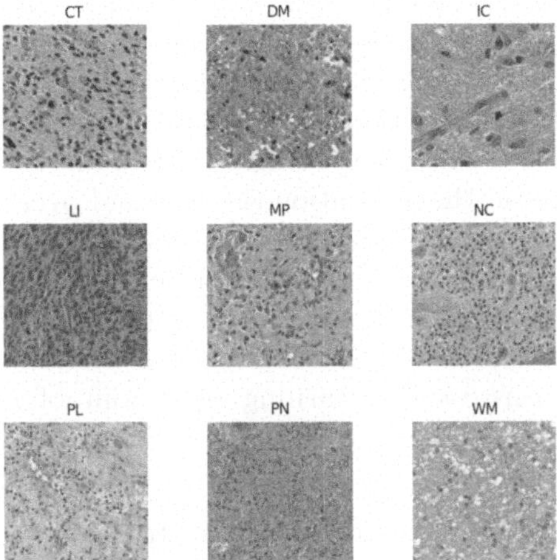

(a) Representative H&E-stained image patches from the BraTS-Path 2025 dataset, showing the nine annotated glioblastoma tumour sub-regions.

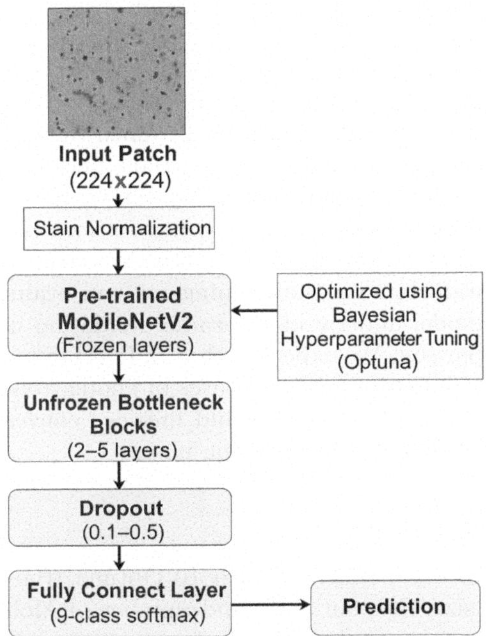

(b) Overview of the MobileNetV2 pipeline for glioblastoma sub-region classification, employing transfer learning, Bayesian optimisation (Optuna), and fine-tuning.

Fig. 1. (a) Example histopathology sub-region patches from the BraTS-Path 2025 dataset. (b) Proposed MobileNetV2 pipeline architecture.

their ImageNet-pretrained weights), and only the final classification layer was replaced and trained on our dataset. This transfer learning approach allows the model to reuse general visual features while learning to distinguish specific tumour patterns. The training of the baseline model used standard hyperparameters without any extensive tuning. We trained the model for a few epochs while monitoring performance on the validation set to avoid overfitting. The baseline model's performance was evaluated on the test set using a comprehensive set of metrics: overall accuracy, class-wise precision and recall, F1-score, specificity for each class, Matthews Correlation Coefficient (MCC), and the Area Under the ROC Curve (AUC). Additionally, we recorded the training and validation loss/accuracy curves to assess the learning behaviour of the models (Fig. 2a, Fig. 2b).

2.3 Hyperparameter Optimisation with Optuna

After establishing the baseline, we sought to improve the model's performance through Bayesian hyperparameter optimisation [13]. We used Optuna, an optimisation framework, to automatically search for the best hyperparameter configuration for our MobileNetV2 model [1]. The optimisation targeted several key hyperparameters simultaneously: the learning rate, batch size, dropout rate in the classifier, and the number of MobileNetV2 layers to unfreeze (for example, how deep into the network fine-tuning should extend). We allowed Optuna to conduct 10 trial experiments, where each trial trained the model with a different combination of these hyperparameters. Each trial's performance was evaluated on the validation set, and the hyperparameter set yielding the highest validation accuracy was selected as the optimal configuration. Using this best-found configuration, we then retrained the model with the chosen layers unfrozen and the optimal hyperparameters on the training set and evaluated it on the test set. This optimised model underwent the same evaluation metrics as the baseline for a direct comparison. We expected that unfreezing more layers would let the model learn more domain-specific features of glioblastoma tissues, and that tuning the learning rate and dropout would improve convergence and prevent overfitting during this more flexible training phase.

2.4 Training Configuration

Bayesian optimisation was performed with 10 Optuna trials, each varying the learning rate, batch size, dropout rate, and number of MobileNetV2 layers to unfreeze. The configuration that achieved the highest validation accuracy was selected for all subsequent experiments. The final hyperparameters were: a learning rate of 1.96×10^{-4}, batch size of 32, dropout rate of 0.12, and 4 unfrozen layers in the MobileNetV2 backbone. These values provided an optimal balance between convergence speed, generalisation, and computational efficiency. The network was trained with the categorical cross-entropy loss function, which is well-suited to multi-class classification. This loss function penalises divergence between predicted probability distributions and the one-hot encoded labels, ensuring the model learns to distinguish effectively across the nine glioblastoma sub-regions. Training and validation loss/accuracy were monitored across epochs to control overfitting and assess convergence behaviour. All histopathology patches were resized to 224 × 224 pixels to match MobileNetV2's input requirements. Pixel intensities were normalised to the [0,1] range by dividing by 255 (min–max scaling). While z-score normalisation is common in natural image pipelines, it was avoided here due to staining variability and background heterogeneity in H&E slides, making standardisation unstable [9]. Min–max scaling was adopted instead, as it preserves stain intensity patterns consistently across the dataset without distorting histological structures.

2.5 K-Fold Cross Validation

To ensure that our results were not dependent on a particular train-test set and to evaluate the model's stability and robustness, 5-fold cross-validation was performed. The entire dataset was re-partitioned into 5 folds, with each fold acting once as the validation set while the remaining 4 served as the training data. All 5 models were trained independently using the best hyperparameters from the Optuna stage. For each fold, metrics were recorded on the validation set: class-wise precision, recall, F1-score, accuracy, macro-average scores, area under the ROC curve (AUC), and Matthews correlation coefficient (MCC). Confusion matrices were also analysed for each fold to identify recurrent misclassification trends. Training and validation accuracy/loss were logged per epoch for all folds to monitor convergence and overfitting.

3 Results

3.1 MobileNetV2 Baseline Model

The MobileNetV2 classifier delivered a weaker performance, reaching a test accuracy of 89.79% and a macro-averaged F1-score of 78.89%. Across the 9 tumour sub-region classes, the model consistently achieved high precision and recall, including in areas typically known to be more difficult. Common classes such as Cellular Tumour and White Matter achieved F1-scores of 0.8958 and 0.8833, respectively, and were see through their Matthews Correlation Coefficients (MCC = 0.86). The model also performed poorly on more subtle or less frequently represented classes. Dense Macrophages and Presence of Lymphocytes, which had lower representation in the dataset, achieved F1-scores of 0.7887 and 0.6415, respectively. This decline in performance was also reflected in their class-wise MCC values, which dropped to 0.7912 and 0.6468, indicating the model's limited ability to generalise to underrepresented tumour subregion.

Microvascular Proliferation and Pseudopalisading Necrosis remained challenging for the baseline model, with F1-scores of only 0.6016 and 0.5378, respectively. Despite being among the more difficult categories, Infiltration into Cortex and Leptomeningeal Infiltration achieved moderately better results, with F1-scores of 0.9120 and 0.8785, and specificity values above 99%. The confusion

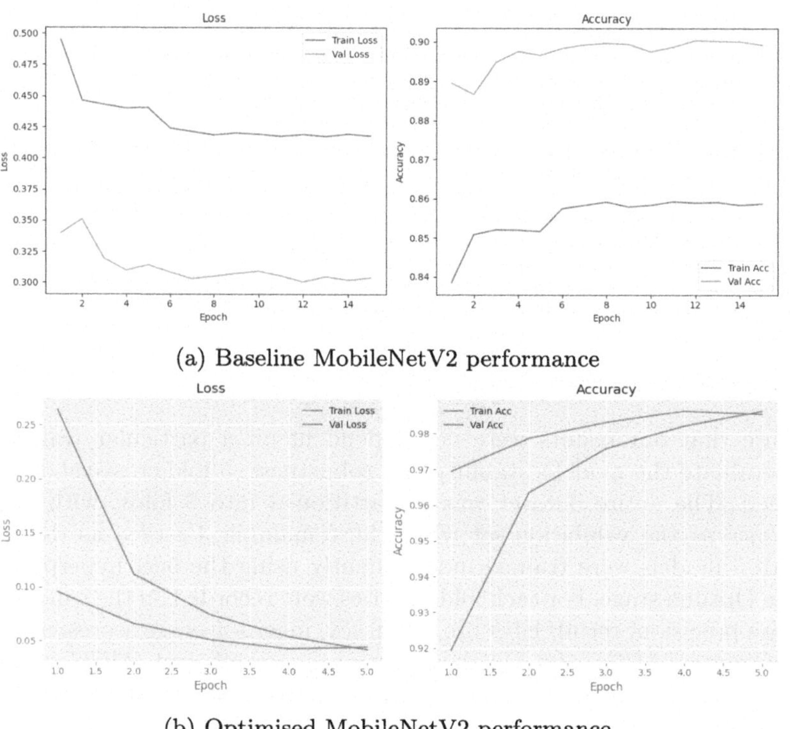

Fig. 2. Training and validation loss and accuracy curves. (a) Baseline MobileNetV2 model. (b) Optimised MobileNetV2 model after Bayesian hyperparameter tuning. The optimised model shows improved convergence and generalisation, with lower loss and higher validation accuracy.

matrix revealed frequent misclassifications, particularly among the CT, NC, and PN classes, which often exhibit similar histological features. This pattern was also reflected in ROC curves, with AUC values varying more widely, though most remained above 0.90. Overall, the baseline model showed reasonable convergence during training but struggled to generalise effectively across all tumour subregions, especially the less represented classes.

3.2 Optimised-Model Optuna

The model was retrained with the optimal hyperparameters from Optuna obtained a macro-averaged F1-score of 95.05% and a validation accuracy of 98.54%. All but one class achieved both precision and recall >87% and even the toughest class (LI) still reached an 82.5% F1 with >99% specificity.Particularly, after optimisation, the recall for DM increased from 0.7226 in the baseline to 0.9835. Improvements in every class were validated by the ROC curve analysis. The model achieved an AUC of 0.9980 for CT and 0.9749 and 0.9910 for MP and PN, respectively, with an AUC for each class exceeding 0.97. The confusion matrix of the optimised model displayed a distinct diagonal trend, with misclassifications decreased by more than 60% when compared to the baseline. The validation accuracy improved gradually over the 5 epochs and stabilised with a narrow generalisation gap, suggesting reduced overfitting due to the use of dropout and fine-tuned layers.

Table 1. Performance comparison of Baseline and optimised MobileNetV2 models.

Metric	Baseline MobileNetV2 (%)	Optimised MobileNetV2 (Optuna) (%)
Test Accuracy	89.79	98.54
Macro Precision	84.92	94.16
Macro Recall	75.08	96.16
Macro F1-Score	78.89	95.05
Global MCC	86.00	98.01

3.3 K-Fold Cross-Validation

The improved model's generalisability was validated by cross-validation. Over the 5 folds, the average test accuracy was 98.72%. The macro-averaged F1-scores for each fold ranged from 96.4% to 96.6%. Minority classes were consistently predicted with high precision, and no fold had a discernible decline in performance. The confusion matrices remained stable across folds, with occasional misclassifications between DM and CT, and between PN and NC—likely due to their morphological similarity. These misclassifications were small and did not recur in the same fold, suggesting random fluctuation rather than a systematic flaw in the model. All classes and folds combined have an average AUC of 0.987. In every fold, MCC values stayed over 0.97. These findings show a great capacity for generalisation and consistent performance across several dataset partitions.

3.4 Bras-PATH Testing Phase Results

When evaluated on the official BraTS-Path 2025 testing dataset, the proposed MobileNetV2 model achieved an overall F1-score of 0.3902 and MCC of 0.5092. Although these results are significantly lower than those obtained during internal validation, they nonetheless demonstrate that the model retains a moderate level of discriminative power across unseen data. This outcome highlights the inherent challenge of generalising histopathological models beyond the curated training distribution, particularly when external slides exhibit variations in staining, resolution, and tissue morphology that differ from the internal dataset.

4 Discussion

In order to minimise the time and variability associated with manual annotation, the goal of this work was to create a model that could automatically identify glioblastoma sub-regions in H&E-stained histology slides. Although these comments are essential for diagnosis and treatment planning, they can be labour-intensive and unreliable in practice. The final model, which was developed using MobileNetV2 and refined using Bayesian optimisation, produced robust and consistent outcomes for each of the 9 tumour classes. The macro-averaged F1-score was 95.05%, while the overall test accuracy was 98.54%. Performance significantly improved in classes where the baseline performed poorly, like Dense Macrophages (DM) and Presence of Lymphocytes (PL), which increased to F1-scores of 0.98 and 0.97, respectively. Despite being one of the hardest to categorise, leptomeningeal infiltration (LI) achieved an F1 of 0.8250 with over 99% specificity, demonstrating that the model could still accurately detect minority traits.

Despite testing using 5-fold cross-validation, external data will be required to assess the model's ability to handle variability in the real world. The model's

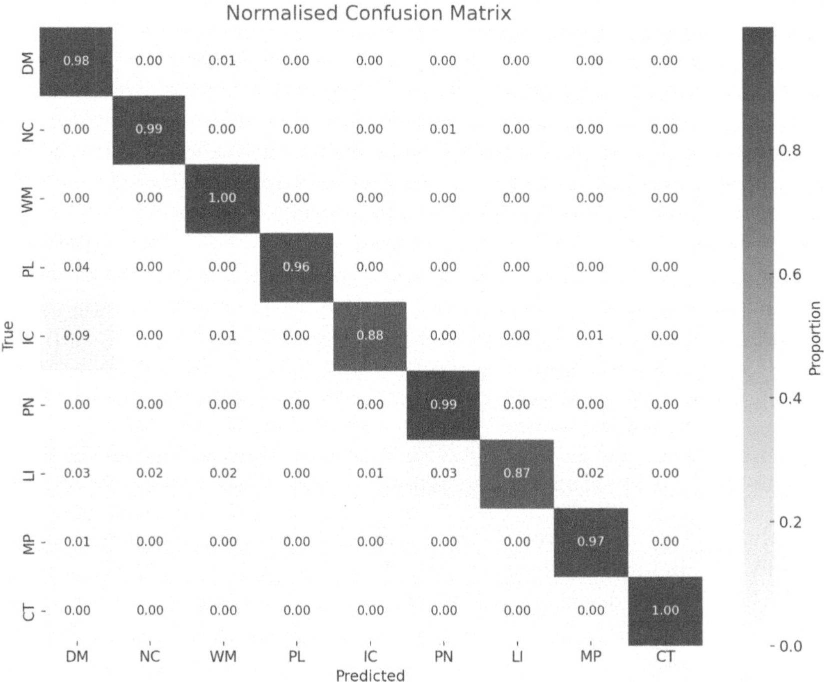

Fig. 3. Confusion matrix of the optimised MobileNetV2 model, illustrating per-class classification accuracy across all glioblastoma sub-regions. The matrix shows strong diagonal dominance, with minimal misclassifications between histologically similar classes (e.g., CT vs. DM and PN vs. NC).

prediction process may also be clarified by looking into technologies like Grad-CAM, which highlights the areas of an image that most affected the model's choice to provide visual explanations. However, if deep learning is improved with the right focus on structure and optimisation, these results offer strong evidence that it can enhance the consistency, speed, and accessibility of histological tumour segmentation for therapeutic use.

The discrepancy between the internal and testing-phase results may be attributed to domain shift—differences in tissue preparation, scanner characteristics, or colour profiles between the challenge dataset and the training images. These factors can significantly influence pixel-level representations, thereby reducing the model's ability to generalise. Furthermore, the model was optimised primarily on internal validation folds, which might have led to slight overfitting to intra-dataset features. Despite this, the consistent internal performance indicates strong learning capacity, suggesting that integrating colour normalisation, data augmentation, or domain adaptation techniques could help bridge this gap in future iterations (Fig. 3 and Table 1).

5 Conclusion

This work developed a lightweight deep learning model based on transfer learning to answer the demand for scalable and accurate classification of glioblastoma sub-regions in histology slides. Without depending on computationally demanding infrastructures, the model achieved high performance across all 9 classes using a MobileNetV2 backbone and Bayesian hyperparameter tuning (Optuna). Its ability to segregate intricate tumour regions using a single, effective network confirms that deploying simplified deep learning techniques to difficult histopathological problems is feasible. Beyond its functionality, the model's usefulness is found in its ease of use. Compared to bigger ensemble models, its speed and compactness make it far more appropriate for inclusion into actual digital pathology operations. This is especially important in clinical or resource-constrained settings when speed, consistency, and reproducibility are just as important as accuracy. This process can help pathologists, standardise analysis, and facilitate larger-scale cancer morphology investigations by decreasing the need for manual annotation.

The results demonstrate a substantial performance gain from these steps – the optimised model achieves a high overall accuracy of 98.5% on the BraTS-Path 2025 dataset and strong precision/recall across all tumour classes. This study shows that even a compact CNN architecture, when properly tuned and validated, can effectively classify complex histopathological images.

Future research should evaluate the model's handling of external datasets with differences in staining, scanner type, or sample quality, even though internal results are encouraging. To help clinical users better understand the model's decision-making process, future research should also look into interpretability tools. However, this study provides a solid foundation by demonstrating that effective models can satisfy the accuracy requirements of contemporary pathology while being deployable and easily scalable with proper optimisation.

Acknowledgements. This work used the BraTS-Path 2025 dataset provided via the Synapse platform. We acknowledge the organisers for data access and challenge resources, and cite the required references as per the data usage policy.

Conflict of Interest. The authors declare that they have no conflict of interest.

References

1. Akiba, T., Sano, S., Yanase, T., Ohta, T., Koyama, M.: Optuna: a next-generation hyperparameter optimization framework. In: Proceedings of the 25th ACM SIGKDD International Conference on Knowledge Discovery and Data Mining, pp. 2623–2631 (2019)
2. Bakas, S., et al.: BraTS-Path challenge: assessing heterogeneous histopathologic brain tumor sub-regions. arXiv preprint arXiv:2405.10871 (2024)
3. Beutel, J., Kundel, H.L., Van Metter, R.L.: Handbook of medical imaging. Society of Photo Optical (2000)
4. Campanella, G., et al.: Clinical-grade computational pathology using weakly supervised deep learning on whole slide images. Nat. Med. **25**(8), 1301–1309 (2019)
5. Chen, J., et al.: Transunet: Transformers make strong encoders for medical image segmentation. arXiv preprint arXiv:2102.04306 (2021)
6. Coudray, N.: Classification and mutation prediction from non-small cell lung cancer histopathology images using deep learning. Nat. Med. **24**(10), 1559–1567 (2018)
7. Hatamizadeh, A., et al.: UNETR: transformers for 3D medical image segmentation. In: Proceedings of the IEEE/CVF winter conference on applications of computer vision, pp. 574–584 (2022)
8. Karargyris, A., et al.: Federated benchmarking of medical artificial intelligence with MedPerf. Nat. Mach. Intell. **5**, 799–810 (2023). https://doi.org/10.1038/s42256-023-00652-2
9. Patil, A., et al.: Fast, self supervised, fully convolutional color normalization of H and E stained images. arXiv preprint arXiv:2011.15000 (2020). https://arxiv.org/abs/2011.15000
10. Ronneberger, O., Fischer, P., Brox, T.: U-Net: Convolutional networks for biomedical image segmentation. In: International Conference on Medical image computing and computer-assisted intervention, pp. 234–241. Springer (2015)
11. Sandler, M., Howard, A., Zhu, M., Zhmoginov, A., Chen, L.C.: Mobilenetv2: Inverted residuals and linear bottlenecks. In: Proceedings of the IEEE conference on computer vision and pattern recognition, pp. 4510–4520 (2018)
12. Sandler, M., Howard, A.G., Zhu, M., Zhmoginov, A., Chen, L.: Inverted residuals and linear bottlenecks: Mobile networks for classification, detection and segmentation. CoRR **abs/1801.04381** (2018). http://arxiv.org/abs/1801.04381
13. Wu, J.: Hyperparameter optimization for machine learning models based on Bayesian optimization. J. Electron. Sci. Technol. **17**(1), 26–40 (2019)

Patch-Level Brain Tumor Sub-region Classification Using Foundation Models Under Long-Tailed Data Distributions

Luis Carlos Rivera Monroy[1,2(✉)], Martin Mayr[2,3], Leonid Mill[1,2], Harald Köstler[3], and Andreas Maier[2,3]

[1] MIRA Vision Microscopy GmbH, Göppingen, Germany
luis.rivera@fau.de
[2] Pattern Recognition Lab, Friedrich-Alexander-Universität Erlangen-Nürnberg, Erlangen, Germany
[3] Erlangen National High Performance Computing Center (NHR@FAU), Friedrich-Alexander-Universität Erlangen-Nürnberg, Erlangen, Germany

Abstract. Accurate patch-level classification of glioblastoma subregions is essential for diagnosis but challenged by tumor heterogeneity and extreme class imbalance. We propose an ensemble framework that uses feature embeddings from four foundation models: UNI, Virchow, Gigapath and Midnight. Each embedding is partitioned into fixed-size chunks to preserve morphological detail and enable localized modeling. Dedicated XGBoost classifiers are trained on each chunk using balanced sample weights to mitigate class imbalance. A shared chunk selection mechanism ensures consistency between training and validation sets and prevents data leakage. Chunk-level predictions are fused via simple averaging into a unified probability vector. To enhance detection of rare subregions we apply rare-class boosting by scaling their predicted probabilities before re-normalization. Per-class decision thresholds are optimized on the validation set to maximize macro-F1 score improving sensitivity to underrepresented patterns. The pipeline achieves a global-averaged F1 score of 0.76 and a Matthews correlation coefficient of 0.70 demonstrating robustness under domain shift and severe label imbalance. Our approach highlights the value of feature chunking ensemble fusion and adaptive post-processing in integrating foundation models for digital pathology. The method provides a reproducible and effective solution for sub-region analysis in glioblastoma histology.

Keywords: Glioblastoma · Foundation models · Feature fusion · Ensemble learning

1 Introduction

Glioblastoma is a highly aggressive and heterogeneous primary brain tumor, and its diagnosis and treatment planning rely on accurate identification of distinct

S. Bakas et al. (Eds.): MICCAI 2025, LNCS 16377, pp. 213–222, 2026.
https://doi.org/10.1007/978-3-032-16370-7_19

histopathological sub-regions. These regions, such as pseudopalisading necrosis, microvascular proliferation, and cellular tumor, carry different biological and clinical implications. However, distinguishing them remains a complex task due to morphological overlap and limited inter-observer agreement among pathologists [9,13,14].

In recent years, artificial intelligence methods have shown promise in supporting sub-region classification by leveraging large annotated datasets of histology images [1,2,5,12]. Foundation models trained on diverse pathology datasets are increasingly used to extract meaningful representations from tissue images. These models offer rich feature embeddings, but their integration into robust classification systems remains an open question [10].

In this work, we explore different strategies to combine feature representations obtained from several foundation models trained on histopathology data. We evaluate how the individual models behave and interact when used together, and we investigate how their combination influences performance in the context of glioblastoma sub-region classification [16,18].

During development, we observed that the use of common data augmentations, such as image rotations, flipping, brightness changes, or added noise, often degraded the quality of the extracted features. These augmentations, while standard in many computer vision tasks, appeared to introduce unwanted variability that negatively affected performance in our setting [4,15].

Our final model combines features from four foundation models that were found to be complementary. We apply a gradient boosting approach based on XGBoost, followed by a classifier that aggregates the predictions from the individual trees. This design balances interpretability, performance, and computational efficiency [6]. At the time of writing, the final model is still under training, but preliminary results on the validation set indicate a global-averaged F1 score of 0.76 and a Matthews correlation coefficient (MCC) of 0.70.

This study highlights the potential of combining pretrained feature spaces for histopathology classification tasks and provides practical insights into the design of ensemble systems for sub-region analysis in glioblastoma [2,5,7].

2 Methods

2.1 Dataset Description

The BraTS-Path 2024 Challenge provides a large-scale, multi-institutional histopathology dataset for patch-level classification of glioblastoma sub-regions [3,7]. Glioblastoma, the most common malignant primary brain tumor in adults, is marked by poor prognosis (median survival: 12–18 months) and pronounced heterogeneity at both molecular and histopathological levels. Capturing this heterogeneity is critical for diagnosis, treatment planning, and outcome prediction.

The dataset consists of hematoxylin and eosin (H&E)-stained, formalin-fixed, paraffin-embedded (FFPE) whole slide images (WSIs) sourced from TCGA-GBM and TCGA-LGG collections in The Cancer Imaging Archive (TCIA). Only IDH-wildtype glioblastomas (WHO Grade 4), as reclassified under the 2021

WHO CNS tumor guidelines, are included. Cases not meeting current molecular criteria were excluded to ensure diagnostic consistency.

Expert neuropathologists annotated nine histologic sub-regions across multiple institutions, following a harmonized protocol:

- Cellular Tumor (CT)
- Pseudopalisading Necrosis (PN)
- Microvascular Proliferation (MP)
- Geographic Necrosis (NC)
- Cortical Infiltration (IC)
- White Matter Penetration (WM)
- Leptomeningeal Infiltration (LI)
- Dense Macrophages (DM)
- Presence of Lymphocytes (PL)

Each WSI was partitioned into 512×512 pixel patches, labeled based on the dominant histologic pattern or marked as background when no structure was discernible. This patch-level granularity supports detailed analysis of intratumoral heterogeneity and inter-class confusion.

The dataset is divided as follows:

- **Training:** 824,663 patches from 192 slides
- **Validation:** 298,533 patches from 18 slides
- **Test:** Over 600,000 patches from 40 slides

While participants may incorporate external data for pretraining or augmentation, all reported results must be based solely on the BraTS-Path 2025 validation dataset to ensure a standardized and fair evaluation.

This dataset offers a realistic benchmark reflecting variability in staining protocols, scanners, and institutional practices, enabling development and assessment of robust deep learning models for histomorphological classification in glioblastoma.

It is important to emphasize that all model development, hyperparameter tuning, and threshold optimization were exclusively performed on the provided labeled training and internal validation sets. The official BraTS-Path blind validation set was never accessed during development and is reserved solely for final evaluation by the challenge organizers.

2.2 Proposed Approach

An overview of the classification pipeline is shown in Fig. 1. The method combines embeddings from four foundation models: **UNI** [11], **Virchow** [17], **Giga-Path** [19], and **Midnight** [8]. Each embedding vector, derived from patch-level representations of whole-slide images, encodes local tissue morphology. Given the heterogeneity in embedding dimensions across models, global pooling is avoided to preserve fine-grained spatial detail. Instead, each embedding is divided into non-overlapping chunks of size 512. Each chunk contains a unique, contiguous

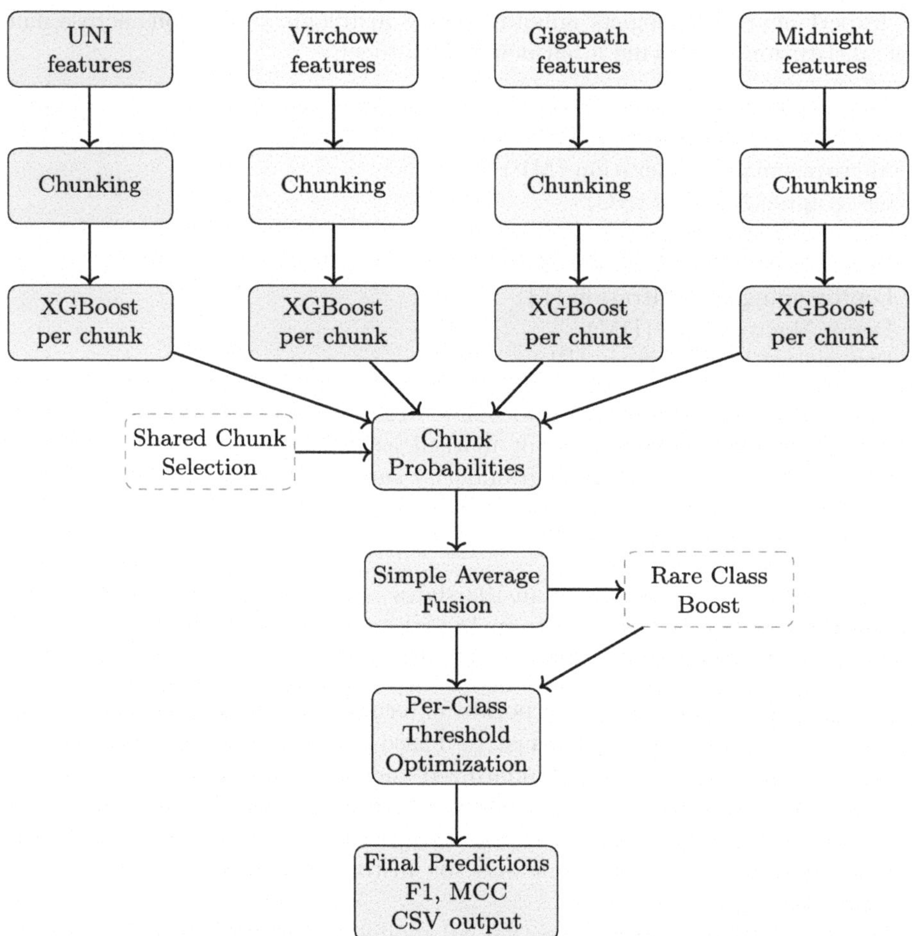

Fig. 1. Overview of the proposed ensemble classification pipeline based on chunked feature processing, simple averaging, and rare-class boosting. The pipeline starts with four distinct sources of precomputed features: UNI, Virchow, Gigapath, and Midnight. Each feature set is partitioned into fixed-size chunks, enabling memory-efficient training of independent XGBoost classifiers. Chunk-level probability vectors generated by these classifiers are filtered, retaining only chunks shared between training and validation datasets to ensure consistency. The retained chunk-level predictions are then averaged into a single class probability estimate. Rare-class boosting uniformly increases probabilities for underrepresented classes to improve detection sensitivity. Per-class decision thresholds optimized on the validation set convert the final probabilities into discrete class predictions. Outputs include predictions, performance metrics (macro-F1, global-F1, and MCC), and CSV files for submission.

segment of the embedding vector, ensuring that no feature dimension is repeated across chunks. If the final segment is shorter than 512, it is zero-padded to reach the required length. This design preserves fine-grained morphological information, facilitates interpretability at the sub-vector level, and guarantees consistency across embeddings of heterogeneous dimensionality.

For each foundation model, we followed the preprocessing protocols recommended by the original authors, which typically include image resizing, normalization, and patch extraction. This ensured compatibility with each model's training distribution; please refer to the respective model descriptions for further details.

Data Splits and Evaluation Protocol. Two labeled subsets are used: a large training set for base model development and a smaller labeled subset, `Validation-Data-384-Collated-JPG`, referred to as the *validation set.* This set supports threshold optimization, performance assessment, and reproducibility checks. The official BraTS-Path validation set, which is unlabeled, is not used during development and is reserved for final submission.

Feature extraction was performed on NVIDIA H100 GPUs in our internal environment, enabling efficient large-scale embedding generation. For the testing phase, where resources were more constrained, we further optimized the extraction pipeline to run fully offline, using the latest PyTorch improvements. These optimizations reduced feature extraction time to under one minute per patch while maintaining consistency with the original model outputs.

Chunk-Level Base Learners. For each feature source $s \in \{\text{UNI}, \text{Virchow}, \text{GigaPath}, \text{Midnight}\}$ and chunk index c, a dedicated **XGBoost** classifier [6] is trained on the c-th chunk of the embedding from s. The output is a class probability vector $\mathbf{p}_{s,c} \in \mathbb{R}^9$, corresponding to the nine diagnostic sub-regions.

To address extreme class imbalance, balanced sample weights are applied:

$$w_i = \frac{N}{K \cdot N_{y_i}}, \tag{1}$$

where N is the total number of samples, $K = 9$, and N_{y_i} is the count of samples in class y_i. This ensures minority classes contribute proportionally during training.

Shared Chunk Selection and Reproducibility. To maintain consistency between training and validation, only chunks for which models were successfully trained in both phases are retained. Let $\mathcal{C}_{\text{train}}$ and $\mathcal{C}_{\text{val}}$ denote the sets of chunk identifiers (s, c), where s indexes the foundation model and c the chunk index, that are available in the training and validation splits, respectively. The shared chunk set is defined as:

$$\mathcal{C}_{\text{shared}} = \mathcal{C}_{\text{train}} \cap \mathcal{C}_{\text{val}}. \tag{2}$$

In practice, this means that only chunks (s, c) for which an XGBoost model could be successfully trained in both training and validation splits are retained. If a given chunk is unavailable in either split (e.g., due to dimensional incompatibility or insufficient samples), it is excluded from $\mathcal{C}_{\text{shared}}$. This ensures that predictions are always based on a consistent set of chunks across training and evaluation, preventing data leakage and improving reproducibility.

Simple Average Fusion with Rare-Class Boosting. Chunk-level probability vectors from the selected models are combined using simple averaging:

$$\mathbf{q}_i = \frac{1}{M} \sum_{m=1}^{M} \mathbf{p}_{m,i}, \tag{3}$$

where $M = |\mathcal{C}_{\text{shared}}|$.

To improve detection of underrepresented classes, a rare-class boosting step is applied. Classes with fewer than 50 training samples are scaled uniformly by a factor $\beta = 2.5$:

$$\mathbf{q}'_i = \mathbf{q}_i \odot \mathbf{r}, \quad \text{where} \quad r_c = \begin{cases} \beta & \text{if } c \in \mathcal{R}, \\ 1 & \text{otherwise}, \end{cases} \tag{4}$$

and $\mathcal{R}$ is the set of rare classes. The result is re-normalized:

$$\mathbf{q}_i^{\text{final}} = \frac{\mathbf{q}'_i}{\|\mathbf{q}'_i\|_1}. \tag{5}$$

The boosting factor was determined empirically: we evaluated values in the range $[0, 5]$ on the internal validation set, and observed that $\beta = 2.5$ consistently provided a modest but stable improvement in macro-F1. Smaller values yielded negligible gains, while larger values often degraded performance by overcompensating probabilities of rare classes.

Advantages and Limitations.

- **Advantages**
  - *Robustness to class imbalance:* Achieved through balanced weighting, rare-class boosting, and threshold optimization.
  - *Preservation of local structure:* Chunking retains fine-grained morphological information that might be lost in global pooling.
  - *Improved generalization:* Shared chunk filtering and adaptive post-processing enhance stability under domain shift.
- **Limitations**
  - *Computational cost:* Training multiple chunk-specific models increases memory and time requirements.
  - *Chunking sensitivity:* Performance may vary with chunk size and alignment relative to discriminative features.
  - *Fixed fusion weights:* Simple averaging assumes equal reliability across models and chunks, without learned weighting.

To support transparency and reproducibility, the complete feature extraction and training pipeline has been implemented in a modular framework. The code and configuration files will be released upon publication of this manuscript at: https://github.com/luiscarm9/BRATS_2025_Pathology_LME, enabling other researchers to reproduce our experiments and extend the methodology to related histopathology tasks.

3 Results and Discussion

3.1 Results

We evaluated a wide range of modeling strategies for patch-level classification of glioblastoma sub-regions using precomputed embeddings from foundation models. A consistent finding across all experiments was the detrimental effect of data augmentations. We tested multiple augmentation techniques including rotation, flipping, JPEG compression, brightness adjustments, stain normalization, and Gaussian noise. In every case, models trained on augmented features underperformed compared to those using the original embeddings. On average, the global F1 score decreased by approximately 10% points. As a result, all subsequent experiments were conducted using non-augmented features only.

We explored several modeling approaches:

- MLP classifiers applied to individual or concatenated feature vectors
- Trainable projection of features into a shared latent space with learned fusion weights
- Classical machine learning methods such as k-nearest neighbors and per-source XGBoost models
- Linear combination layers for fusing model outputs
- The proposed ensemble method based on chunked XGBoost classifiers and probability fusion

Approaches involving MLPs or encoder-based projections exhibited strong overfitting. Performance on frequent classes improved rapidly during training, while predictions for rare classes deteriorated significantly after the first epoch. This behavior was especially pronounced under extreme class imbalance. Additionally, domain shift between training and validation splits led to poor generalization in many configurations.

The highest-performing non-ensemble model projected Virchow and UNI features into a shared latent space with learned combination weights. On the external BraTS-Path validation set, this approach achieved a global F1 score of 0.79 and an MCC of 0.73. However, when evaluated on the small internal labeled validation set (used for threshold optimization and macro-F1 computation), its macro-F1 score dropped to 0.51, reflecting poor sensitivity to rare sub-regions.

In contrast, the proposed ensemble framework achieved a global F1 score of 0.76 and an MCC of 0.70 on the external validation set. While slightly lower than the best non-ensemble submission in terms of global metrics, it demonstrated significantly more balanced class-wise performance and greater robustness to distribution shifts. On the internal validation set, it reached a macro-F1 score above 0.61, the highest among all configurations tested, highlighting its superior sensitivity to rare and underrepresented sub-regions. This configuration was therefore selected as our final method, after which the complete internal labeled set was used for training to maximize data utilization before submission. A summary of the comparative performance across configurations is presented in Fig. 2.

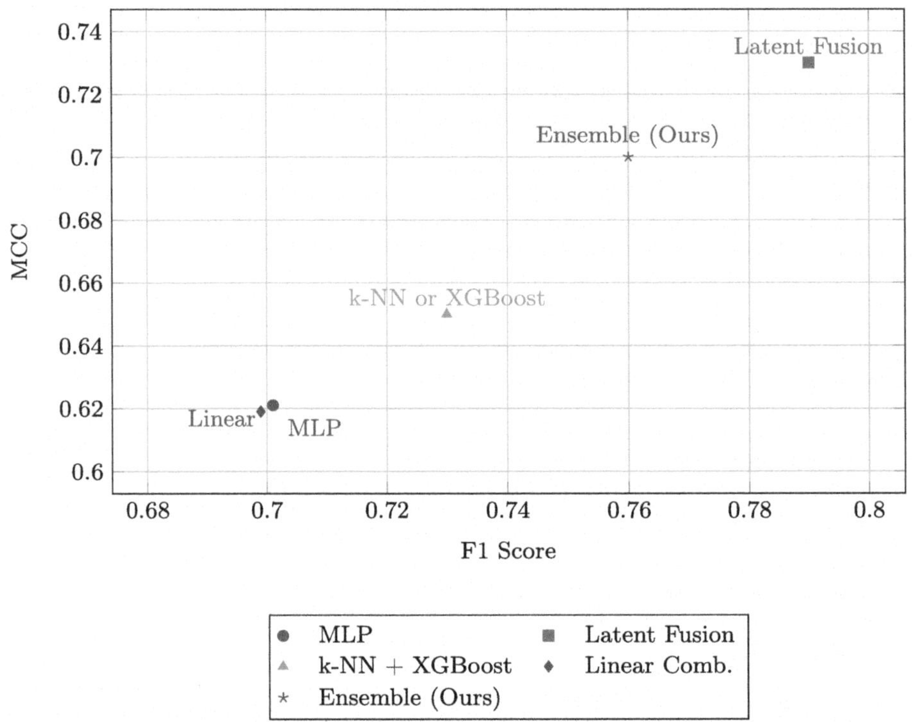

Fig. 2. Performance comparison of model variants. Scatter plot of F1 Score versus Matthews Correlation Coefficient (MCC) for five model configurations evaluated on the BraTS-Path validation set. Each point is labeled and color-coded for clarity.

The final results of our approach on the blind validation phase yielded an F1-score of 0.5934 ± 0.0299 and a Matthews Correlation Coefficient (MCC) of 0.6447 ± 0.0299. This phase was carried out entirely offline by the challenge organizers on a private, unreleased dataset comprising over one million regions. Participants had no access to this dataset, ensuring an unbiased and standardized evaluation across all submitted methods.

3.2 Discussion

The results highlight the challenges inherent in histopathological classification under extreme label imbalance and domain variability. The consistent degradation caused by data augmentations suggests that foundation model embeddings are sensitive to perturbations that may disrupt their learned semantic structure. This contrasts with typical end-to-end deep learning pipelines, where augmentation usually improves generalization.

The overfitting observed in MLP-based and projection-based models underscores the risk of high-capacity architectures in imbalanced settings. Optimization driven by micro-averaged metrics can produce misleadingly high scores while failing to detect clinically critical but rare patterns. The latent space model, despite achieving the highest global F1, performed worse than random guessing on several minority classes, revealing a critical flaw in its generalization capability.

Our ensemble approach prioritizes stability, fairness, and reproducibility. By partitioning embeddings into chunks and training dedicated XGBoost models, we preserve fine-grained morphological information. The shared chunk selection mechanism ensures consistency between training and validation and prevents data leakage. The use of rare-class boosting and per-class threshold optimization directly addresses the long-tailed nature of the label distribution, enhancing sensitivity to underrepresented but diagnostically significant sub-regions.

Although the ensemble model achieves a slightly lower global F1 than the best alternative, its balanced performance and robustness to domain shift make it a more reliable choice for real-world deployment. The design aligns with clinical requirements where missing a rare but aggressive feature can have serious consequences. For these reasons, we selected the ensemble method for final submission, confident in its ability to generalize to unseen data in the BraTS-Path 2025 Challenge.

Acknowledgments. The authors gratefully acknowledge the scientific support and HPC resources provided by the Erlangen National High Performance Computing Center (NHR@FAU) of the Friedrich-Alexander-Universität Erlangen-Nürnberg (FAU). The hardware is funded by the German Research Foundation (DFG).

References

1. Abdel-Nabi, H., et al.: A comprehensive review of the deep learning-based tumor analysis approaches in histopathological images: segmentation, classification and multi-learning tasks. Clust. Comput. **26**(5), 3145–3185 (2023)
2. Aboian, M., et al.: Miccai 2025 lighthouse challenge: brain tumor segmentation cluster of challenges (brats) (2025). https://doi.org/10.5281/ZENODO.13981215, https://zenodo.org/doi/10.5281/zenodo.13981215
3. Bakas, S., et al.: Brats-path challenge: assessing heterogeneous histopathologic brain tumor sub-regions (2024). https://doi.org/10.48550/ARXIV.2405.10871, https://arxiv.org/abs/2405.10871

4. Buslaev, A., Iglovikov, V.I., Khvedchenya, E., Parinov, A., Druzhinin, M., Kalinin, A.A.: Albumentations: fast and flexible image augmentations. Information **11**(2), 125 (2020)
5. Campanella, G., et al.: Clinical-grade computational pathology using weakly supervised deep learning on whole slide images. Nat. Med. **25**(8), 1301–1309 (2019). https://doi.org/10.1038/s41591-019-0508-1, http://dx.doi.org/10.1038/s41591-019-0508-1
6. Chen, T., Guestrin, C.: Xgboost: A scalable tree boosting system. In: Proceedings of the 22nd ACM SIGKDD International Conference on Knowledge Discovery and Data Mining, KDD 2016, pp. 785–794. ACM, August 2016.https://doi.org/10.1145/2939672.2939785, http://dx.doi.org/10.1145/2939672.2939785
7. Karargyris, A., et al.: Federated benchmarking of medical artificial intelligence with medperf. Nature Machine Intelligence **5**(7), 799–810 (2023). https://doi.org/10.1038/s42256-023-00652-2, http://dx.doi.org/10.1038/s42256-023-00652-2
8. Karasikov, M., et al.: Training state-of-the-art pathology foundation models with orders of magnitude less data. arXiv preprint arXiv:2504.05186 (2025), https://arxiv.org/abs/2504.05186
9. Louis, D.N., et al.: The 2021 who classification of tumors of the central nervous system: a summary. Neuro Oncol. **23**(8), 1231–1251 (2021)
10. McGenity, C., et al.: Artificial intelligence in digital pathology: a systematic review and meta-analysis of diagnostic test accuracy. npj Digit. Med. **7**(1) (2024). https://doi.org/10.1038/s41746-024-01106-8, http://dx.doi.org/10.1038/s41746-024-01106-8
11. Moor, M., et al.: Foundation models for generalist medical artificial intelligence. Nature **616**(7956), 259–265 (2023)
12. Morales, S., Engan, K., Naranjo, V.: Artificial intelligence in computational pathology – challenges and future directions. Digit. Sig. Process. **119**, 103196 (2021). https://doi.org/10.1016/j.dsp.2021.103196, http://dx.doi.org/10.1016/j.dsp.2021.103196
13. Network, T.C.G.A.R.: Comprehensive, integrative genomic analysis of diffuse lower-grade gliomas. New England J. Med. **372**(26), 2481–2498 (2015). https://doi.org/10.1056/nejmoa1402121, http://dx.doi.org/10.1056/NEJMoa1402121
14. Price, M., et al.: Cbtrus statistical report: primary brain and other central nervous system tumors diagnosed in the united states in 2017–2021. Neuro-Oncol. **26**(Supplement_6), vi1–vi85 (2024). https://doi.org/10.1093/neuonc/noae145, http://dx.doi.org/10.1093/neuonc/noae145
15. Shorten, C., Khoshgoftaar, T.M.: A survey on image data augmentation for deep learning. J. Big Data **6**(1) (2019). https://doi.org/10.1186/s40537-019-0197-0, http://dx.doi.org/10.1186/s40537-019-0197-0
16. Supriyadi, M.R., et al.: A systematic literature review: exploring the challenges of ensemble model for medical imaging. BMC Med. Imaging **25**(1) (2025). https://doi.org/10.1186/s12880-025-01667-4, http://dx.doi.org/10.1186/s12880-025-01667-4
17. Vorontsov, E., et al.: A foundation model for clinical-grade computational pathology and rare cancers detection. Nat. Med. **30**(10), 2924–2935 (2024)
18. Xiong, C., Chen, H., Sung, J.J.Y.: A survey of pathology foundation model: progress and future directions (2025). https://doi.org/10.48550/ARXIV.2504.04045, https://arxiv.org/abs/2504.04045
19. Xu, H., et al.: A whole-slide foundation model for digital pathology from real-world data. Nature **630**(8015), 181–188 (2024)

GAMMA-Net: Gated Attention Multi-scale Modular Architecture

Madhav Arora[1], Aniket Negi[1], Ayush Thakur[1], Syed Rameem Zahra[2], and Ankur Gupta[1(✉)]

[1] Netaji Subhas University of Technology, New Delhi 110078, India
agupta4@cs.iitr.ac.in

[2] Centre for Artificial Intelligence and Machine Learning, SKUAST-K, Srinagar, J&K 190025, India
syed.zahra@skuastkashmir.ac.in

Abstract. The accurate histological classification of diffuse gliomas is challenging due to tumor heterogeneity and severe class imbalance in medical datasets. This paper presents our methodology for the pathology task of the BraTS-Lighthouse 2025 Challenge, which introduces a novel hybrid ensemble approach combining deep learning with classical machine learning. We found extreme class imbalance and used a two-stage data balancing strategy: using StyleGAN2-ADA for image augmentation, followed by random oversampling of the minority classes in the feature space. We then extracted a rich 4096-dimensional feature vector, by concatenating feature embeddings extracted independently from two pre-trained Vision Transformer based foundation models, UNI2-h and Virchow-2. Our classification system consists of two arms: a deep learning arm featuring a Gated Attention Multi-Layer Perceptron (GA-MLP) which contains stacked attention blocks, and a classical arm comprising an ensemble of K-Nearest Neighbors, a calibrated Random Forest, and an XGBoost classifier. The GA-MLP is trained using a composite loss function, comprising of Focal Loss and F1 Loss. The final predictions are generated by a weighted soft-voting mechanism between the two arms. This strategy utilizes the distinct inherent strengths of each arm to improve diagnostic performance and consistency for glioblastoma multiforme, with the overarching objective of enhancing patient outcomes.

Keywords: Ensemble Learning · Histopathology · Glioblastoma Multiforme · Vision Transformer · Gated Attention · Generative Adversarial Networks

1 Introduction

Glioblastoma multiforme (GBM) is the most malignant and aggressive subtype of glioma and is the most common primary brain tumor in adults. It remains an

M. Arora and A. Negi—These authors contributed equally.

S. Bakas et al. (Eds.): MICCAI 2025, LNCS 16377, pp. 223–233, 2026.
https://doi.org/10.1007/978-3-032-16370-7_20

incurable disease with a median survival of 15 months, even with treatment [9]. Treatment has been challenging due to its highly infiltrative nature, genetic diversity, and the protective role of the blood-brain barrier (BBB) [13].

In response to these clinical exigencies, the Brain Tumor Segmentation Challenge (BraTS) has established itself as the leading benchmarking initiative over the past decade. The BraTS-Lighthouse 2025 Challenge builds upon this foundation by introducing novel tasks designed to address pressing, unresolved clinical questions. Among these, Task 10, *Assessing the Heterogeneous Histologic Landscape of Glioma*, shifts the focus from radiographic imaging to the underlying cellular architecture of the tumor.

This initiative tasks the research community with the development of sophisticated computational models capable of performing automated analysis and classification of complex microscopic glioma environment within histopathological slides. This focus on the histological landscape is intended to bridge the explanatory gap between macroscopic radiophenotypes and microscopic determinants of tumorigenesis and therapeutic resistance. The successful development of such quantitative histopathology tools has the potential for a more precise prognostication and the formulation of personalized therapeutic regimens, thus offering a pathway to improved clinical outcomes for patients affected by this aggressive malignancy.

2 Dataset Specification

This study utilizes publicly available H&E-stained FFPE digitized tissue sections from the TCGA-GBM and TCGA-LGG datasets within The Cancer Imaging Archive [2]. This comprises a retrospective, multi-institutional collection of patients with newly diagnosed diffuse gliomas. The provided tissue samples have been updated to align with the latest WHO criteria, focusing on GBMs, and include annotations from specialized neuropathologists who have meticulously identified and segmented distinct histological regions into smaller units or patches. These patches are then categorized according to specific histological traits into nine regions of interest, which are shown in Fig. 1.

3 Methods

3.1 Data Augmentation and Sampling

The dataset revealed a significant imbalance in the class distribution, with the PL class having the fewest images at 1,998, contrasting with the NC class, which had the most, with 259,329 images total. As a result, data augmentation became necessary to counteract this imbalance and avoid the model from becoming biased towards the over-represented classes. To achieve this, we used StyleGAN2-ADA[1] [10], which is known to deliver outstanding results even when the number of images is limited.

[1] https://github.com/dvschultz/stylegan2-ada-pytorch.

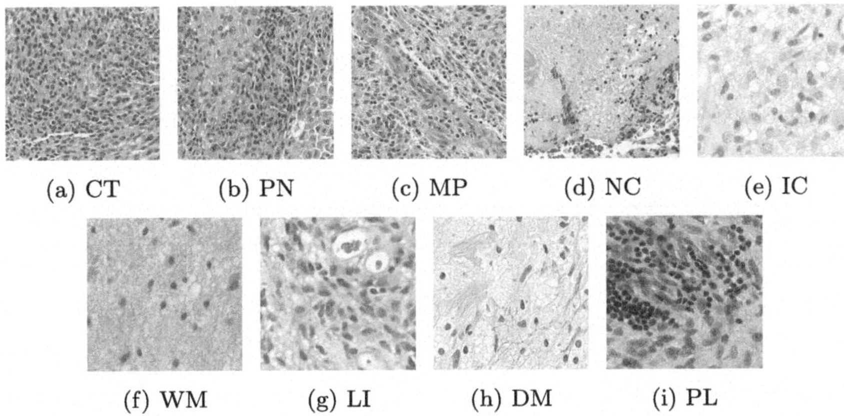

Fig. 1. Regions of interest included in the study: (a) (CT) presence of cellular tumor, (b) (PN) pseudopalisading necrosis, (c) (MP) areas abundant in microvascular proliferation, (d) (NC) geographic necrosis, (e) (IC) infiltration into the cortex, (f) (WM) penetration into white matter, (g) (LI) leptomeningial infiltration, (h) (DM) regions with dense macrophages, and (i) (PL) presence of lymphocytes.

Table 1. Class-wise image count before and after augmentation.

Class	Best FID	Ticks	Original	Generated	Sub-sampled	Total Count
CT	–	–	250,370	0	0	250,370
PN	13.144	770	38,821	200,000	77,642	116,463
MP	19.97	260	21,349	200,000	42,698	64,047
NC	–	–	259,329	0	0	259,329
IC	12.92	670	126,773	125,000	0	126,773
WM	8.5	650	56,067	200,000	56,067	112,134
LI	19.20	310	6,419	200,000	12,838	19,257
DM	11.30	930	4,359	200,000	8,718	13,077
PL	15.55	370	1,998	200,000	3,996	5,994
Total	–	–	765,485	1,325,000	201,959	967,444

Table 1 provides a detailed breakdown of the image counts for each class, both prior to and following augmentation. This score is listed alongside the training checkpoint at which it was achieved, measured in ticks, where each tick represents the processing of 4,000 images.

In addition to the counts, the table quantitatively summarizes the performance of the generator by presenting the optimal Fréchet Inception Distance (FID) [8] of the generated images vis-à-vis the real images for each of the augmented class, formally defined in Eq.(1).

$$\mathrm{FID}(\mathcal{X}_r, \mathcal{X}_g) = \|\mu_r - \mu_g\|_2^2 + \mathrm{Tr}\left(\Sigma_r + \Sigma_g - 2\left(\Sigma_r \Sigma_g\right)^{1/2}\right) \tag{1}$$

To enhance the generalization performance of the model, the training dataset was enriched with synthetic examples. Subsequently, to counteract the risk of the model learning spurious features from the generative process (i.e., GAN artifacts), we implemented an undersampling technique on the synthetic data subset. The specifics of this synthesis-constrained data augmentation strategy are formally described in Algorithm 1.

Algorithm 1: SYNCAA: SYNthetic Capacity-Aware Augmentation

Input: Number of real samples $N_{\text{real}} \in \mathbb{N}$
Total synthetic pool size $N_{\text{synth}} \in \mathbb{N}_0$
Synthetic sample set $\mathcal{S}_{\text{all}} = \{s_1, s_2, \ldots, s_{N_{\text{synth}}}\}$
Real sample set $\mathcal{R} = \{r_1, r_2, \ldots, r_{N_{\text{real}}}\}$
Output: Augmented dataset $\mathcal{D}_{\text{aug}}$

```
1  Function GenerateAugmentedDataset(N_real, N_synth, S_all, R):
2      if N_real < 5 × 10^4 then
3          N_synth^max ← min(N_synth, 2 · N_real);
4      else
5          if 5 × 10^4 ≤ N_real < 10^5 then
6              N_synth^max ← min(N_synth, N_real);
7          else
8              N_synth^max ← 0;
9      S_aug ~ U(S_all, N_synth^max) ;   /* uniform sample w/o replacement */
10     D_aug ← R ∪ S_aug ;               /* form final dataset */
11     return D_aug;
```

Hence, in each training iteration, the SYNCAA algorithm ensured that only a subset of the synthetic data was incorporated, based on the real data availability for each class. As shown in Table 1, this resulted in a carefully subsampled synthetic set per class, balancing the dataset without overexposing the model to generated content. The final dataset used for training thus comprised both real and selectively curated synthetic examples, promoting diversity while mitigating the risk of overfitting to GAN-induced artifacts.

3.2 Feature Extraction

The feature extraction protocol commenced with a standardized preprocessing pipeline to prepare the image patches for model input. Each patch was first resized to 256×256 pixels and subsequently center-cropped to 224×224 pixels. These processed patches served as input to two state-of-the-art Vision Transformer (ViT) [7] based foundation models, **UNI2-h** [4] and **Virchow-2** [14].

Embeddings were independently derived from each model and then concatenated, fusing their complementary feature representations into a single, composite 4096-dimensional feature vector, as shown in Eq.(2). This procedure was systematically applied to all image patches, and the resulting set of high-dimensional feature descriptors was persisted for subsequent downstream classification analyses.

$$\left.\begin{array}{l} \mathbf{f}_{\text{Uni}} \in \mathbb{R}^{d_1}, \quad \mathbf{f}_{\text{Virchow}} \in \mathbb{R}^{d_2} \\ \mathbf{f}_{\text{concat}} = \begin{bmatrix} \mathbf{f}_{\text{Uni}} \\ \mathbf{f}_{\text{Virchow}} \end{bmatrix} \in \mathbb{R}^{d_1+d_2} \end{array}\right\} \quad \text{where } d_1 = 1536 \text{ and } d_2 = 2560 \tag{2}$$

3.3 Gated Attention Multi-scale Modular Architecture (GAMMA-Net)

The proposed framework is a hybrid architecture that leverages both deep neural attention mechanisms and classical ensemble learning to robustly perform classification on high-dimensional feature representations. As illustrated in Fig. 2, the model is composed of two parallel inference pathways: a deep learning-based Gated Attention Multi-Layer Perceptron (GA-MLP) and a classical soft-voting ensemble arm.

The GA-MLP is specifically engineered to emphasize salient features through gated attention mechanisms, thereby improving discriminative capacity in imbalanced data scenarios. In parallel, the classical ensemble integrates complementary decision boundaries from traditional models to enhance generalization. This dual-path strategy culminates in a final weighted soft-voting ensemble that fuses predictions from both arms to yield a generalized probabilistic output.

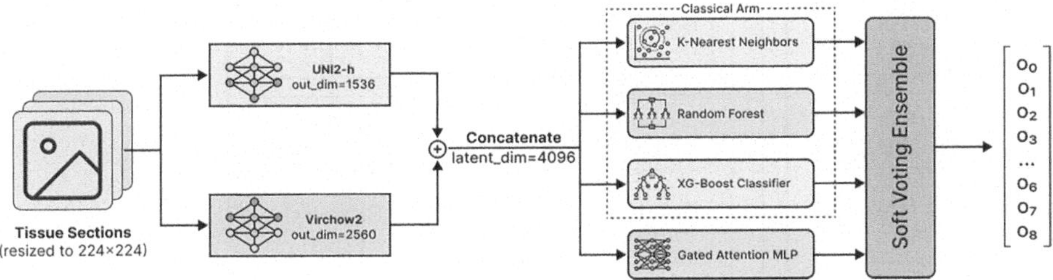

Fig. 2. Architectural representation of GAMMA-Net.

Gated Attention Multi-layer Perceptron (GA-MLP). To effectively identify salient patterns within the high-dimensional feature space, a Multi-Layer Perceptron was designed to integrate a dedicated attention mechanism for enhanced feature learning prior to classification. The initial component is a feature extractor composed of two cascaded residual block modules. Each block is engineered to mitigate the vanishing gradient problem by creating two parallel pathways: a main transformation path, $F(x)$, and a skip connection, $H(x)$.

The skip connection uses a linear projection to align tensor dimensions or an identity mapping if dimensions are unchanged. The outputs are combined through element-wise addition, allowing the network to learn modifications to an identity function. The output y of a block for an input x is formally defined in Eq. (3).

$$y = ReLU(F(x) + H(x)) \tag{3}$$

This process transforms the initial 4096-dimensional input vector into an abstract 256-dimensional feature space. The resulting 256-dimensional feature vector, which we'll denote as z, is then passed to a separate attention head. This head consists of a compact two-layer MLP with a final Sigmoid activation, which generates a data-dependent attention mask, M_{att}. This mask re-calibrates the features through element-wise multiplication, effectively amplifying salient features. The re-weighted feature vector, z_{att}, is computed as shown in Eq. (4).

$$\begin{aligned} M_{\text{att}} &= \sigma\left(W_2 \cdot \text{ReLU}\left(W_1 z + b_1\right) + b_2\right) \\ z_{\text{att}} &= z \odot M_{\text{att}} \end{aligned} \tag{4}$$

The architecture of GA-MLP is shown in Fig. 3.

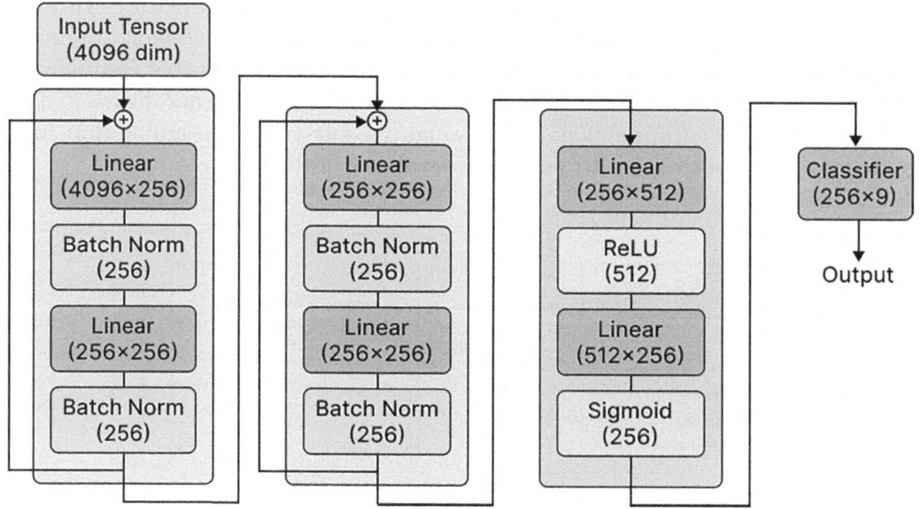

Fig. 3. Architecture of GA-MLP.

Composite Attention Loss. To effectively optimize the training of the Gated Attention MLP, we introduce a tailored objective function termed the **Composite Attention Loss**. This criterion is specifically designed to address challenges arising from severe class imbalance and to enhance sensitivity to minority classes. It achieves this by integrating two complementary components: Focal Loss ($\mathcal{L}_{\text{FL}}$) and Soft F1 Loss ($\mathcal{L}_{\text{F1}}$).

The combined objective is expressed as a weighted sum of the two loss terms, as defined in Eq. (5).

$$\mathcal{L}_{\text{total}} = \alpha \cdot \mathcal{L}_{\text{FL}} + \beta \cdot \mathcal{L}_{\text{F1}} \tag{5}$$

where the weighting coefficients $\alpha = 0.7$ and $\beta = 0.3$ regulate the influence of each loss component on the overall training dynamics.

The constituent loss functions are formally defined in Eq. (6):

$$\mathcal{L}_{\mathrm{FL}} = -\sum_{i=1}^{N} \nu \cdot (1 - \hat{y}_i)^{\delta} \cdot y_i \log(\hat{y}_i)$$
$$\mathcal{L}_{\mathrm{F1}} = 1 - \frac{2\sum_{i=1}^{N} y_i \hat{y}_i}{\sum_{i=1}^{N} y_i + \sum_{i=1}^{N} \hat{y}_i} \tag{6}$$

Here, $y_i \in \{0, 1\}$ denotes the ground truth label, while $\hat{y}_i \in [0, 1]$ represents the predicted probability for sample i. The Focal Loss term includes the modulation factor $(1 - \hat{y}_i)^{\delta}$, which adaptively down-weights well-classified examples, thereby focusing learning on harder cases. The scalar ν serves as a normalization constant to stabilize training. The Soft F1 Loss directly optimizes for the F1 score by penalizing imbalances between precision and recall.

Classical Arm. To further support the Gated Attention Multi-Layer Perceptron, we employed a soft-voting ensemble of classical machine learning models. It consisted of probabilities from K-Nearest Neighbors [6] (P_{KNN_i}), a calibrated Random Forest [3] (P_{RF_i}), and an XGBoost classifier [5] (P_{XGB_i}) for each image (i). This ensemble was trained on the same 4096-dimensional feature vectors. The probabilistic outputs of these models were then combined for each image using a soft vote according to Eq. (7).

$$P_{\mathrm{classical}_i} = \frac{1}{3}(P_{RF_i} + P_{KNN_i} + P_{XGB_i}) \tag{7}$$

Final Ensemble Voting. The resulting probability distribution is representative of the decision made with equal participation of the three classical models. It is then integrated with the output of the Gated MLP in a weighted soft vote. This creates a hybrid prediction for each fold, balancing the predictive strengths of both deep learning and classical approaches, as shown in Eq. (8).

$$P_{\mathrm{ensemble}_i} = w_{\mathrm{mlp}} \cdot P_{MLP_i} + (1 - w_{\mathrm{mlp}}) \cdot P_{\mathrm{classical}_i} \tag{8}$$

Finally, a single robust prediction for each sample is produced by averaging the ensemble probabilities of all N_f folds, as described in Eq. (9). The class with the highest averaged probability is selected as the final output.

$$P_{\mathrm{final}} = \frac{1}{N_f} \sum_{i=1}^{N_f} P_{\mathrm{ensemble}_i} \tag{9}$$

4 Results

4.1 Experimental Setup

The framework was trained and tested with Python 3.12 using PyTorch version 2.6 on an Ubuntu 24.04 LTS Server having 1024 GB of shared system memory, an AMD EPYC 7742 64-Core Processor, and a single NVIDIA A100-SXM4-40 GB GPU having 40 GB of VRAM. The model was trained using K-Fold Cross Validation over 5 folds. The classical models were taken from the CuML library with CUDA support to reduce the training time, and fully utilize the GPU. The GA-MLP was optimized with the AdamW [11] optimizer, for 100 epochs at most to reach a favorable overall performance. This was complemented by Early Stopping [12] regularization based on the progression of validation loss across ten successive epochs. The learning rate was initialized as 10^{-4} and fixed during the training phase with a batch size of 64. The weights for the GA-MLP (w_{mlp}) were found using the hyperparameter searching tool, optuna [1] over 50 trials.

4.2 Cross-Validation Performance

The proposed hybrid ensemble was first evaluated using 5-fold cross-validation on the training data. The results, summarized in Table 2, indicate a high level of consistency and accuracy across all folds.

The validation loss values for the MLP component remained tightly grouped, ranging from 0.1427 to 0.1473, with an average of 0.1450 and a standard deviation of 0.0020. This suggests stable learning and minimal overfitting across different splits of the dataset. The Hybrid F1-Macro score exhibited similarly strong performance, with values consistently above 0.993, yielding an average of 0.9950 and a standard deviation of 0.0012. The Hybrid Matthews Correlation Coefficient (MCC) also remained close to perfect, with an average of 0.9970 and a standard deviation of 0.0007, underscoring the reliability of the ensemble in capturing balanced predictions, even in the presence of potential class imbalance (Fig. 4).

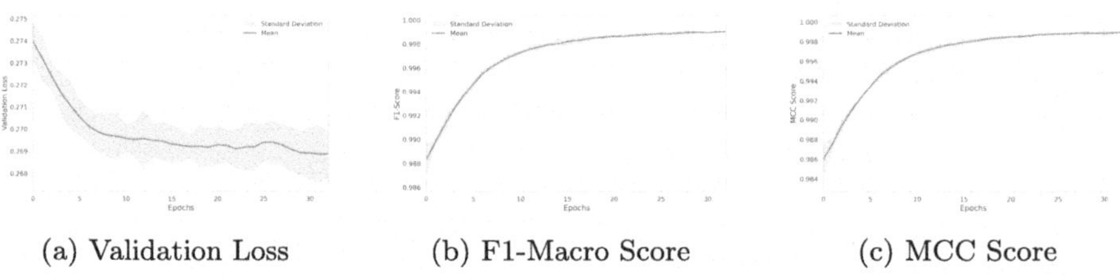

(a) Validation Loss (b) F1-Macro Score (c) MCC Score

Fig. 4. Training Progress as visualized by the validation loss, F1 and MCC scores during 5-fold cross validation.

4.3 Blind Validation Results

To further evaluate generalization performance, the ensemble model was tested on the official blind validation set. On this unseen dataset, the model achieved a global F1-score of 0.79 and a Matthews Correlation Coefficient (MCC) of 0.735. These results confirm that the model retains strong predictive capabilities

Table 2. 5-Fold Cross-Validation performance of the hybrid ensemble on the training data.

Fold	Validation Loss (MLP)	Hybrid F1-Macro	Hybrid MCC
1	0.1465	0.9957	0.9972
2	0.1427	0.9954	0.9974
3	0.1432	0.9964	0.9979
4	0.1453	0.9937	0.9965
5	0.1473	0.9938	0.9961
Average	**0.1450 ± 0.0020**	**0.9950 ± 0.0012**	**0.9970 ± 0.0007**

under realistic conditions and generalizes well beyond the training distribution. Despite the natural performance drop compared to cross-validation, the ensemble demonstrates competitive effectiveness when applied to unseen data.

4.4 Testing Results

The final testing results for the challenge are mentioned in Table 3.

Table 3. Final Test Results

	MCC Score	F1 Score
mean	0.592	0.489
std	0.0055	0.0205

5 Discussion

In this work, we proposed a hybrid classification framework that unifies a deep Gated Attention Multi-Layer Perceptron (GA-MLP) with a classical ensemble of tree-based and instance-based learners. The primary motivation behind this dual-armed architecture was to capitalize on the complementary strengths of deep learning and traditional machine learning: while GA-MLP leverages attention mechanisms to isolate salient patterns in high-dimensional embeddings, the classical ensemble adds interpretability and robustness, especially in low-data regimes.

Despite achieving near-perfect cross-validation performance, our method exhibited a significant drop on the blind test set, suggesting a domain shift between training and evaluation distributions. We hypothesize that heavy reliance on StyleGAN2-ADA for synthetic minority class augmentation, although necessary for class balancing, may have induced dataset-specific overfitting.

Although our SYNCAA algorithm aimed to mitigate GAN-induced artifacts through sub-sampling and capacity-aware constraints, some residual distributional artifacts may have persisted.

To further counter class imbalance, we introduced a composite loss function for the GA-MLP, combining Focal Loss and Soft F1 Loss. This improved minority class sensitivity during training, though the domain shift likely limited its effectiveness at generalization time. Interestingly, omitting Soft MCC Loss–despite its popularity in imbalanced learning–proved beneficial, suggesting that more nuanced domain adaptation strategies may be needed.

Nevertheless, the hybrid approach remains promising. Several future directions emerge from our findings. First, replacing the fixed soft-voting scheme with a learnable stacking-based meta-learner could enable more adaptive integration of deep and classical arms. Second, treating the soft-voting weight (w_{mlp}) as a tunable hyperparameter, optimized via nested cross-validation or Bayesian optimization, may improve predictive calibration. Lastly, future augmentation pipelines could explore embedding-space perturbation techniques instead of generative sampling, preserving semantic structure while avoiding domain drift.

Overall, our work highlights the challenges of generalization under domain shift in biomedical image classification, and demonstrates the potential of ensemble learning as a viable strategy for high-dimensional and imbalanced datasets.

Acknowledgments. The authors would like to express their sincere gratitude to the **Centre of Excellence (CoE) in Artificial Intelligence (AI)**, Netaji Subhas University of Technology (NSUT), New Delhi, for their invaluable support throughout the course of this research. Data used in this publication were obtained as part of the challenge project through **Synapse ID (syn64153130)**.

Disclosure of Interests. *The authors declare that they have no competing financial or non-financial interests that could have appeared to influence the work reported in this article.* All analyses were conducted independently of any commercial or personal affiliations, and no funding sources had any role in the design, execution, or interpretation of the findings. The models and methods described in this work were developed solely for academic research purposes, and none of the authors hold patents, stock ownership, or other financial ties related to the technologies discussed herein.

References

1. Akiba, T., Sano, S., Yanase, T., Ohta, T., Koyama, M.: Optuna: a next-generation hyperparameter optimization framework. In: Proceedings of the 25th ACM SIGKDD International Conference on Knowledge Discovery & Data Mining, pp. 2623–2631 (2019)
2. Bakas, S., et al.: Brats-path challenge: assessing heterogeneous histopathologic brain tumor sub-regions (2024)
3. Breiman, L.: Random forests. Mach. Learn. **45**(1), 5–32 (2001)
4. Chen, R.J., et al.: Towards a general-purpose foundation model for computational pathology. Nature Med. (2024)

5. Chen, T., Guestrin, C.: Xgboost: a scalable tree boosting system. In: Proceedings of the 22nd ACM SIGKDD International Conference on Knowledge Discovery and Data Mining, KDD 2016, pp. 785–794. ACM, New York, NY, USA (2016). https://doi.org/10.1145/2939672.2939785, https://doi.org/10.1145/2939672.2939785
6. Cover, T., Hart, P.: Nearest neighbor pattern classification. IEEE Trans. Inf. Theory **13**(1), 21–27 (1967). https://doi.org/10.1109/TIT.1967.1053964
7. Dosovitskiy, A., et al.: An image is worth 16x16 words: transformers for image recognition at scale (2021). https://arxiv.org/abs/2010.11929
8. Heusel, M., Ramsauer, H., Unterthiner, T., Nessler, B., Hochreiter, S.: Gans trained by a two time-scale update rule converge to a local nash equilibrium. In: Advances in Neural Information Processing Systems, vol. 30 (2017)
9. Kanderi, T., Munakomi, S., Gupta, V.: Glioblastoma multiforme. StatPearls [Internet], StatPearls Publishing, Treasure Island (FL), updated 2024 may 6 edn. (2025), Accessed via NCBI Bookshelf
10. Karras, T., Aittala, M., Hellsten, J., Laine, S., Lehtinen, J., Aila, T.: Training generative adversarial networks with limited data. In: Proceedings of NeurIPS (2020)
11. Loshchilov, I., Hutter, F.: Decoupled weight decay regularization (2019). https://arxiv.org/abs/1711.05101
12. Prechelt, L.: Early stopping-but when? In: Neural Networks: Tricks of the Trade, pp. 55–69. Springer (2002)
13. Wu, W., et al.: Glioblastoma multiforme (gbm): an overview of current therapies and mechanisms of resistance. Pharmacol. Res. **171**, 105780 (2021)
14. Zimmermann, E., et al.: Virchow2: scaling self-supervised mixed magnification models in pathology. arXiv preprint arXiv:2408.00738 (2024)

Challenge 11 – BraTS-PRO

A Siamese Vision Transfer Architecture for Prediction of Brain Tumour Responses during Therapy

Xiaohong W. Gao[1](✉), Chia-Hui Chien[1], Guan-Lin Liu[1], and Jyh-Cheng Chen[2]

[1] Department of Computer Science, Middlesex University, Hendon, London NW4 4BT, UK
x.gao@mdx.ac.uk

[2] Department of Biomedical Imaging and Radiological Sciences, National Yang Ming Chiao Tung University, Taipei, Taiwan

Abstract. This paper presents the results of prediction of therapeutic responses for patients who undergo chemo or radio therapy for the treatment of brain tumour. This work is in response to Task 11 of 2025 BraTS Brain Tumor Progression Challenge organized in conjunction with MICCAI 2025 (https://conferences.miccai.org/2025/en/). In this competition, a Siamese Vision Transformer (SViT) is applied, which allows the inferences between baseline state, i.e. after tumour resection or initial treatment and later tumour development. The backbone model is CMT-Ti. Inspired by the work of MuSiC_ViT for x-ray chest disease detection, this SViT system accomplishes four classification of therapeutic responses, which are Complete Response (CR), Partial Response (PR), Stable Disease (SD) and Progressive Disease (PD). Overall, based on the available training dataset with 91 patients, 90% accuracy can be achieved. For the test dataset, the model SViT has achieved top 2 performance for Task 11.

Keywords: Siamese Neural network · Vision Transformers · BraTS challenges · Brain Tumour Therapy

1 Introduction

1.1 A Subsection Sample

This 2025 BraTS Challenge is the continuation of previous competitions [1–4] and has attracted significant numbers of participants. Technically, the Task-11 of the Challenge in essence is a classification problem to identify the status of response after a patient has undergone a therapy. The challenge here is that this response is related to the baseline tumour status, i.e. after initial tumour resection or therapy. Hence, a Siamese comvolutional neural network (CNN) appears to be appropriate, which is designed to compare the similarity between two inputs. Within this architecture, shared weights are used, implying the same neural network processes both inputs in parallel, learning comparable representations. In addition, a Vision Transformer (ViT) refers to a deep learning architecture that adapts the transformer model, originally designed for natural language

S. Bakas et al. (Eds.): MICCAI 2025, LNCS 16377, pp. 237–245, 2026.
https://doi.org/10.1007/978-3-032-16370-7_21

processing, to image data. Instead of using convolutional layers like CNNs, ViTs treat images as sequences of patches, enabling them to capture long-range dependencies and global context more effectively. When CNN meets ViT (CMT-Tiny), a lightweight network is created to take advantage of both CNN and ViT, transforming into a compact, efficient model for image classification and related tasks [5].

2 Methodology

2.1 Deep Learning Network

Inspired by the work by Cho et al. [6], a Siamese Vision Transformer (SViT) network is employ for this task as presented with CMT-Ti as backbone model in Fig. 1, the SViT architecture is illustrated and embeds two networks that share the same weights. The loss functions are calculated based on three metrics, attention mechanism that is applied to ViT networks, visual similarity between baseline and follow-ups and anatomic region similarity check disease status.

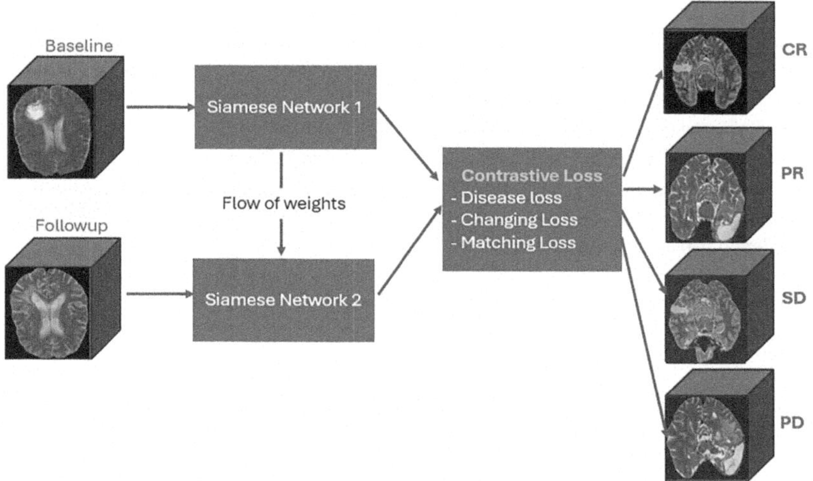

Fig. 1. The architecture of Siamese Vision Transformer (SViT) applied in this study.

In Fig. 1, the SviT network processes a pair of baseline and follow-up images. The forward model employs the architecture of CMTs [5] as an encoder. Dissimilar to a CNN-based model, a vision transformer (ViT) model uses a large reception field [7] thanks to the application of an attention mechanism. While a ViT is mainly trained for capturing global image features, multi-scale features can be obtained via CMT [5] to ensure low-resolution features are captured, which is particularly important for medical images where sub-changes are crucial for accurate diagnosis. Towards this end, CMT ustilises depth-wise convolution and multi-head self-attention to efficiently capture local and global structure information through the integration of CNN and ViT.

Similar to the work conducted in [6], Fig. 1 performs a multi-task learning. One task is to classify a pair of baseline and follow-up 2D images into are no-response/complete-response (CR), no-response/partial-response (PR), normal/stable-disease (SD) and normal/progressive-disease (PD). Another is to compare anatomic region similarities. Two cross-entropy loss functions are calculated to distinguish normal and response classes (i.e., CR, PR, SD and PD labels) from baseline ($\boldsymbol{y_b}$) and follow-up ($\boldsymbol{fu}$) MR brain images.

The overall loss is formulated in Eq. (1) with three loss functions to assess response/no-response classes for each patient, by which the performance is enhanced when factors λ_1, λ_2, and λ_3 were set to 1, 0.1, and 0.01 respectively empirically.

$$\mathcal{L}_{total} = \lambda_1 \mathcal{L}_{response} + \lambda_2 \mathcal{L}_{disease} + \lambda_3 \mathcal{L}_{matching} \quad (1)$$

In Eq. (1), the $\mathcal{L}_{response}$ is calculated in Eq. (2).

$$\mathcal{L}_{response} = CE\Big(y_{response}, S\Big(W_3 f(x_b) \bigoplus f(x_{fu})\Big)\Big) \quad (2)$$

$$\mathcal{L}_{disease} = CE(y_b, S(W_1 f(x_b)) + CE(\Big(y_{fu}, S\big(W_2 f(x_{fu})\big)\Big) \quad (3)$$

In Eqs. (2) and (3), $y_{response}$ indicates the label for the response/no-response classes of image pairs, and $\oplus$ denotes vector-wise concatenation. The weights of W_1, W_2, and W_3 denote fully connected layers.
Where $S(.)$ is the softmax function and is computed using Eq. (4).

$$S(x_i) = \frac{e^{x_i}}{\sum_{k=1}^{K} e^{x_k}}, for\ i = 1, \ldots, K. \quad (4)$$

K refers to the number of data samples.

The cross-entropy (CE) loss function is used to determine the four classes of an MR image pair and is computed as Eq. (5).

$$CE(y, f(x)) = \sum_i y_i \log f(x_i) \quad (5)$$

Similar to the work by Cho et al. [5], the matching loss function denotes to the anatomy-matching module (AMM) that matches the associated features maps from two brain images as presented in Fig. 2. The AMM comprises a feature extraction part (FEP) and a channel recalibration part (CRP). The loss function is calculated in Eq. (6).

$$\mathcal{L}_{matching} = 2 - 2\frac{1}{n}\sum_{i=1}^{n}(K_i \bullet Q_i)/K_i Q_i \quad (6)$$

Where K_i and Qi are the features generated in ViT as key and query focusing on the similar regions through similarity modeling of the K and Q created by the FEP in the two paired images, representing cosine similarity formula. In Eq. (5), n is 4 as shown in Fig. 2 below.

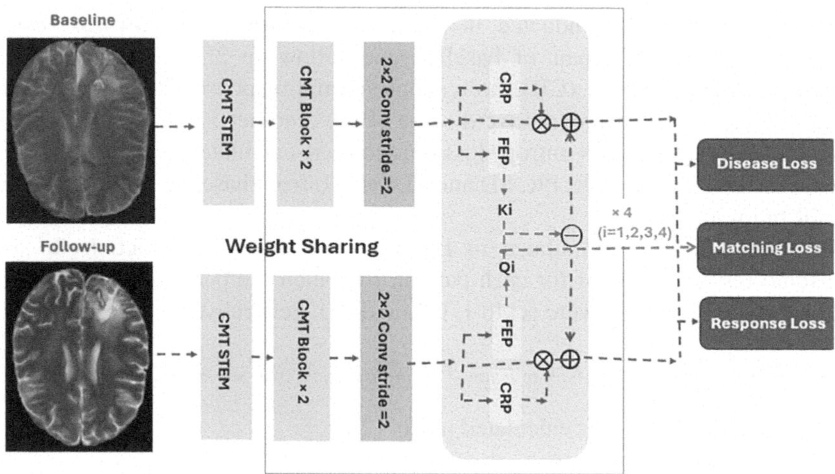

Fig. 2. The workflow of calculation of loss functions for SviT network.

2.2 Datasets

Data are collected from the BraTS 2025 Challenge [1] and are in 3D form of MR images. Due to the variations of volume sizes, e.g. many images have one direction containing only 24 slices, the training and testing take place based on 2D frames. In this study, only registered MR dataset is employed. At each z direction, 3 frames are selected containing the top 3 largest lesions, calculated according to the segmentation masks. For testing with segmentation information, this is estimated based on the gray level intension. Figure 3 demonstrates a sample data set for a patient from 3 direction views, Axial (top), Coronal(middle) and Sagittal (bottom), where the circled 3 frames in each direction are applied for training. If the width or height is less than 100 pixels (1 pixel = 500 μm), then this frame is discarded.

Figure 4 demonstrates the selection of top 3 frames in each direction to be applied for training. For z direction, if the frame numbers are less than 100, the top 3 will be the first 3 frames with the largest sum of pixel values. If the frame numbers are larger than 100, the 3 consecutive frames will bear little differences. Hence the incremental of selection will be the whole number of (Z + 100)/100. For example, if Z = 512, then the incremental will be 6, i.e. the top 3 will be the slices top 1, 7, and 13. In Fig. 3, the segmentation marks are super-imposed with red referring to 'Tumor' and orange 'other lesions (e.g. swelling)' as provided by the dataset.

Figure 5 illustrates the paired samples for training with baseline (SViT Network 1in Fig. 1) and follow-up images (SViT Network 2 in Fig. 1).

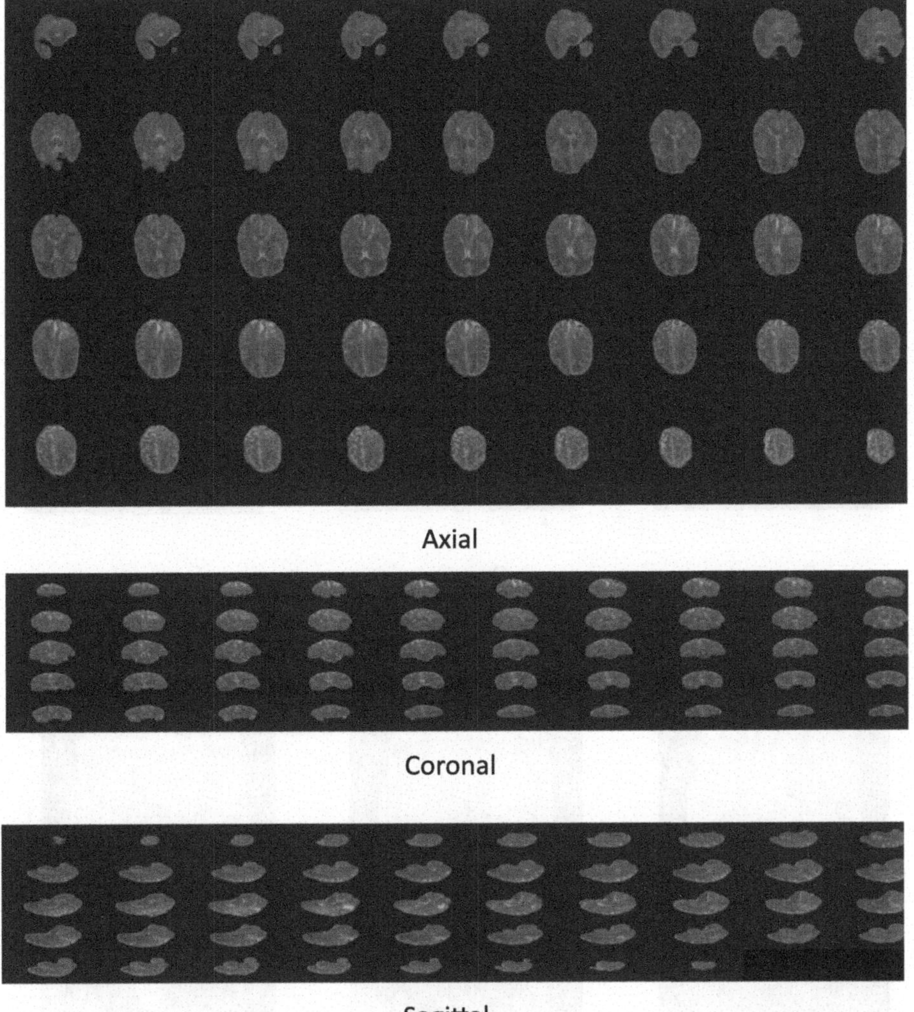

Fig. 3. Three directional view of a 3D T2 MR image. Top: Axial; Middles: Coronal; bottom: Sagittal.

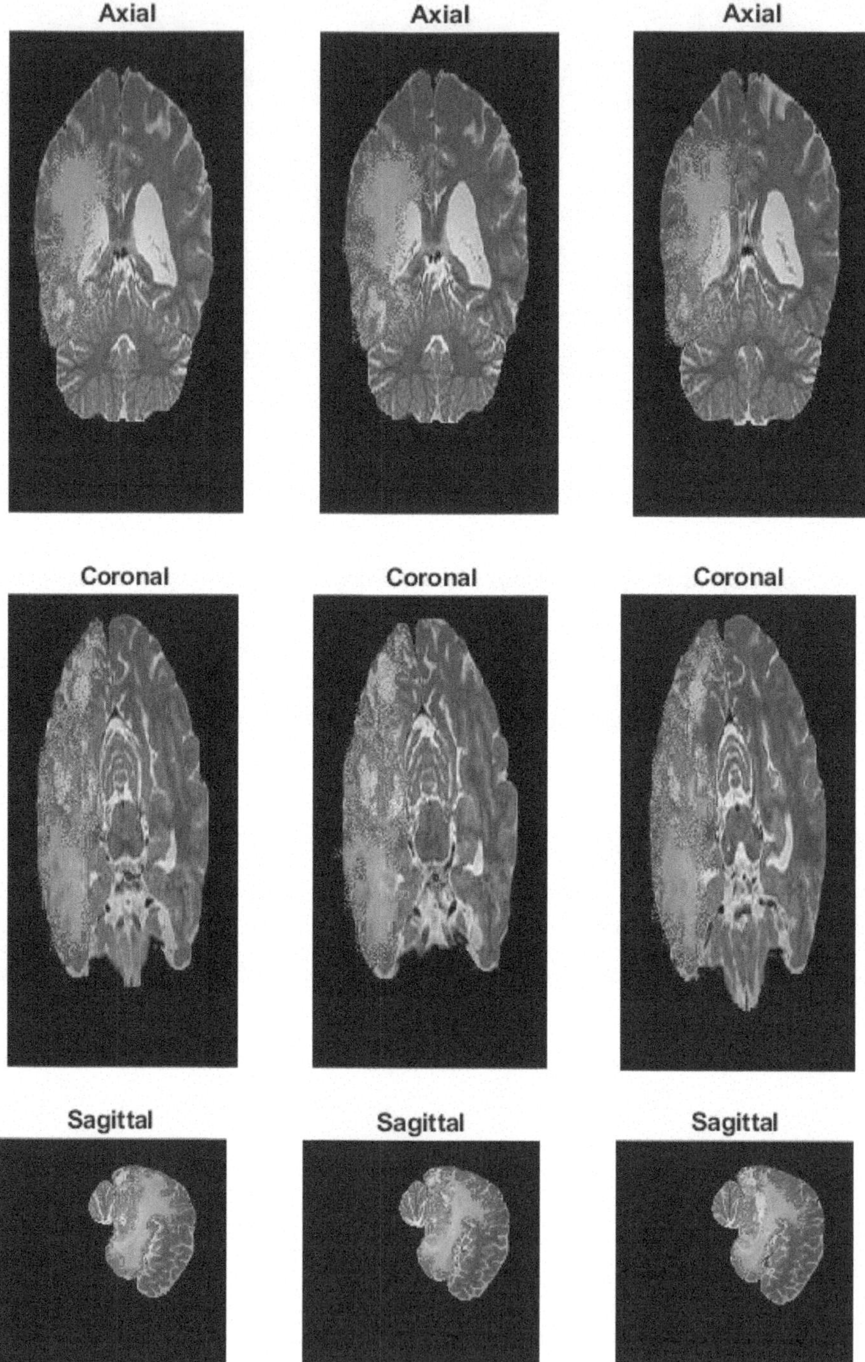

Fig. 4. The selected frames for training and testing from the patient data shown in Fig. 2. The red colour refers to tumour whereas orange the other lesions.

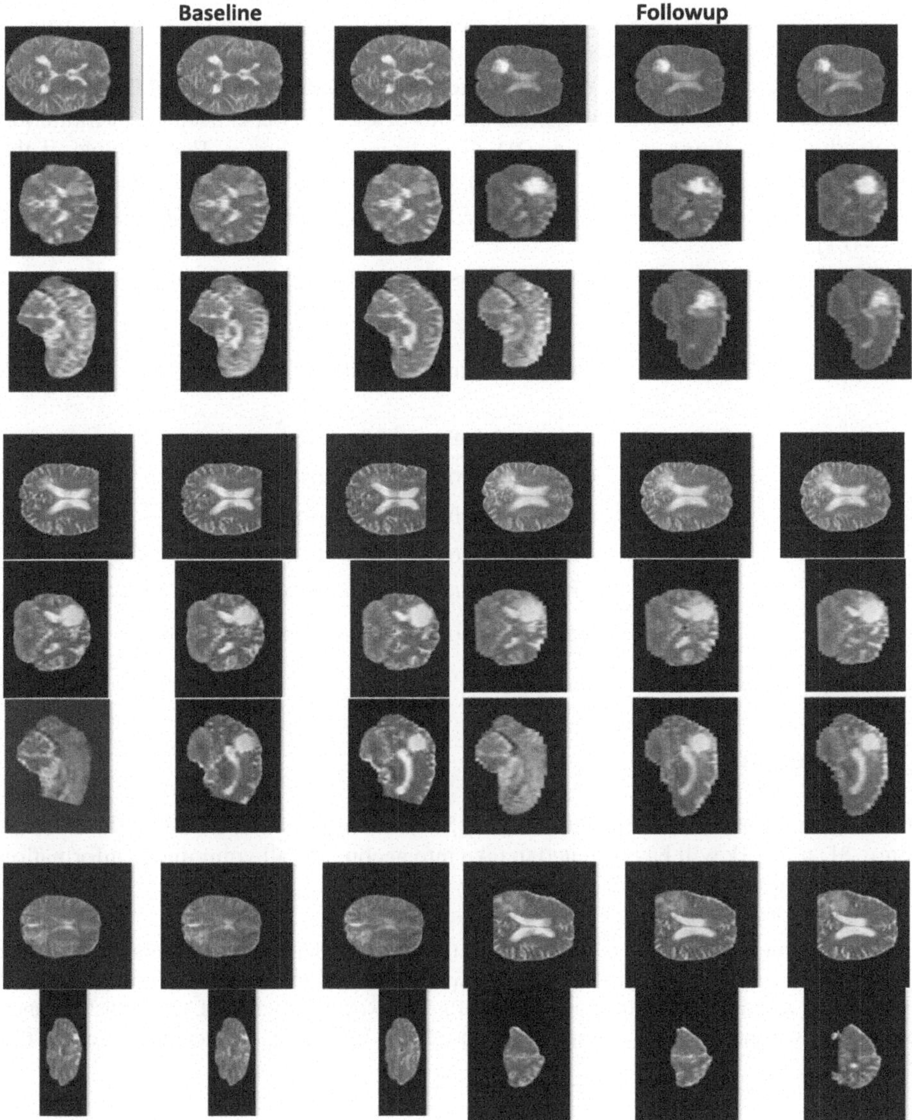

Fig. 5. The illustration of paired sample data for training and testing. The left column is the baseline that applies the Siamese Network 1 in Fig. 1. The right column shows the followup images trained employing the Siamese Network 2 in Fig. 1.

3 Results

From the available datasets from 91 patients, 1432 frames are selected to train the SViT network with a ratio of 80:20 for training and validation. The initial results based on 2D slices appear to be promising with 90% accuracy. The final results are calculated based on all the frames for each subject. For example, if the prediction results of 9 slices are

[2, 3] for 4 classes of [CR, PR, SD, PD] respectively, then the prediction for this patient is PD with the highest probability of [0.22, 0.22, 0.22, 0.33].

If the probabilities of top 2 or more share the same values, a factor of 0.1 is applied to allow the higher weight goes to more serious diseases. This is because of limitation of selections of training and testing 2D slices from 3D volumes. For example, if the probability of 4 classes are [0.3, 0.1, 0.3, 0.3], then the final probability would be [0.3, 0.1, 0.2, 0.4], with the last one (PD) gains 0.1 (+0.1) whereas the neighboring one loses 0.1 (−0.1).

Table 1 provides the final test results based on the test dataset, which ranked **top 2** for this Task 11.

Table 1. The final test results.

	F1	BA	AP
CR	0	0.5	0.0079
PR	0	0.5	0.1847
SD	0.0754	0.4898	0.2663
PD	0.6725	0.4999	0.5123
Mean	0.1870	0.4974	0.2428

4 Conclusion

Due to the limit number of 3D datasets, this SViT network is trained using 2D slices. In future, 3D network will be evaluated to take into account of all voluminous information that a 3D dataset contains.

Acknowledgement. The authors would like to thank the BraTS 2025 organizers for providing not only the valuable dataset but also tireless patient support by answering insightfully all related questions. In addition, the authors are grateful for The Royal Society and The British Council for financial support the early career fellowships (2024–2025) to allow them to participate this competition.

References

1. Suter, Y., et al.: The LUMIERE dataset: longitudinal glioblastoma MRI with expert RANO evaluation. Sci. Data. **9**(1), 768 (2022)
2. HD-GLIO-AUTO.: https://github.com/CCI-Bonn/HD-GLIO-AUTO
3. DeepBraTumIA.: https://www.nitrc.org/projects/deepbratumia/.
4. Kickingereder, P., Isensee, F., et al.: Automated quantitative tumor response assessment of MRI in neuro-oncology with artificial neural networks: a multicentre, retrospective study. Lancet Oncol. **20**(5), 728–740 (2019)

5. Guo, J., et al: CMT: convolutional neural networks meet vision transformers. In: Proceedings of the IEEE/CVF Conference on Computer Vision and Pattern Recognition, pp. 12175–12185 (2022)
6. Cho, K., Kim, J., Kim, K., et al.: MuSiC-ViT: a multi-task Siamese convolutional vision transformer for differentiating change from no-change in follow-up chest radiographs. Med. Image Anal. **89**, 102894 (2023)
7. Dosovitskiy, A., Beyer, L., Kolesnikov, A., et al.: An image is worth 16x16 words: transformers for image recognition at scale. In: 9th International Conference on Learning Representations, ICLR 2021 (2021)

Automated Brain Tumor Response Assessment from Longitudinal Multiparametric MRI Data Using Swin UNETR and a Radiomics Based Classifier

Satyajit Maurya[1], Ewunate Assaye Kassaw[1], Mohammad Tufail Sheikh[1], Amit Mehndiratta[1,2,3,4], and Anup Singh[1,2,3](✉)

[1] Centre for Biomedical Engineering, Indian Institute of Technology Delhi, Delhi, India
anupsm@iitd.ac.in

[2] Yardi School of Artificial Intelligence, Indian Institute of Technology Delhi, Delhi, India

[3] Department of Biomedical Engineering, All India Institute of Medical Science, Delhi, India

[4] Faculty of Medicine and Health, University of New South Wales (UNSW), Sydney, Australia

Abstract. Accurate and consistent response assessment is essential for guiding clinical decisions and optimizing treatment strategies in brain tumor patients. However, current methods for treatment response evaluation rely heavily on manual assessment of Response Assessment in Neuro-Oncology (RANO) criteria, which is time-consuming and prone to inter-observer variability. To address these limitations, we developed a fully automated pipeline combining segmentation and classification models to assess brain tumor response. Initially, Swin UNETR and U-Net models were trained on the BraTS dataset to automatically segment the whole tumor (WT) and enhancing tumor (ET) masks from FLAIR and WT masked T1c MRI sequences, respectively. Following segmentation from the best performing Swin UNETR model, shape-based and first-order radiomic features were extracted from the longitudinal LUMIERE dataset. A classification model utilizing TabM was developed for classifying the tumor treatment response into one of Complete Response (CR), Partial Response (PR), Stable Disease (SD), or Progressive Disease (PD) classes. Median Dice scores of 0.8811 and 0.8754 were obtained for the WT and ET using Swin UNETR models, respectively on the BraTS dataset. Using the extracted radiomic features, the TabM classifier achieved an average five-fold cross-validation balanced accuracy of 0.6415 on the LUMIERE dataset. A balanced accuracy of 0.5118 was obtained on the hidden multi-centric test dataset comprising 1010 cases of 300 patients. These results demonstrate the feasibility of automatically assessing brain tumor treatment response using longitudinal FLAIR and T1c MRI scans.

Keywords: Glioblastoma · Response Assessment in Neuro-Oncology (RANO) criteria · Swin UNETR · TabM

S. Maurya and E. A. Kassaw—Contributed equally with all other contributors.

S. Bakas et al. (Eds.): MICCAI 2025, LNCS 16377, pp. 246–257, 2026.
https://doi.org/10.1007/978-3-032-16370-7_22

1 Introduction

Gliomas and Meningiomas are amongst the most prevalent brain tumors. Gliomas account for almost 80% of all malignant brain tumors [1]. These are associated with high rates of morbidity and mortality [2]. Glioblastoma (GBM) is the most aggressive form of glioma having a median overall survival of only 12–18 months and a five-year survival rate of around 5% [3]. The current standard of care for GBM involves maximal safe resection followed by adjuvant radiotherapy and chemotherapy, typically with temozolomide [4]. Despite advances in brain tumor care, therapeutic efficacy remains limited by the immunosuppressive tumor microenvironment and the restrictive blood-brain barrier, which impedes drug delivery and immune cell infiltration.

A critical and crucial aspect of managing brain tumor patients is the accurate and consistent assessment of their response to treatment. This evaluation guides crucial clinical decisions, such as continuing, modifying, or discontinuing therapies. To standardize the evaluation of treatment response, a set of criteria is essential, particularly in managing high-grade gliomas, where accurate and consistent assessment guides critical clinical decisions. The Macdonald criteria, introduced in 1990 relied on the bidimensional measurements of contrast-enhancing tumor regions [5]. While an important first step, this criterion proved to have significant limitations. For instance, they did not account for non-enhancing tumor components visible on T2-weighted and FLAIR MRI sequences. To address these shortcomings, the international Response Assessment in Neuro-Oncology (RANO) working group was established. The RANO criteria also incorporated the evaluation of non-enhancing T2/FLAIR signal abnormalities and integrated corticosteroid dosage and clinical status to provide a more holistic assessment. While RANO criteria provides a structured framework, its reliance on subjective imaging assessments and T2/FLAIR interpretation underscores the need for advanced criteria to standardize response classification.

The reliance on manual, bidimensional measurements is laborious, susceptible to inter as well as intra-observer variability, and can be inaccurate for the irregularly shaped tumors often seen in gliomas. This has led to a growing recognition of the advantages of volumetric analysis, which provides a more sensitive and reproducible method for quantifying tumor burden. Studies have shown that volumetric measurements can offer improved sensitivity in detecting subtle changes in tumor size over time [6]. Recognizing this, the RANO 2.0 criteria now formally includes volumetric measurements as an optional assessment method. Tumor response can be classified into categories such as complete response (CR), partial response (PR), stable disease (SD), and progressive disease (PD) based on a combination of imaging metrics, clinical status, and corticosteroid dosing. For high-grade gliomas, CR requires complete disappearance of all measurable contrast-enhancing disease, demonstrated on post-radiotherapy MRI with no new lesions and maintained for at least four weeks off corticosteroid therapy. PR is defined by at least a 50% reduction in the sum of products of perpendicular diameters of contrast enhancing lesions or a corresponding volumetric reduction (commonly $\geq$65%). This is accompanied by the additional condition that there is no increase in non-measurable disease, no appearance of new lesions, and no requirement for increased corticosteroid dosing. PD is characterized by a $\geq$ 25% increase in the product of diameters of enhancing lesions or a $\geq$ 40% increase in lesion volume and/or the emergence of new lesions.

SD is designated when the changes in imaging findings do not meet the thresholds for CR, PR, or PD.

A key limitation of conventional RANO assessment is its dependence on manual lesion segmentation and bi-dimensional measurements. To overcome this challenge, some AI-driven approaches have been developed that demonstrate strong concordance with manual RANO classification while automating the measurement of contrast-enhancing lesions [7, 8]. AI-based algorithms, particularly those using deep learning, have demonstrated remarkable potential to automate and standardize the response assessment process [9] [10]. Some studies have aimed to develop end-to-end pipelines for assessing the tumor response [6]. However, these methods are limited either by small dataset sizes and poor classification accuracy, or by not classifying treatment response according to the RANO criteria into four classes [11].

The Swin UNETR [12] architecture emerges as a particularly promising solution, combining Swin Transformers [13] with U-Net [14] models to simultaneously capture local tissue details and global contextual relationships in 3D medical images. Following segmentation, radiomics analysis enables comprehensive tumor characterization through high-throughput extraction of quantitative features. These features encode tumor heterogeneity and tumor microenvironmental properties beyond human visual perception. When coupled with deep learning classifiers, this combined approach (Swin UNETR + radiomics) can offer a robust, data-driven framework for treatment response prediction that addresses the limitations of conventional methods while maintaining clinical interpretability.

This study, therefore, aims to develop and validate a fully automated pipeline for brain tumor response assessment from longitudinal multiparametric MRI data to overcome the subjectivity and labor-intensive nature of current RANO assessment methods utilizing the LUMIERE dataset [15] as part of the 2025 BraTS Brain Tumor Progression Challenge.

2 Materials and Methods

2.1 Data

This study utilized the LUMIERE dataset (n = 91) [15], containing multi-parametric MRI (T1w, T2w, FLAIR, post-contrast T1w (T1c)) with longitudinal acquisitions. Automated segmentations from DeepBraTumIA (https://www.nitrc.org/projects/deepbratumia) and HD-GLIO-AUTO (https://github.com/CCI-Bonn/HD-GLIO-AUTO) models, RANO expert ratings, PyRadiomics-derived features [16], and clinical metadata were available as part of this dataset. Due to observed segmentation inconsistencies in the LUMIERE dataset, we developed a robust deep learning (DL) based segmentation model using the BraTS 2025 Glioma Challenge dataset (comprising 1,251 pre-operative and 1,350 post-operative/post-treatment cases), which provided standardized multi-institutional MRI data with expert-validated ground truth masks for all tumor subcomponents. The proposed DL model was used for segmentation of tumor masks for the LUMIERE dataset. Details of this model are provided in the Sect. 2.2.

Since RANO criteria integrates both qualitative T2w/FLAIR data (for detecting new lesions) and quantitative T1c measurements (for bidimensional/volumetric analysis), our study utilized both FLAIR and T1c sequences. Whole tumor (WT) masks were generated by combining the three tumor subcomponent labels: enhancing tissue (ET), surrounding non-enhancing FLAIR hyperintensity (SNFH), and non-enhancing tumor core (NETC). We developed two separate deep learning models, one for WT segmentation using FLAIR images and the other for ET segmentation using T1c images. The BraTS data was partitioned patient-wise into training (70%) and validation (30%) sets, stratified by pre−/post-operative status. Model performance was evaluated on an independent test set of 271 post-treatment cases from the BraTS dataset, ensuring robust assessment of generalizability.

2.2 DL-Based Segmentation Model Development

The automated tumor segmentation masks provided with the LUMIERE dataset exhibited notable inaccuracies. For instance, in the case of "Patient-048," the DeepBraTumIA tool miscategorized the resection cavity as a necrotic region in the post op scans. Similarly, the HD-GLIO-AUTO tool showed poor performance for the same patient, failing to accurately segment the contrast-enhancing tumor in later follow-ups (e.g., week 49). These limitations necessitated the development of more accurate, dedicated segmentation models. Consequently, we implemented and compared 3D U-Net and 3D Swin UNETR architectures for WT and ET segmentation using the BraTS dataset. To improve ET segmentations, we adopted a cascaded approach inspired by [3], where T1c images were masked using predicted WT outputs. Table 1 summarizes the key training parameters for both U-Net and Swin UNETR models. Figure 1a shows the segmentation model development pipeline. The best performing model determined using Dice score was used for segmenting the tumor sub-components on the LUMIERE dataset for further downstream tasks following some pre-processing steps as discussed in the next sub-section.

Table 1. Training parameters used for U-Net and Swin UNETR architectures.

Parameter Category	Parameter	U-Net	Swin UNETR
Architectural	Input Patch Size	(128, 128, 64)	(128, 128, 64)
	Input Channels	1	1
	Output Channels	1	1
	Channel Sequence	(16, 32, 64, 128, 256)	N/A
	Stride Sequence	(2, 2, 2, 2)	N/A
	Feature Size	N/A	48
	Transformer Depths	N/A	(2, 2, 2, 2)
	Attention Heads	N/A	(3, 6, 12, 24)
Data & Pre-processing	Normalization	Z-Score (zero mean, unit variance)	
	Data Augmentation	Random Flipping, Random Intensity Scaling, Random Intensity Shifting	
Training	Loss Function	Weighted Dice Cross Entropy Loss	

(*continued*)

Table 1. *(continued)*

Parameter Category	Parameter	U-Net	Swin UNETR
	Optimizer	AdamW	
	Initial Learning Rate	1e-4	
	Learning Rate Scheduler	Cosine Annealing	
	Weight Decay	1e-5	
	Batch Size	8	
	Number of Epochs	150	
	Validation Frequency	Every 5 epochs	
Implementation	Hardware	GPU: NVIDIA V100 (32GB 5120 CUDA cores) CPU: 2x Intel Xeon G-6148 (20 cores 2.4 GHz)	

2.3 Radiomics Feature Based DL-Classification Model Development

This analysis utilized the LUMIERE dataset containing 638 longitudinal MRI scans from 91 GBM patients. After applying quality control measures, we excluded 22 scans lacking RANO ratings, 3 duplicate ratings, 14 entries without imaging data, 91 pre-operative studies, and 14 cases missing either T1c or FLAIR sequences. This resulted in 497 qualified scan timepoints. There were also a few cases with only post-op data following the pre-op data that were removed from the analysis. We treated consecutive scans as independent observations, yielding a final cohort of 377 analyzable cases with complete imaging data and RANO assessments.

The LUMIERE dataset exhibited substantial heterogeneity in image dimensions and slice counts across scans. To ensure consistency in our analysis pipeline, we registered the skull-stripped images to the SRI24 atlas templates, aligning FLAIR sequences with the T2w template and T1c sequences with the T1w template resulting in a uniform spatial resolution of 240 × 240 × 155 as shown in Fig. 1b. Finally, median-based intensity normalization was applied to standardize signal variations across the dataset.

The registered FLAIR and T1c images were processed through segmentation models to generate the WT and ET masks. From these masks, 14 shape-based and 18 first-order radiomic features were extracted (using PyRadiomics [16]) at both baseline and follow-up time points, yielding a total of 128 features per case. These features were used to classify treatment response into one of four RANO categories: CR, PR, SD, or PD. For the classification model development, an 80–20 stratified K-fold cross validation split for training and validation was used (Fig. 1c). The capability to capture key features from complex tabular data makes TabM the best for analyzing such datasets [17]. The AdamW optimizer was used to minimize a cross-entropy loss, and the training performance was evaluated using balanced accuracy. Rigorous parameter tuning was performed using Optuna [18]. Synthetic Minority Over-sampling Technique (SMOTE) was used to address the data imbalance issue (CR: 26, PD: 241, PR: 20, SD: 90).

3 Results

3.1 Segmentation Model Performance

Swin UNETR outperformed U-Net for segmenting both the WT and ET masks on the BraTS 2025 Glioma Challenge dataset. Moreover, using WT masked T1c images with Swin UNETR showed improved dice results compared to when using the T1c images directly. Table 2 presents the segmentation model performance results.

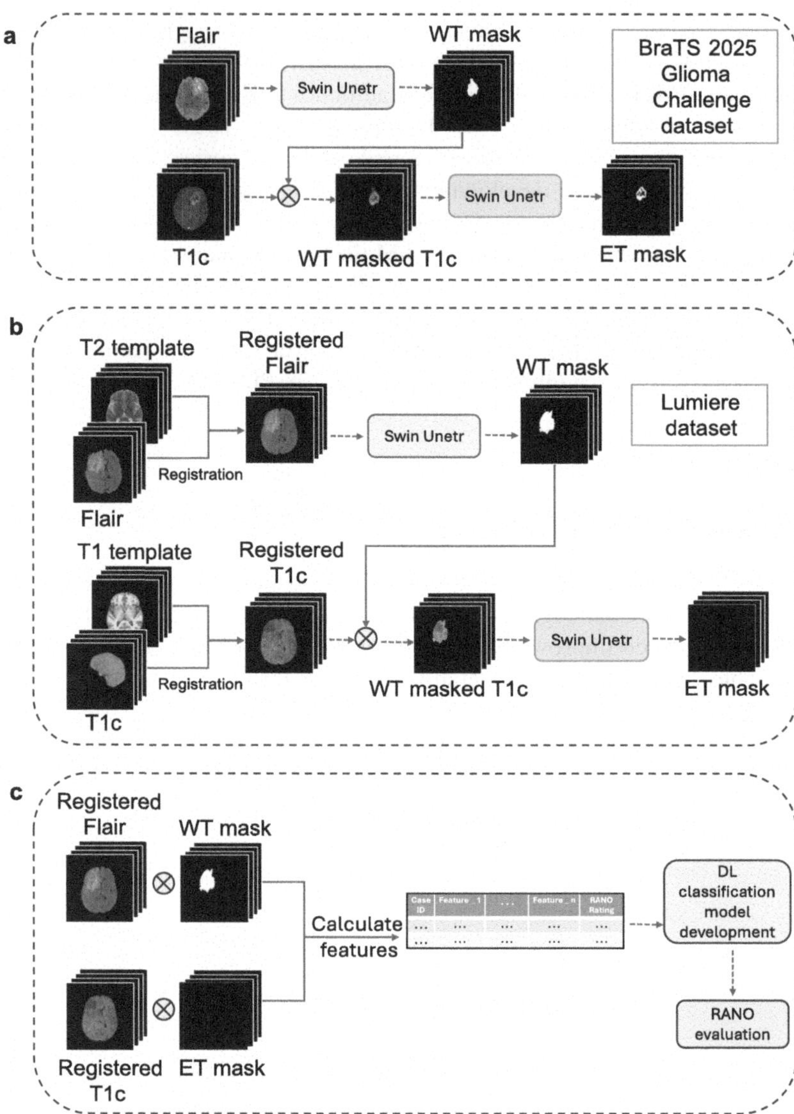

Fig. 1. The overall study design, (a) segmentation model development using the BraTS dataset, (b) Whole Tumor and Enhancing Tumor mask prediction on the LUMIERE data using the developed model from (a), and (c) radiomic feature extraction using the Lumiere data and development of the classification methods.

Table 2. Dice scores of the developed segmentation models.

Architecture	Segmentation	Metrics	Original data	Masked data
U-Net	WT	Validation Dice	0.8652	
		Test dice	0.7337 ± 0.2859	
		Median Test dice	0.8586	
	ET	Validation Dice	0.6934	0.7121
		Test dice	0.6372 ± 0.3317	0.6360 ± 0.3356
		Median test dice	0.7838	0.7948
Swin Unetr	WT	Validation Dice	**0.887**	
		Test dice	**0.7636 ± 0.2773**	
		Median test dice	**0.8811**	
	ET	Validation Dice	0.7637	**0.7944**
		Test dice	0.6832 ± 0.3317	**0.7632 ± 0.2850**
		Median test dice	0.8254	**0.8754**

Using the corresponding best performing models the WT and ET masks were predicted on the LUMIERE dataset. Figure 2 shows the sample images along with the overlaid segmentation masks (for Patient-018), the tumor progression and the corresponding RANO ratings. Following this, the radiomic features were obtained corresponding to WT and ET masked FLAIR and T1c images, respectively. These features were then used for classification model development as discussed in the following sub section.

3.2 Classification Model Performance

Using the Optuna parameter tuning, the following parameters were obtained for the best performance with TabM: number of bins – 25, embedding vector dimensionality – 27, learning rate - 0.00158, L2 regularization of 0.000148, 113 ensembled sub-models, dropout of 0.3068, 191 neurons in each block, and 2 sequential blocks in the model's main backbone. Using these parameters, an average balanced accuracy of 0.6415 was obtained with five-fold cross validation. Next, the model was trained on the whole dataset and the model weights were saved for inference. Using these saved model weights, a balanced accuracy of 0.6482 was obtained on the hidden challenge validation dataset comprising of 14 cases from 6 patients. On the hidden test set (comprising 1010 cases from 300 patients), the developed model scored a mean balanced accuracy of 0.5118, an F1 score of 0.2532 and an average precision of 0.30.

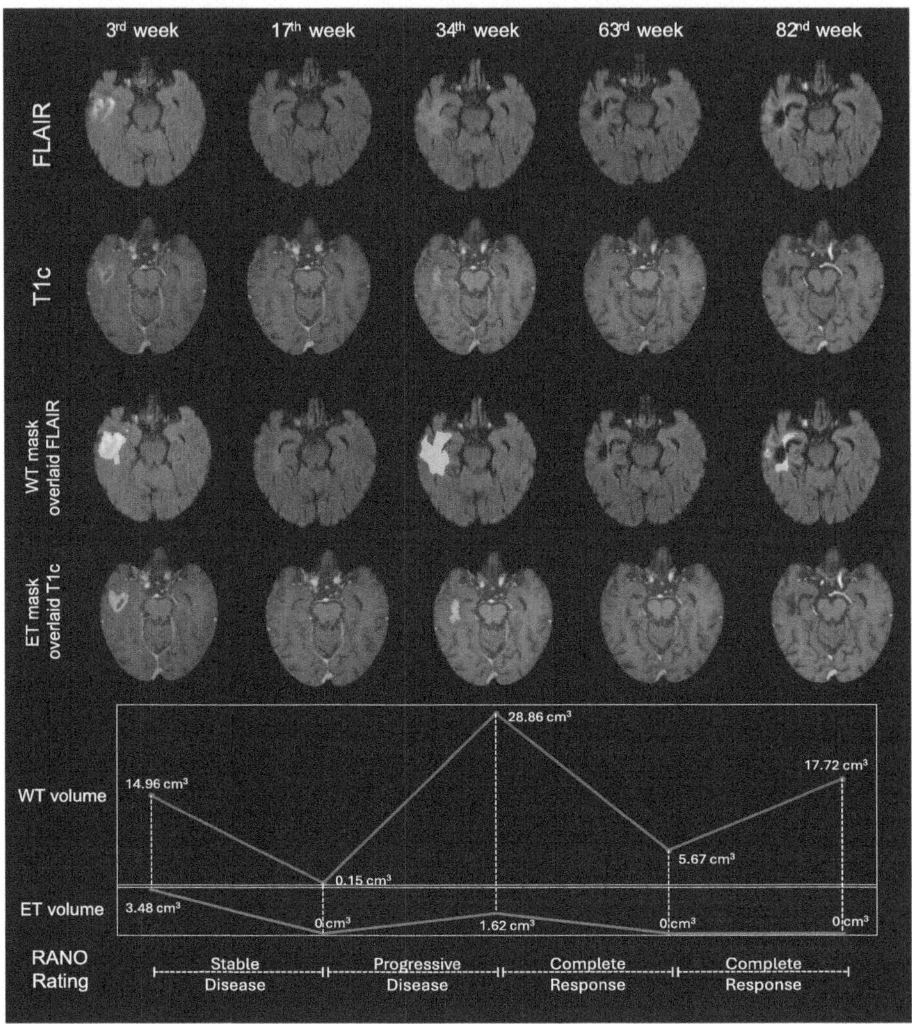

Fig. 2. Segmentation masks overlaid on the corresponding images along with the tumor subcomponent volume and the RANO ratings.

4 Discussion

In this study an automated pipeline for determining the RANO rating from longitudinal MRI scans was developed using a DL-based segmentation model and a radiomics based DL classifier. Swin UNETR and U-Net models were used for segmenting the tumor subcomponents from longitudinal MRI data. The results (Table 2) showed that the Swin UNETR model outperformed U-Net for both WT and ET segmentations using the BraTS 2025 Glioma Challenge dataset. Hierarchical Swin Transformer blocks used in Swin UNETR effectively capture both the global and local image context information [12].

This is advantageous over the U-Net model that is based on convolutional operations limited for taking into consideration the long-range data dependencies. Median dice scores of 0.8811 and 0.8254 were obtained for WT and ET segmentation, respectively on the original FLAIR and T1c images. Additionally, an improvement in dice score was obtained by using a cascaded method, in which the WT predictions were used to mask the T1c images to obtain the ET masks. This improved the median dice score from 0.8254 to 0.8754. Most of the other brain structures that could be falsely detected as ET were removed using this cascaded approach. Using a similar approach, the study [3] had obtained a median dice score of 0.839 on the BraTS'21 hidden test data.

The final goal of this study was to automate the RANO response assessment. This was achieved by extracting the shape-based (using WT and ET masks) and the first-order radiomic features (using FLAIR and T1c images) from the LUMIERE dataset. Features were extracted both for the baseline and the follow-up timepoints. This was aimed towards capturing quantitative changes indicative of response. The LUMIERE dataset is highly imbalanced with respect to its classes. SMOTE oversampling technique was used to balance data classes. In our experiments, we found that without using SMOTE, with TabM classifier, the average five-fold cross validation balanced accuracy was considerably lower at 0.5266. Using the same classifier combined with SMOTE, an average five-fold cross validation balanced accuracy of 0.6415 was obtained on the LUMIERE dataset. A previous study has reported a balanced accuracy of 0.51 using the same dataset [19]. On the 1010 hidden test cases, the model obtained a balanced accuracy of 0.5118. This value was considerably lower than those obtained during training and validation. A probable reason for this discrepancy could be: a) the training dataset was smaller, consisting of only 377 cases from 91 subjects, and b) the model may have lower generalizability because it was trained on single-centric data while being tested on multi-centric data.

The developed automated method presented in this study directly addresses the limitations of the bi-dimensional manual RANO assessments that are prone to inter as well as intra-observer variability while being time intensive. The fully automated pipeline of this study was able to output the RANO classification within 5.58 mins for a single case that includes baseline and follow-up scans using the specified hardware mentioned in Table 1. By automating both segmentation and classification, our approach offers a more reproducible and efficient alternative.

Although encouraging, the balanced accuracy that was attained also emphasizes how difficult automated RANO assessment is. Due to data restrictions in the challenge testing set, our model was unable to fully incorporate the RANO criteria, which are complex and include not only changes in tumor size but also clinical status and corticosteroid dosage. The recent RANO 2.0 update further refines these criteria, emphasizing volumetric measurements as an option and providing more specific guidance on handling non-enhancing disease and pseudoprogression. Future iterations of our pipeline should aim to incorporate these updated guidelines and additional clinical data to improve classification accuracy.

There may be major advantages to incorporating such an automated technology into the therapeutic workflow. For neuroradiologists and oncologists, it could be a decision-support tool that offers quick, numerical evaluations of therapy response. This might result in quicker and better-informed clinical judgments, which could enhance patient outcomes.

5 Limitations and Future Directions

This study has some limitations. The classification analysis was conducted on a relatively small and heterogeneous dataset (LUMIERE). While we employed robust cross-validation and a separate test set, validation on a larger, multi-institutional dataset is necessary to ensure the generalizability of our findings.

Future work should focus on several key areas. First, integrating the full spectrum of RANO 2.0 criteria, including clinical data and corticosteroid usage, is crucial for developing a more clinically relevant tool. Second, investigating the model's ability to differentiate true progression from pseudoprogression which is a major challenge in neuro-oncology, would be a significant advancement. Lastly, feature selection techniques such as MRMR (Minimum Redundancy Maximum Relevance), and LASSO (Least Absolute Shrinkage and Selection Operator) can be explored to check for model performance improvements.

6 Conclusion

In summary, this work shows that a fully automated pipeline for evaluating brain tumor response from longitudinal MRI data is both feasible and promising. Combining a Swin UNETR model for precise segmentation with a tuned DL classifier based on texture features for RANO classification, we have created a tool to improve the effectiveness of treatment response assessment in neuro-oncology.

Acknowledgements. This work was supported by the Indian Council of Medical Research (ICMR) under the project 'Centre for Advanced Research in Quantitative Imaging and Al Modeling for Early Diagnostics and Prognostic Monitoring in Oncology' (Project No. CAR-2024-01-000187). The authors thank High Performance Computing (HPC) facility of Indian Institute of Technology Delhi for computational resources. The authors are also grateful to the BraTS Challenge organizers for making the dataset available to the research community.

References

1. Ostrom, Q.T., Bauchet, L., Davis, F.G., et al.: The epidemiology of glioma in adults: a "state of the science" review. Neuro-Oncology. **16**(7), 896–913 (2014)
2. Yadav, V.K., Sharma, S., Maurya, S., et al.: Presence of fragmented Intratumoral thrombosed microvasculature in the necrotic and Peri-necrotic regions on SWI differentiates IDH wild-type glioblastoma from IDH mutant grade 4 astrocytoma. J. Magn. Reson. Imaging.
3. Maurya, S., Kumar Yadav, V., Agarwal, S., Singh, A.: Brain Tumor Segmentation in mpMRI Scans (BraTS-2021) Using Models Based on U-Net Architecture. In: International MICCAI Brainlesion Workshop, pp. 312–323. Springer (2021)
4. Fernandes C, Costa A, Osório L, et al. Current standards of care in glioblastoma therapy. Exon Publ. Published online 2017:197–241.

5. Chinot, O.L., Macdonald, D.R., Abrey, L.E., Zahlmann, G., Kerloëguen, Y., Cloughesy, T.F.: Response assessment criteria for glioblastoma: practical adaptation and implementation in clinical trials of antiangiogenic therapy. Curr. Neurol. Neurosci. Rep. **13**(5), 347 (2013)
6. Kickingereder, P., Isensee, F., Tursunova, I., et al.: Automated quantitative tumour response assessment of MRI in neuro-oncology with artificial neural networks: a multicentre, retrospective study. Lancet Oncol. **20**(5), 728–740 (2019)
7. Chang, K., Beers, A.L., Bai, H.X., et al.: Automatic assessment of glioma burden: a deep learning algorithm for fully automated volumetric and bidimensional measurement. Neuro-Oncology. **21**(11), 1412–1422 (2019)
8. Nalepa, J., Kotowski, K., Machura, B., et al.: Deep learning automates bidimensional and volumetric tumor burden measurement from MRI in pre-and post-operative glioblastoma patients. Comput. Biol. Med. **154**, 106603 (2023)
9. Vollmuth, P., Foltyn, M., Huang, R.Y., et al.: Artificial intelligence (AI)-based decision support improves reproducibility of tumor response assessment in neuro-oncology: an international multi-reader study. Neuro-Oncology. **25**(3), 533–543 (2023)
10. Rudie, J.D., Calabrese, E., Saluja, R., et al.: Longitudinal assessment of posttreatment diffuse glioma tissue volumes with three-dimensional convolutional neural networks. Radiol. Artif. Intell. **4**(5), e210243 (2022)
11. Suter, Y., Schuhmacher, F., Ermis, E., et al.: Towards Radiomics-based automated disease progression assessment for glioblastoma patients. In: International MICCAI Brainlesion Workshop, pp. 36–47. Springer (2023)
12. Hatamizadeh, A., Nath, V., Tang, Y., Yang, D., Roth, H.R., Xu, D.: Swin unetr: Swin transformers for semantic segmentation of brain tumors in mri images. In: International MICCAI Brainlesion Workshop, pp. 272–284. Springer (2021)
13. Liu, Z., Lin, Y., Cao, Y., et al.: Swin transformer: hierarchical vision transformer using shifted windows. In: Proceedings of the IEEE/CVF International Conference on Computer Vision, pp. 10012–10022 (2021)
14. Ronneberger, O., Fischer, P., Brox, T.: U-net: convolutional networks for biomedical image segmentation. Lect Notes Comput Sci (including Subser Lect Notes Artif Intell Lect Notes Bioinformatics). **9351**, 234–241 (2015). https://doi.org/10.1007/978-3-319-24574-4_28
15. Suter, Y., Knecht, U., Valenzuela, W., et al.: The LUMIERE dataset: longitudinal glioblastoma MRI with expert RANO evaluation. Sci. Data. **9**(1), 768 (2022)
16. Van Griethuysen, J.J.M., Fedorov, A., Parmar, C., et al.: Computational radiomics system to decode the radiographic phenotype. Cancer Res. **77**(21), e104–e107 (2017)
17. Gorishniy, Y., Kotelnikov, A., Babenko, A.: Tabm: Advancing tabular deep learning with parameter-efficient ensembling. arXiv Prepr arXiv, 241024210. Published online (2024)
18. Akiba, T., Sano, S., Yanase, T., Ohta, T., Koyama, M.: Optuna: A next-generation hyperparameter optimization framework. In: Proceedings of the 25th ACM SIGKDD International Conference on Knowledge Discovery & Data Mining, pp. 2623–2631 (2019)
19. Matoso, A., Passarinho, C., Loureiro, M.P., Moreira, J.M., Figueiredo, P., Nunes, R.G.: Towards a deep learning approach for classifying treatment response in glioblastomas. arXiv Prepr arXiv, 250418268. Published online (2025)

RECAP-Net: RANO Ensemble for Classification of Active Progression

Vansh Kakkar, Deepak, Harshanth Raja, Harshdip Saha, and Ankur Gupta(✉)

Department of Computer Engineering, Netaji Subhas University of Technology, New Delhi 110078, India
agupta4@cs.iitr.ac.in

Abstract. Glioblastoma is an aggressive brain tumor requiring accurate monitoring of treatment response. This work addresses the 2025 BraTS Tumor Progression Challenge task of classifying glioblastoma treatment response using longitudinal magnetic resonance imaging scans based on standardized assessment criteria. We propose RECAP-Net, an end-to-end deep learning pipeline combining spectral-normalized generative adversarial network-based augmentation, Swin UNETR based custom segmentation and an ensemble of three-dimensional convolutional neural network architectures (ResNet, DenseNet, EfficientNet). Multimodal pre- and post-treatment Magnetic Resonance Imaging volumes and segmentation masks are preprocessed and fed into the model. Our approach captures tumor progression over time and handles class imbalance effectively. Experimental results demonstrate high accuracy and robustness, supporting its utility for automated treatment assessment in clinical neuro-oncology.

Keywords: Brain MRI · RANO · Ensemble · Soft-Voting · Swin UNETR · Resnet · EfficientNet · DenseNet · Tumor Progression

1 Introduction

Glioblastoma (GBM) [1] is the most aggressive primary brain tumor in adults, with median survival under 15 months despite intensive treatment. Assessing therapy response remains a major clinical challenge, addressed in practice by the Response Assessment in Neuro-Oncology (RANO) [2] criteria, which categorize response as complete (CR), partial (PR), stable (SD), or progressive disease (PD) based on imaging and clinical features. Most automated tumor analysis methods focus on single time-point segmentation, overlooking the longitudinal nature of disease progression [3]. To address this, the 2025 BraTS-PRO Challenge introduced a task to classify tumor response from paired pre- and post-therapy MRIs, optionally using tumor segmentations. Our approach leverages multi-modal 3D MRIs, fused segmentations from HD-GLIO-AUTO [4] and DeepBraTumIA [5], and a deep learning ensemble trained on harmonized data.

S. Bakas et al. (Eds.): MICCAI 2025, LNCS 16377, pp. 258–269, 2026.
https://doi.org/10.1007/978-3-032-16370-7_23

2 Dataset Specifications

We utilized the LUMIERE dataset [6], curated for the BraTS-PRO 2025 challenge to support research in longitudinal monitoring of glioma patients. It consists of MRI scans from 91 patients, totaling 616 volumes, with each subject contributing 2–4 timepoints. Each volume is paired with expert-assigned RANO response labels and automatically generated tumor segmentations. The dataset spans diverse institutions, scanners, and imaging protocols, promoting robust model generalization.

2.1 Imaging Modalities and Preprocessing

Each scan includes four standard MRI sequences: T1-weighted (T1), contrast-enhanced T1-weighted (T1ce), T2-weighted (T2), and FLAIR. These modalities are crucial for highlighting distinct tumor subregions—T1ce emphasizes enhancing regions, FLAIR captures edema, and T2 visualizes cystic or necrotic areas. For every baseline–follow-up scan pair, both the original and affine-registered volumes are provided, with follow-ups aligned to baseline scans to reduce inter-scan spatial variability.

2.2 Segmentations

Tumor segmentation masks are generated using two independent tools—HD GLIO–AUTO and DeepBraTumIA—and include three classes: background (0), peritumoral edema (1), and enhancing tumor core (2). These segmentations are available for both baseline and follow-up scans in original and registered spaces, enabling modeling of tumor morphology across time. While the provided labels cover edema and enhancing regions, other clinically important subregions such as necrosis and the postoperative resection cavity were not included in the dataset annotations. This exclusion reflects the design of the dataset and its alignment with RANO criteria.

2.3 Annotation Protocol and Labeling

Each scan pair is labeled according to expert RANO evaluations, with response categories mapped to numerical classes: 0 for CR, 1 for PR, 2 for SD, and 3 PD. Labels are provided for every baseline-follow-up pair, with multiple such pairs possible per patient. All annotations, including image paths and labels, are stored in a JSON file (`patients.json`), which serves as the reference during training. During evaluation, follow-up labels and segmentations are withheld to simulate real-world inference.

3 Methodology

3.1 Data Preprocessing and Augmentation

Robust neuro-oncology models need careful preprocessing and class-aware augmentation. Our pipeline applies intensity normalization, spatial harmonization, and synthetic data generation to counter class imbalance. Data follow the BraTS directory structure with registered baseline and follow-up MRIs (T1, T1ce, T2, FLAIR) and segmentations. RANO labels range from 0–3. Before spatial operations, each modality was normalized independently in its native space to preserve intensity distribution. Normalization uses z-scores over brain voxels:

$$I_{\text{norm}}(x) = \frac{I(x) - \mu}{\sigma} \tag{1}$$

where μ, σ are mean and std within the brain, with $\sigma > 10^{-8}$ for stability. Since organizers provided pre-aligned volumes (follow-ups affine-registered to baselines), we applied only cropping and padding to achieve a uniform tensor size. Eight modalities (4 baseline + 4 follow-up) plus two tumor masks were concatenated into a 10-channel tensor of shape $(10, 256, 256, 256)$, saved as `.npy` files for efficient 3D batching. Using a fixed $256 \times 256 \times 256$ resolution standardized the input space and removed non-brain regions while retaining essential anatomy (Table 1).

Algorithm 1 Cropping and Padding for Uniform Tensor Size

Input: Pre-aligned volume V with shape (C, H, W, D)
Output: Standardized tensor $\hat{V}$ with shape $(C, 256, 256, 256)$
Target size = 256 for each spatial dimension
foreach *spatial dimension* $s \in \{H, W, D\}$ **do**
  if $s > 256$ **then**
    Center-crop V along s to size 256
  end
  else if $s < 256$ **then**
    Symmetrically pad V with zeros along s to size 256
  end
end
return standardized tensor $\hat{V}$ of shape $(C, 256, 256, 256)$

Table 1. Channel mapping of input tensor

Channel Index	Content
0–3	Baseline T1, T1ce, T2, FLAIR
4–7	Follow-up T1, T1ce, T2, FLAIR
8	Baseline tumor mask
9	Follow-up tumor mask

The dataset is imbalanced (3:2:1:1 across RANO classes). Standard flips are anatomically invalid, so we designed a two-stage augmentation. First, a conditional 3D SN-GAN [7] trained on 8-channel temporal MRIs generated realistic longitudinal tumor progressions. By training on the complete longitudinal scan data, the GAN learned to generate realistic and anatomically consistent progressions of tumor appearance over time, directly addressing the dynamic nature of the data. Second, our pre-trained Swin UNETR (Sect. 3.5) produced baseline and follow-up tumor masks for each GAN output. Thus, every synthetic 8-channel scan gained 2 masks, forming a full 10-channel tensor.

The GAN uses a 3D generator with four transposed conv blocks, BN, ReLU, and dropout. The discriminator applies spectral norm and projection-based conditioning. Training uses BCE loss, label smoothing (0.9 for real; [0,0.1] for fake), and a 2:1 generator-discriminator update ratio.

$$\mathcal{L}_D = -\mathbb{E}_{x,y}\left[\log D(x,y)\right] - \mathbb{E}_{z,y}\left[\log(1 - D(G(z,y),y))\right] \tag{2}$$

$$\mathcal{L}_G = -\mathbb{E}_{z,y}\left[\log D(G(z,y),y)\right] \tag{3}$$

Here, $\mathcal{L}_D$ and $\mathcal{L}_G$ are discriminator and generator losses. x is a real MRI, $z \sim \mathcal{N}(0,1)$ a latent vector, y the class label, and $G(z,y)$ the synthetic sample. $D(x,y)$ outputs the probability of realness. The generator maximizes realism, while the discriminator distinguishes real vs synthetic. GANs train for 10 epochs, batch size 4, using Adam [8] with lr 1×10^{-4} (G) and 2×10^{-4} (D). We generate enough samples to reach 230 per class, sampling latent vectors from $\mathcal{N}(0,1)$. Visual checks confirm realism. Quantitative results: 3D-SSIM 0.92 ± 0.03, KL-divergence 0.037 ± 0.004. Dice score improves from $0.842 \rightarrow 0.868$ (+2.6%). Overall, the pipeline standardizes multi-modal MRI, balances classes via SN-GAN augmentation, and yields realistic, scalable data for neuro-oncology deep learning (Table 2).

Table 2. Class distribution before and after augmentation

Class	Original Count	Augmented Count	Total
0 (CR)	26	204	230
1 (PR)	20	210	230
2 (SD)	85	145	230
3 (PD)	230	0	230

3.2 Model Architecture Overview

Our approach employs a sophisticated ensemble learning framework that combines three state-of-the-art 3D convolutional neural network architectures to achieve robust classification of brain tumor response patterns. The ensemble integrates 3D variants of ResNet-18 [9], DenseNet-121 [10], and EfficientNet-B0 [11], implemented using the MONAI framework. These three architectures were selected for their diverse feature extraction philosophies: ResNet's residual connections combat vanishing gradients, DenseNet's feature reuse enhances efficiency, and EfficientNet's compound scaling provides a strong performance baseline. This diversity was hypothesized to create a more robust ensemble by capturing complementary data patterns.

3.3 Preprocessing and Channel Augmentation

The 10-channel input tensor, comprising eight MRI modalities of baseline and follow-up scans and two segmentation masks, was augmented to a 15-channel tensor to explicitly highlight temporal changes. This augmentation step is applied *after* all volumes have been resampled and z-score normalized (as described in Sect. 3.1), and *before* the tensor is passed into the ensemble classifiers. Specifically, we compute voxel-wise difference maps between baseline and follow-up scans for each modality and the tumor mask, as specified in Eq. (4) and Eq. (5).

$$D_m(x) = I_{m,f}(x) - I_{m,b}(x), \quad m \in \{\mathrm{T1}, \mathrm{T1ce}, \mathrm{T2}, \mathrm{FLAIR}\} \tag{4}$$

$$D_{\mathrm{mask}}(x) = M_f(x) - M_b(x) \tag{5}$$

The resulting five channels are concatenated with the original 10 channels to yield a 15-channel tensor of shape $(15, 256, 256, 256)$. These difference maps explicitly direct the model to focus on regions of temporal change, which is essential for robust RANO assessment.

Algorithm 2 Class-Balanced Augmentation via Conditional 3D SN-GAN

Input: Imbalanced dataset $\mathcal{D} = \{(x_i, y_i)\}_{i=1}^{N}$, where $y_i \in \mathcal{C} = \{0, 1, 2, 3\}$
Output: Balanced dataset $\mathcal{D}'$ with $T = 230$ samples per class
Latent vector $z \sim \mathcal{N}(0, \mathbf{I})$, target count $T = 230$
Preprocessing: Resize all x_i to $\mathbb{R}^{10\times256\times256\times256}$
Model Initialization:
Generator $G : (\mathbb{R}^{100}, \mathcal{C}) \rightarrow \mathbb{R}^{10\times256\times256\times256}$ Discriminator $D : (\mathbb{R}^{10\times256\times256\times256}, \mathcal{C}) \rightarrow [0, 1]$
Training: Train (G, D) on $\mathcal{D}_{\mathrm{train}}$ via conditional spectral normalization
foreach $c \in \{0, 1, 2\}$ **do**
  $n_c \leftarrow \mathtt{count}(\{y_i = c\})$ **if** $n_c < T$ **then**
    $N_{\mathrm{gen}} \leftarrow T - n_c$ **for** $i = 1$ **to** N_{gen} **do in parallel**
      Sample $z_i \sim \mathcal{N}(0, \mathbf{I})$ $\tilde{x}_i \leftarrow G(z_i, c)$ Store $\tilde{x}_i$ as `fake_`i`.npy` in class c folder
    end
  end
end
foreach $c \in \mathcal{C}$ **do**
  $\mathcal{D}'_c \leftarrow \mathcal{D}^{\mathrm{orig}}_c$ **if** $c \in \{0, 1, 2\}$ **then**
    $\mathcal{D}'_c \leftarrow \mathcal{D}'_c \cup \tilde{\mathcal{D}}_c$
  end
end
return $\mathcal{D}' = \bigcup_{c\in\mathcal{C}} \mathcal{D}'_c$

3.4 Segmentation Strategy and Evaluation

To enhance tumor response classification, we tested several 3D segmentation models—3D CNN (baseline), UNetR [12], SegResNet [13], and Swin UNETR [14]—via the MONAI framework. All were fine-tuned on the Lumiere dataset with annotations from HD-GLIO-AUTO and DeepBraTumIA for

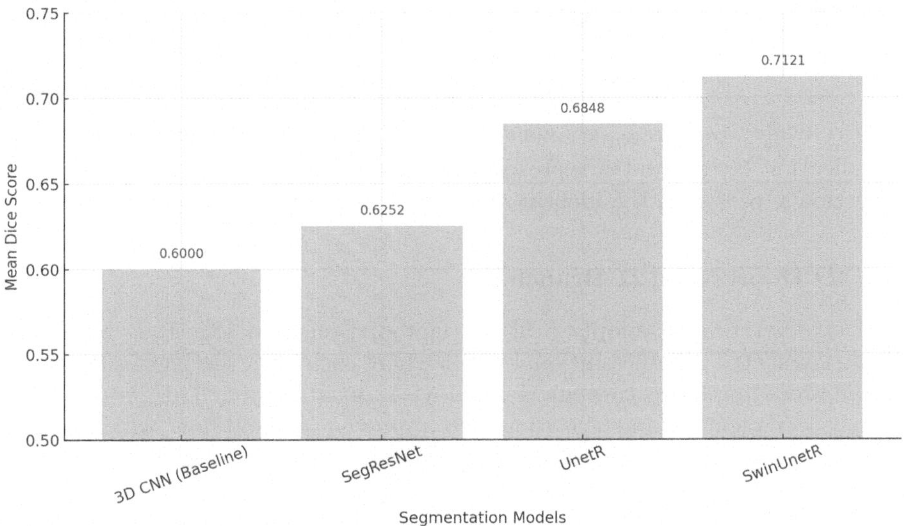

Fig. 1. Average Dice Scores of 3D Segmentation Models on the Lumiere dataset.

anatomical consistency. Swin UNETR was trained with four input modalities (T1, T1ce, T2, FLAIR) to generate a unified segmentation map. Performance was measured by Dice Similarity Coefficient. As shown in Fig. 1, Swin UNETR achieved the best Dice (0.7121), outperforming other models across baseline and follow-up scans. Hence, we adopted it to generate segmentation masks, which were then added as channels to the classification pipeline, improving tumor morphology and progression modeling.

The Swin UNETR mapping is expressed in Eq. (6):

$$S(x) = D\left(T\left(P(x)\right) \oplus E(x)\right) \tag{6}$$

where x is the MRI volume, $P(x)$ its patch embedding, and $T(\cdot)$ the Swin Transformer encoder. $E(x)$ are encoder features preserved for skip connections, $\oplus$ is concatenation, and $D(\cdot)$ the decoder reconstructing the final mask $S(x)$. This combines transformer-based global context with U-Net-style localization for accurate segmentation.

3.5 3D ResNet-18 Branch

The ResNet branch of our ensemble employs a 3D adaptation of ResNet-18. This model incorporates 3D residual blocks composed of two stacked 3D convolutions with identity skip connections. These residual pathways facilitate uninterrupted gradient flow during backpropagation, enabling effective training of deeper architectures. The structure is well-suited for capturing both low-level anatomical cues and complex tumor progression dynamics across time.

The operation within each residual block is formalized by Eq. (7):

$$\mathbf{y} = \sigma\left(\mathrm{BN}_2\left(\mathrm{Conv}_2\left(\sigma\left(\mathrm{BN}_1\left(\mathrm{Conv}_1(\mathbf{x})\right)\right)\right)\right)\right) + \mathbf{x} \tag{7}$$

Here, Conv_1 and Conv_2 are 3D convolutional layers, BN_1 and BN_2 are batch normalization layers, and σ represents the ReLU activation function. The skip connection $\mathbf{x}$ preserves the identity mapping, promoting stable training.

3.6 3D DenseNet-121 Branch

The DenseNet branch adopts a 3D variant of DenseNet-121. It is built from densely connected 3D convolutional layers where each layer receives feature maps from all preceding layers through channel-wise concatenation. This promotes feature reuse, efficient parameterization, and improved gradient flow, which are particularly advantageous for capturing subtle spatial changes indicative of tumor progression.

The forward computation at the ℓth layer is described by Eq. (8):

$$\mathbf{x}_\ell = \mathrm{ReLU}\left(\mathrm{BN}_\ell\left(\mathrm{Conv}_\ell\left([\mathbf{x}_0, \mathbf{x}_1, \ldots, \mathbf{x}_{\ell-1}]\right)\right)\right) \tag{8}$$

Here, $[\cdot]$ denotes channel-wise concatenation of all preceding outputs. Batch normalization and ReLU activation enhance training stability and non-linearity, while the dense connectivity facilitates hierarchical learning across volumetric scans.

3.7 3D EfficientNet-B0 Branch

The EfficientNet branch leverages a 3D adaptation of EfficientNet-B0. This architecture uses compound scaling to jointly optimize depth, width, and resolution. It features mobile inverted bottleneck (MBConv) blocks enhanced with Squeeze-and-Excitation (SE) mechanisms for adaptive recalibration of feature channels.

The MBConv operation is expressed as Eq. (9):

$$\mathbf{y} = \mathbf{x} + \mathrm{SE}\left(\mathrm{BN}_3\left(\mathrm{DWConv}\left(\mathrm{BN}_2\left(\mathrm{Swish}\left(\mathrm{BN}_1\left(\mathrm{Conv}_{\mathrm{exp}}(\mathbf{x})\right)\right)\right)\right)\right)\right) \tag{9}$$

In this formulation, $\mathrm{Conv}_{\mathrm{exp}}$ is a pointwise 3D convolution for expanding channels, DWConv is a depthwise separable 3D convolution, and $\mathrm{SE}(\cdot)$ denotes the squeeze-and-excitation module. The non-linearity used is Swish ($x \cdot \mathrm{sigmoid}(x)$), which improves model expressiveness. The residual connection is retained when input and output dimensions align.

3.8 Ensemble Model and Fusion Strategy

The core of our architecture is defined by the `Brats3DEnsemble` class, which orchestrates the integration of ResNet, DenseNet, and EfficientNet in a parallel processing pipeline. Each model processes the input volume independently, producing a vector of class logits or probabilities. These outputs are then combined

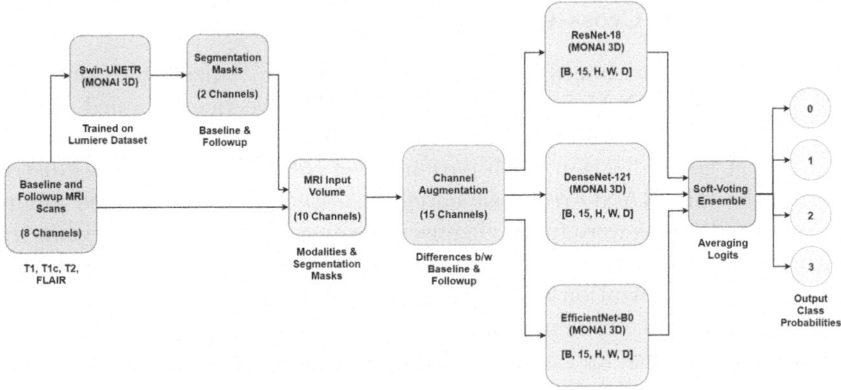

Fig. 2. Ensembled model architecture

through logit averaging [15], leveraging the diversity of model architectures to reduce predictive variance and enhance generalization.

Formally, the individual prediction from the m-th model is given in Eq. (10):

$$\mathbf{p}^{(m)} = f^{(m)}(\mathbf{x}) \tag{10}$$

where $f^{(m)}$ denotes the m-th model, $\mathbf{x}$ is the input volume, and $\mathbf{p}^{(m)}$ is the corresponding output logits.

The final ensemble prediction is computed according to Eq. (11):

$$\mathbf{p}_{\text{ensemble}} = \frac{1}{M} \sum_{m=1}^{M} \mathbf{p}^{(m)} \tag{11}$$

where M is the total number of models in the ensemble. This fusion mechanism encourages complementary learning and results in more stable and accurate classification performance across diverse response types (Fig. 2).

4 Results and Discussion

4.1 Experimental Setup

All experiments were conducted on a high-performance Linux-based workstation featuring dual NVIDIA A100 GPUs (80 GB each), 512 GB RAM, and AMD EPYC 7763 CPUs. The training pipeline was built using PyTorch 2.1 [16], with MONAI [17], TorchIO [18], and NumPy handling medical image preprocessing, augmentation, and tensor operations. Input data consisted of paired baseline-follow-up MRI volumes across four modalities (T1, T1ce, T2, FLAIR), optionally concatenated with segmentation masks to form 10-channel 3D tensors. Stratified tumor-centered patches of size 96×96×96 were extracted, and on-the-fly augmentations (affine, intensity shifts, elastic deformations, modality dropout, & tumor-masked cutmix [19]) were applied using TorchIO.

4.2 Training and Cross-validation

All three 3D CNN backbones in our ensemble were initialized with pre-trained weights from the MONAI framework [20], which have been trained on large-scale medical imaging datasets. A 5-fold stratified cross-validation strategy ensured robust generalization, with patient-level splits preserving class distribution across the four RANO response categories. Each fold was trained independently, and predictions were fused via ensemble averaging. Mixed precision training with PyTorch AMP and GradScaler reduced memory usage and improved training speed. Optimization utilized the AdamW optimizer with cosine annealing and warm restarts, gradient clipping (1.0), and label smoothing [21] ($\epsilon = 0.1$) to enhance convergence and address class imbalance. Early stopping (patience: 5 on 15–20 epochs) based on validation F1-score was applied.

4.3 Evaluation and Inference

Performance was assessed using a comprehensive suite of metrics, including F1 score, accuracy, AUROC, per-class precision/recall, and confusion matrices. Metrics were computed independently for each fold and then aggregated to report mean, standard deviation, and confidence intervals, offering statistical insight into model robustness. Model checkpoints were saved based on validation F1-score, with final predictions averaged across folds.

4.4 Performance Analysis

The results, summarized in Tables 3, 4, 5 and visualized in Fig. 3, highlight RECAP-Net's effectiveness in response classification across diverse clinical presentations. On the augmented Lumiere training data (Table 3), the model achieved high and consistent scores across all metrics. Performance on the BraTSPRO 2025 validation set (Table 4) demonstrated strong generalization, particularly for SD and PD classes. Results on the final testing phase dataset (Table 5) further confirmed RECAP-Net's stability across all RANO categories.

Table 3. Quantitative Comparison of Models on the Augmented Lumiere Dataset

Model	Balanced Accuracy	F1 Score	TPR	TNR	Precision	AUROC
ResNet-10	0.8710	0.8740	0.8780	0.8820	0.8730	0.8790
ResNet-18	0.8860	0.8850	0.8920	0.8910	0.8840	0.8900
DenseNet-121	0.8980	0.9000	0.9060	0.9110	0.8970	0.9110
EfficientNet-B0	0.9160	0.9180	0.9200	0.9270	0.9150	0.9280
RECAP-Net	**0.9400**	**0.9460**	**0.9510**	**0.9550**	**0.9420**	**0.9600**

Table 4. Validation performance metrics across RANO response categories.

Category	TP	FP	FN	TN	Bal. Acc	F1	TPR	TNR	AP	ROC-AUC
Complete Response	0	0	1	13	0.50	0.00	0.00	1.00	0.071	0.50
Partial Response	0	0	2	12	0.50	0.00	0.00	1.00	0.143	0.50
Stable Disease	3	6	1	4	0.575	0.462	0.75	0.40	0.321	0.575
Progressive Disease	2	3	5	4	0.429	0.333	0.286	0.571	0.471	0.429

Table 5. Testing Phase Results

Category	F1-Score	Balanced Accuracy	Average Precision
CR	0.0000	0.5000	0.0056
PR	0.2222	0.4825	0.1698
SD	0.0000	0.4992	0.2811
PD	0.5767	0.5034	0.5406
Mean	**0.1997**	**0.4963**	**0.2493**

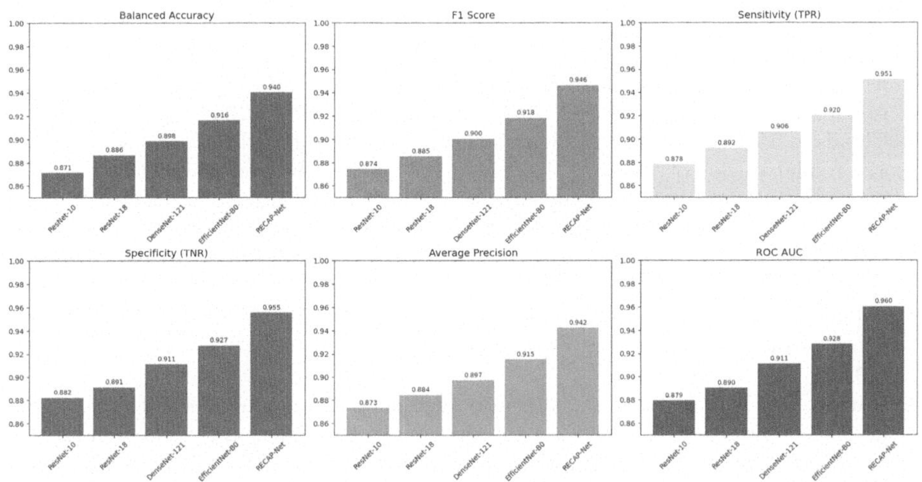

Fig. 3. Visual comparison of *RECAP-Net* with other 3D CNN architectures.

Acknowledgments. The authors would like to express their sincere gratitude to the **Centre of Excellence (CoE) in Artificial Intelligence (AI)**, Netaji Subhas University of Technology (NSUT), New Delhi, for their invaluable support throughout the course of this research. Data used in this publication were obtained as part of the challenge project through **Synapse ID (syn64153130)**.

Disclosure of Interests. *The authors declare that they have no competing financial or non-financial interests that could have appeared to influence the work reported in this article.*

References

1. Lan, Z., Li, X., Zhang, X.: Glioblastoma: an update in pathology, molecular mechanisms and biomarkers. Int. J. Mol. Sci. **25**(5), 3040 (2024)
2. Raman, F., et al.: Evaluation of rano criteria for the assessment of tumor progression for lower-grade gliomas. Cancers **15**(13), 3274 (2023)
3. Kickingereder, P., Isensee, F., et al.: Automated quantitative tumor response assessment of mri in neuro-oncology with artificial neural networks: a multicentre, retrospective study. Lancet Oncol. **20**(5), 728–740 (2019)
4. HD-GLIO-AUTO. https://github.com/CCI-Bonn/HD-GLIO-AUTO. Accessed 18 June 2025
5. DeepBraTumIA. https://www.nitrc.org/projects/deepbratumia/. Accessed 18 June 2025
6. Suter, Y., Knecht, U., Valenzuela, W., Notter, M., Hewer, E., Schucht, P., Wiest, R., Reyes, M.: The lumiere dataset: Longitudinal glioblastoma mri with expert rano evaluation. Sci. Data **9**(1), 768 (2022)
7. Miyato, T., Kataoka, T., Koyama, M., Yoshida, Y.: Spectral normalization for generative adversarial networks. In: International Conference on Learning Representations (ICLR) (2018)
8. Kingma, D.P., Ba, J.: Adam: a method for stochastic optimization. arXiv preprint arXiv:1412.6980 (2014)
9. Ayyachamy, S., Alex, V., Khened, M., Krishnamurthi, G.: Medical image retrieval using resnet-18. In: Medical imaging 2019: imaging informatics for healthcare, research, and applications, vol. 10954, pp. 233–241. SPIE (2019)
10. Chhabra, M., Kumar, R.: A smart healthcare system based on classifier densenet 121 model to detect multiple diseases. In: Mobile radio communications and 5G networks: proceedings of second MRCN 2021, pp. 297–312. Springer (2022)
11. Kansal, K., Chandra, T.B., Singh, A.: Resnet-50 vs. efficientnet-b0: multi-centric classification of various lung abnormalities using deep learning. Procedia Comput. Sci. **235**, 70–80 (2024)
12. Gillot, M., et al.: Automatic multi-anatomical skull structure segmentation of cone-beam computed tomography scans using 3d unetr. PLoS ONE **17**(10), e0275033 (2022)
13. Ruthra, E., Ruhan Bevi, A.: 3d auto segmentation module for ischemic stroke lesions from monai. In: 2023 First International Conference on Advances in Electrical, Electronics and Computational Intelligence (ICAEECI), pp. 1–5. IEEE (2023)
14. Hatamizadeh, A., Nath, V., Tang, Y., Yang, D., Roth, H.R., Xu, D.: Swin unetr: swin transformers for semantic segmentation of brain tumors in mri images. In *International MICCAI brainlesion workshop*, pp. 272–284. Springer (2021)
15. Lakshminarayanan, B., Pritzel, A., Blundell, C.: Simple and scalable predictive uncertainty estimation using deep ensembles. Advances in Neural Information Processing Systems, 30 (2017)
16. Paszke, A., et al.: Pytorch: an imperative style, high-performance deep learning library. Advances in Neural Information Processing Systems, 32 (2019)
17. Jorge Cardoso, M., Li, W., Brown, R., et al.: Monai: an open-source framework for deep learning in healthcare. Comput. Sci. Eng. **25**(2), 18–29 (2023)
18. Pérez-García, F., Sparks, R., Ourselin, S.: Torchio: a python library for efficient loading, preprocessing, augmentation and patch-based sampling of medical images in deep learning. Comput. Methods Programs Biomed. **208**, 106236 (2021)

19. Yun, S., Han, D., Oh, S.J., Chun, S., Choe, J., Yoo, Y.: Cutmix: regularization strategy to train strong classifiers with localizable features. In: Proceedings of the IEEE/CVF International Conference on Computer Vision, pp. 6023–6032 (2019)
20. MONAI Consortium. MONAI: Medical Open Network for AI (2023). https://monai.io/. Accessed 15 Sept 2025
21. Szegedy, C., Vanhoucke, V., Ioffe, S., Shlens, J., Wojna, Z.: Rethinking the inception architecture for computer vision. In: *Proceedings of the IEEE Conference on Computer Vision and Pattern Recognition*, pp. 2818–2826 (2016)

Challenge 12 – AIMS-TBI

Automated Identification of Moderate-to-Severe Traumatic Brain Injury Lesions (AIMS-TBI) 2025 MICCAI Challenge

Evelyn Deutscher[1(✉)], Nicholas J. Tustison[2], Adrian Onicas[3], Elisabeth A. Wilde[3,4,5], Matthew Pease[6], Spyridon Bakas[7], and Emily L. Dennis[3,4]

[1] Cognitive Neuroscience Unit, School of Psychology, Deakin University, Melbourne, Australia
edeutscher@deakin.edu.au

[2] Department of Radiology and Medical Imaging, University of Virginia, Charlottesville, VA, USA

[3] Traumatic Brain Injury and Concussion Center, Department of Neurology, University of Utah, Salt Lake City, UT, USA

[4] George E. Wahlen Veterans Affairs Salt Lake City Healthcare System, Salt Lake City, UT, USA

[5] H. Ben Taub Department of Physical Medicine and Rehabilitation, Baylor College of Medicine, Houston, TX, USA

[6] Department of Neurosurgery, Indiana University, Bloomington, IN, USA

[7] Division of Computational Pathology, Indiana School of Medicine, Indianapolis, IN, USA

Abstract. T1-weighted (T1-w) anatomical magnetic resonance imaging (MRI) enable us to identify injuries (e.g., extent, location, type of lesion, size etc.) within the brains of individuals with moderate-to-severe traumatic brain injury (ms-TBI). Lesion segmentation is a key step prior to running advanced neuroimaging analyses (such as connectomics, tractography); however, to date, no automated lesion segmentation tools have been developed for T1-w images of patients with ms-TBI. To find a solution to this, we established this second edition of the MICCAI challenge with two key improvements. First, the number of images available for training was increased. All images were shared through the Enhancing NeuroImaging Genetics through Meta-Analysis (ENIGMA) Brain Injury working group. Overall, 1100 T1-w scans from individuals with ms-TBI across 12 sites. Data from 875 images underwent manual lesion segmentation using a team of 13 manual raters. For these analyses, 552 images were used in the training dataset, 100 for validation, and 223 for the final test set. Secondly, the metrics used to rank teams based on performance were improved to better reflect the dual nature of the detection and segmentation task at hand by looking at the accuracy of images with visible lesions, and those without visible lesions separately. During the validation phase, 19 submissions were received, and 9 teams submitted the final test set.

Keywords: brain MRI · lesion · traumatic brain injury · segmentation

S. Bakas et al. (Eds.): MICCAI 2025, LNCS 16377, pp. 273–281, 2026.
https://doi.org/10.1007/978-3-032-16370-7_24

1 Introduction

Moderate to Severe Traumatic Brain Injury (msTBI) is caused by external forces (eg: traffic accidents, falls, sports) causing the brain to move rapidly within the skull, resulting in complex pathophysiological changes. Primary injuries arising from the initial forces (e.g., haematoma, hemorrhages, and contusions) (Mckee & Daneshvar, 2015), subsequently induce a cascade of secondary injuries (e.g., gliosis, encephalomalacia, (Maas et al., 2022)) that can include life threatening disorders such as raised intracranial pressure, requiring acute surgical intervention (Bullock et al., 2006). Each of these primary, secondary, and surgery related processes can cause structural deformation in the brain. Each patient with msTBI has a unique accumulation of these structural changes, contributing to extremely heterogeneous lesions, considered a hallmark of msTBI (Covington & Duff, 2021).

In addition to heterogeneity in neuropathology, long-term functional outcomes after msTBI also vary widely. To better understand this variability, researchers and clinicians are increasingly looking to advanced neuroimaging approaches including personalised connectomics and single-subject profiling (Imms et al., 2022; Zeiler et al., 2021). However, these advanced analyses are underpinned by a series of image processing steps including registration, normalization, and parcellation, which are vulnerable to producing errors in the presence of ms-TBI lesions which disrupt tissue boundaries and intensity profiles (Diamond et al., 2020; King et al., 2020). T1-weighted (T1w) MRI scans form the foundation for many advanced imaging pipelines, are used directly to calculate brain morphometrics, and therefore present a starting point for mitigating the influence of lesion induced errors in advanced neuroimaging. A critical first step is the reliable identification and segmentation of lesions on T1w images.

While a multitude of automated lesion segmentation tools have been developed (Gryska et al., 2021), the majority are optimised for use in other common brain pathologies such as stroke (Bey et al., 2024; Pustina et al., 2016), multiple sclerosis (Spampinato et al., 2025; Dereskewicz et al., 2025), and brain tumor (Andrearczyk et al., 2024; LaBella et al. 2024), these tools do not translate well to identifying msTBI lesions due to substantial differences in pathology. The automated identification of traumatic brain injury lesions challenge (AIMS-TBI) was developed to address this gap. The AIMS-TBI challenge leverages data shared within the Enhancing NeuroImaging Genetics through Meta-Analysis (ENIGMA) Consortium (Thompson et al., 2022) Traumatic Brain Injury working group, specifically, the Pediatric msTBI and Adult msTBI subgroups.

The goal of AIMS-TBI is to generate algorithms that can accurately detect and segment 3D lesions, defined as structural damage visible on T1-w MRI due to TBI that may include contusions, hemorrhage, hematoma, encephalomalacia, gliosis, white matter lesions, and surgical drainage tracts.

The inaugural AIMS-TBI Challenge was held at the 2024 MICCAI conference (Deutscher et al., 2025; https://doi.org/10.31234/osf.io/mw5zx_v1). The final AIMS-TBI 2024 dataset comprised a total of 764 images, including 388 images for training, 101 for validation, and 275 for testing. In the validation phase of the challenge, 12 submissions were uploaded, with 5 teams submitting final models in the test stage. The best performing model achieved an average Dice score of 0.61. This result represented a successful first challenge, yet also highlighted substantial room for improvement. The

2025 challenge boasts a larger training dataset and improved metrics to better understand model performance

2 Methods

2.1 Data Collation

Images used in the creation of the AIMS-TBI challenge were shared across 12 institutions within the ENIGMA Brain Injury working group. Table 1 provides an overview of the original data collection sites. From the 1,100 T1-weighted (T1-w) MRI images collated from individuals with ms-TBI, a total of 875 of those were made available for the purposes of this challenge (age mean = 29.3 years (SD = 18.5), range = 5.83–85 years, 325 female). TBI severity was defined using either 1) the Mayo classification system (Malec et al., 2007) or a Glasgow Coma Scale score (Teasdale & Bennett, 1974) at the time of hospital admission; 2) loss of consciousness 30 min or greater; and 3) post-traumatic amnesia >24 h (Rabinowitz & Levin, 2014). T1-w images from all patients were collected across injury phases (from acute to chronic) with time since injury ranging from 0–5801.78 weeks (mean = 196.7 weeks (SD = 436). Informed consent was provided by participants in accordance with local ethics guidelines.

2.2 Data Preparation

Prior to undergoing the initial automated lesion segmentation, images were resampled to dimensions 256 x 256, and a voxel size of 1mm^3 isotropic. Images were defaced using *pydeface* (Gulban et al., 2022), and lesions smaller than 10 voxels were excluded. No further image processing was performed.

2.3 Initial Automated Lesion Segmentation

As an initial step in creating the AIMS-TBI24 dataset, a vanilla u-net was trained on the ATLAS v2.0 dataset using the ANTsPy/ANTsPyNet packages, and further trained on a preliminary set of 200 completed manual segmentations from the AIMS-TBI dataset. Training scripts are available (https://github.com/ntustison/ANTsXNetTraining/blob/main/Lesions/). Although useful in identifying large lesions (reflecting the nature of stroke data), the automatically generated masks still required substantial manual edits and thorough review of all other brain regions to ensure that no smaller lesions were missed.

2.4 Manual Lesion Segmentation

Training. A total of 13 raters completed training prior to beginning lesion segmentation. Training included two training seminars, reading protocol documents, and completing segmentations on a small training dataset of 14 images. Annotators achieved a minimum Dice score of 0.6 (compared to a ground truth segmentation provided by one of the expert raters) on the training set of images, before moving onto complete segmentations on the challenge dataset.

Lesion Segmentation. During the manual segmentation, images were excluded if the rater deemed the image quality to be substantially impacted by factors such as ringing, wraparound, motion or susceptibility, or other artifacts. A total of 57 images were excluded during this stage. Manual segmentation and editing of the initial automated manual lesion segmentations was performed in ITK-snap (www.itksnap.org). For all images a binary lesion mask was created. For patients with no visible lesions, the lesion mask file was empty. The manual masks were created in a sequential process whereby, one primary rater reviewed the initial automated lesion segmentation result and performed manual edits. Next, a second rater reviewed the edited mask created by the first rater and provided additional edits if necessary. And finally, third and final expert rater reviewed the lesion segmentation, provided minor edits if necessary, and approved the segmentations for inclusion in the challenge dataset (any minor edits were communicated back to the primary raters to improve their following segmentations)

Publication of Testing, Training, and Validation Datasets. The final AIMS-TBI 2024 dataset comprised a total of 875 images, split into 552 for training, 100 for validation and 223 for testing. Data were anonymized by stripping identifying information from the header and assigning each scan with a new randomized ID shuffled across sites. Participating teams agreed to use the data only for challenge purposes prior to receiving access to the de-identified data via Box. During training, participating teams could download both the T1-w images and corresponding binary lesion masks, available in neuroimaging informatics technology initiative (NIfTI) image format. During the validation phase, teams uploaded their code as docker container submissions via the Grand Challenge website where they could view rankings and make multiple submissions but had no access to data. The final date for submissions of the test phase was 31st August 2025. The final test has been created to mirror a real-world distribution capturing variances in lesion heterogeneity, whilst also considering the balance of class distribution across training, validation, and testing environments. This strategy aims to create a realistic training and testing environment to develop algorithms capable of identifying heterogeneous lesion types present in real world ms-TBI research data sets. We have ensured that the training and test sets have similar distributions with regard to age, sex, time since injury, and scan manufacturer. All data in the test set were new, unseen data.

Up to 10% missing data was accepted, with scores calculated across the remaining data. Beyond 10% missing data, the scores for missing cases were incorporated into calculations.

As our intention is primarily to create a working lesion segmentation tool applicable to varied real-world ms-TBI datasets, participants were allowed to use additional training data from publicly available datasets and their own institutions to further complement the challenge data.

Table 1. Breakdown of relevant demographic, clinical, and scan characteristics of challenge data

	Training	Validation	Test	Overall
N (Total)	552	100	223	875
N lesion +ve (%)	322 (58.3)	53 (53)	149 (66.8)	524 (59.9)

(continued)

Table 1. *(continued)*

	Training	Validation	Test	Overall
n females (%)	215 (38.9)	37 (37)	73 (32.7)	325 (37.1)
Age (min – max, years)	6.08–85	8–69	5.8–70	5.83–85
TSI (min-max, weeks)	0–5801.78	1.71–1419.60	0.85–3215.33	0–5801.78
Scan Manufacturer [n(%)]				
Philips	167 (30.3)	9 (9)	48 (21.5)	224 (25.6)
GE	113 (20.5)	44 (44)	81 (36.3)	238 (27.2)
Siemens	272 (49.3)	47 (47)	94 (42.2)	413 (47.2)

Note. TSI = time since injury. GE = General Electric. Lesion +ve = T1w images with visible lesions present

2.5 Algorithm Performance Assessment

Metrics. Performance of the submitted algorithms was assessed using four metrics. The metrics chosen were selected to assess both lesion detection accuracy and lesion segmentation accuracy. Formulas 1 and 2 show the calculation of each metric, where the number of true-positives, false-positives, true-negatives and false negatives, are denoted by TP, FP, TN and FN respectively.

Balanced Accuracy:

$$BA = \frac{1}{2}\left(\frac{TP}{TP + FN} + \frac{TN}{TN + FP}\right) \tag{1}$$

Dice similarity coefficient- DSC (voxel-wise):

$$DSC = \frac{2TP}{2TP + FN + FP} \tag{2}$$

Three DSC scores were calculated for each team; (1) DSC for lesions, used only images with visible lesions, (2) the DSC for no lesion was calculated from all images with no visible lesions where the ground truth lesion masks were empty, (3) An overall DSC score was calculated by averaging DSC scores across all images (lesions and no lesions).

Ranking Methods. To identify the algorithm with the best overall performance with respect to both lesion detection accuracy and lesion segmentation accuracy, average scores were computed for each of the four metrics. The teams received a rank of 1 through N (number of teams participating) for each of the four metrics with rank 1 for DSC and BA score given to the team with the highest values. These four ranks were summed and the team with the largest total sum received first place.

3 Results

In the validation phase of the challenge, 19 submissions were uploaded to the docker. At the test stage, 9 teams submitted their final algorithms. Table 2 lists overall rankings and metric scores for participating teams at completion of the test phase (Fig. 1).

Table 2. Rankings and individual scores across teams

Ranking	Team	Balanced accuracy	Overall Dice	Dice lesions	Dice no lesion
1	iMedIA_2025	0.8924	0.6371	0.4904	0.9324
2	AIMHI-MEDAI	0.8622	0.6305	0.4805	0.9324
3	NIC-VICOROB	0.8554	0.6351	0.4941	0.9189
4	SpaceCY*	0.8383	0.6176	0.5149	0.8243
5	jianghaotian0001*	0.8585	0.6085	0.5013	0.8243
6	Biomedia-GV	0.8451	0.5973	0.4711	0.8514
7	Süsü	0.7549	0.4963	0.2759	0.973
8	Team Dolphin	0.8044	0.5658	0.491	0.7162
9	Team CVHCI	0.7245	0.5179	0.3322	0.8919

* No paper submitted

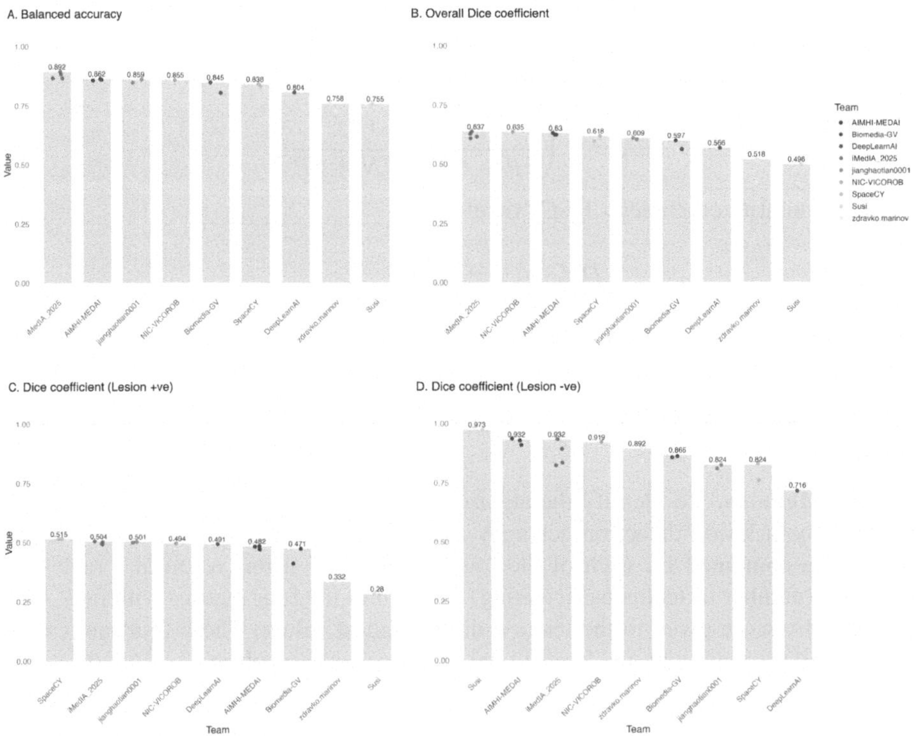

Fig. 1. Rankings and individual scores from the test phase across teams. Bars show the maximum performance metric of each team across submissions. Lesion +ve = T1w images with visible lesions present; Lesion -ve = T1w images without visible lesions

4 Discussion

The AIMS-TBI challenge presents an extremely complex lesion detection and segmentation task. Given the immense heterogeneity among lesion size, location, and appearance in ms-TBI, automated algorithms continue to struggle to achieve accurate segmentation. While several teams reached impressive segmentation scores during the validation phase of this challenge, the final results on the test set leave significant room for improvement. The reliable, automatic detection and segmentation of ms-TBI lesions in T1w images is an important step towards mitigating lesion induced errors in advanced neuroimaging pipelines. The AIMS-TBI authorship team is dedicated to generating a reliable and accurate tool for performing automated lesion segmentation in ms-TBI lesions, as a result, we have highlighted current limitations and future improvements which will be addressed in time for submission at next year's 2026 MICCAI conference.

4.1 Limitations

The AIMS-TBI challenge dataset was specifically designed to represent real-world scenarios, such that the exact type of lesions occurring across training, validation and test sets were not balanced exactly. Whilst this design is justified in respect to developing a tool that will be applicable to a range of real-world ms-TBI research, we acknowledge that this likely plays a part in reduced accuracy in the test data, potentially as a result of models overfitting to the lesions present in the training and validation datasets. Additionally, one of the main limitations of this challenge is that the lesion masks created represent a ground truth binary mask only. The varied pathological appearance of ms-TBI lesions may lend themselves more naturally to a multi-class segmentation challenge.

4.2 Future Improvements

Future iterations of the AIMS-TBI challenge will re-design the binary lesion masks to represent a multi class lesion segmentation challenge. This improved challenge design will enable the development of algorithms capable of distinguishing between different lesion characteristics (e.g.: contusions, haemorrhage and encephalomalacia) and it's hoped would subsequently improve overall detection and segmentation accuracy across images.

5 Conclusion

Following last year's challenge, AIMS-TBI25 was yet again a successful event at MICCAI 2025. With a larger dataset and improved metrics, AIMS-TBI25 provides a deeper understanding of the difficulties faced by the competing teams and their algorithms. There remains a critical gap in the field of ms-TBI research due to the absence of a reliable and accurate lesion segmentation tool for use on T1w images from individuals with a ms-TBI. AIMS-TBI is determined to develop a solution to this in future challenges.

Acknowledgements. This work was supported by NIH R01NS122184 to ELD and EAW. We gratefully acknowledge the contributions of the lesion raters – Courtney McCabe, Jamie Johnson, Emma Read, Ella Sybrowsky, Elizabeth Hovenden, Madi Reading, Dayna Thayn, Finian Keleher, Jake Mitchell, Hannah Lindsey, and Morgan Hafen.

Disclosure of Interest. The authors report that they have no relevant conflicting interests.

References

Andrearczyk, V., et al.: Automatic detection and multi-component segmentation of brain metastases in longitudinal MRI. Sci. Rep. **14**(1), 31603 (2024)

Bey, P., et al.: A lesion-aware automated processing framework for clinical stroke magnetic resonance imaging. Hum. Brain Mapp. **45**(9), e26701 (2024)

Covington, N.V., Duff, M.C.: Heterogeneity is a hallmark of traumatic brain injury, not a limitation: a new perspective on study design in rehabilitation research. Am. J. Speech Lang. Pathol. **30**(2S), 974–85 (2021)

Dereskewicz, E., et al.: FLAMeS: a robust deep learning model for automated multiple sclerosis lesion segmentation. medRxiv, 2025-05 (2025)

Deutscher, E., Tustison, N., Wilde, E., Caeyenberghs, K., Dennis, E.L.: Automated Identification of Moderate-to-Severe Traumatic Brain Injury Lesions (AIMS-TBI) MICCAI 2024 Challenge (2025). https://doi.org/10.31234/osf.io/mw5zx_v1

Diamond, B.R., Donald, C.L.M., Frau-Pascual, A., Snider, S.B., Fischl, B., Dams-O'Connor, K., et al.: Optimizing the accuracy of cortical volumetric analysis in traumatic brain injury. MethodsX **7**, 100994 (2020)

Gryska, E., Schneiderman, J., Björkman-Burtscher, I., Heckemann, R.A.: Automatic brain lesion segmentation on standard magnetic resonance images: a scoping review. BMJ Open. **11**(1), e042660 (2021). https://doi.org/10.1136/bmjopen-2020-042660

Gulban, O.F., Nielson, D., lee, J., Poldrack, R., Gorgolewski, C., Vanessasaurus, et al.: poldrack-lab/pydeface: PyDeface v2.0.2 [Internet]. Zenodo (2022). https://zenodo.org/records/6856482. [cited 2025 Sep 24]

Imms, P., Clemente, A., Deutscher, E., Radwan, A.M., Akhlaghi, H., Beech, P., et al.: Exploring personalised structural connectomics for moderate-to-severe traumatic brain injury. Netw. Neurosci. 1–50 (2022)

King, D.J, Novak, J., Shephard, A.J., Beare, R., Anderson, V.A., Wood, A.G.: Lesion induced error on automated measures of brain volume: data from a pediatric traumatic brain injury cohort. Front. Neurosci. **14**, 491478 (2020)

LaBella, D., et al.: Brain tumor segmentation (brats) challenge 2024: Meningioma radiotherapy planning automated segmentation. arXiv e-prints, arXiv-2405 (2024)

Maas, A.I.R., et al.: Traumatic brain injury: Progress and challenges in prevention, clinical care, and research. Lancet Neurol. **21**(11), 1004–1060 (2022). https://doi.org/10.1016/S1474-4422(22)00309-X

Malec, J.F., et al.: The mayo classification system for traumatic brain injury severity. J. Neurotrauma. **24**(9), 1417–1424 (2007)

Mckee, A.C., Daneshvar, D.H.: The neuropathology of traumatic brain injury. Handb. Clin. Neurol. **127**, 45–66 (2015)

Pustina, D., Coslett, H.B., Turkeltaub, P.E., Tustison, N., Schwartz, M.F., Avants, B.: Automated segmentation of chronic stroke lesions using LINDA: lesion identification with neighborhood data analysis. Hum. Brain Mapp. **37**(4), 1405–1421 (2016)

Rabinowitz, A.R., Levin, H.S.: Cognitive sequelae of traumatic brain injury. Psychiatr. Clin. **37**(1), 1–11 (2014)

Spampinato, M.V., et al.: Cross-sectional validation of an automated lesion segmentation software in multiple sclerosis: comparison with radiologist assessments. Am. J. Neuroradiol. **46**(7), 1510–1516 (2025)

Teasdale, G., Jennett, B.: Assessment of coma and impaired consciousness: a practical scale. The lancet **304**(7872), 81–84 (1974)

Thompson, P.M., Jahanshad, N., Ching, C.R.K., Salminen, L.E., Thomopoulos, S.I., Bright, J., et al.: ENIGMA and global neuroscience: a decade of large-scale studies of the brain in health and disease across more than 40 countries. Transl. Psychiatry **10**(1), 100 (2020)

Zeiler, F.A., Mathieu, F., Monteiro, M., Glocker, B., Ercole, A., Cabeleira, M., et al.: Systemic markers of injury and injury response are not associated with impaired cerebrovascular reactivity in adult traumatic brain injury: a collaborative European neurotrauma effectiveness research in traumatic brain injury (CENTER-TBI) study. J. Neurotrauma **38**(7), 870–878 (2021)

Not All Ensembles Are Equal: A Short Study on Moderate to Severe Traumatic Brain Injury Segmentation Methods

Zdravko Marinov[1](✉), Jens Kleesiek[2,3], and Rainer Stiefelhagen[1]

[1] Karlsruhe Institute of Technology, Karlsruhe, Germany
zdravko.marinov@kit.edu
[2] Institute for AI in Medicine, University Hospital Essen, Essen, Germany
[3] Cancer Research Center Cologne Essen (CCCE), University Medicine Essen, Essen, Germany

Abstract. Lesion segmentation in Moderate to Severe Traumatic Brain Injury (msTBI) is challenging due to the wide variability in lesion size, location, and appearance. The AIMS-TBI Segmentation Challenge 2025 provided a benchmark for evaluating methods on T1-weighted MRI data. In our submission, we focus on a deliberately simple approach: training standard U-Net models without pretraining or external datasets, and exploring how postprocessing and ensembling strategies can improve performance. We find that an ensemble of just two models yields consistent gains over single models, and that performance can be further improved by applying a two-stage ensembling scheme: first at the level of lesion detection (presence vs. absence), and then at the level of segmentation map aggregation. Our results demonstrate that high-quality msTBI lesion segmentation does not necessarily require large-scale pretraining or complex networks. Instead, careful ensemble design and simple postprocessing are effective levers for boosting performance in the challenge setting.

Keywords: Traumatic Brain Injury · T1-weighted MRI · Ensembling

1 Introduction

Moderate to Severe Traumatic Brain Injury (msTBI) is a leading cause of long-term neurological disability worldwide, typically resulting from high-impact events such as road traffic accidents, falls, or sports collisions. These injuries trigger a cascade of complex pathophysiological processes. Primary insults, including hematomas, hemorrhages, and contusions, arise at the moment of impact [21], while secondary injuries such as gliosis and encephalomalacia evolve in the days to weeks following trauma [18]. Acute complications like raised intracranial pressure often necessitate surgical intervention [2]. Together, these processes produce widespread and heterogeneous structural alterations in the brain, a hallmark feature of msTBI [3] as seen in Fig. 1.

S. Bakas et al. (Eds.): MICCAI 2025, LNCS 16377, pp. 282–291, 2026.
https://doi.org/10.1007/978-3-032-16370-7_25

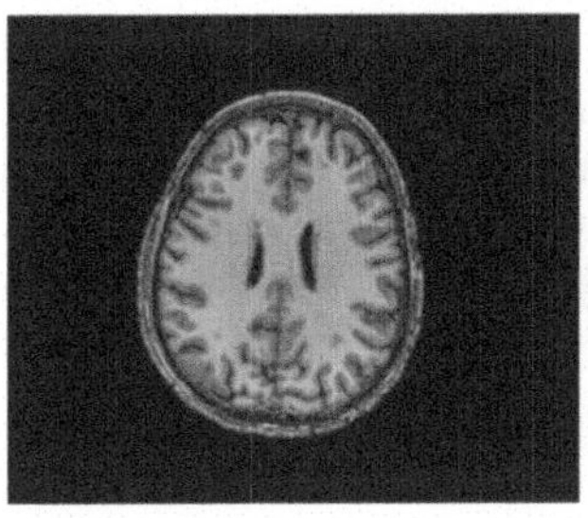
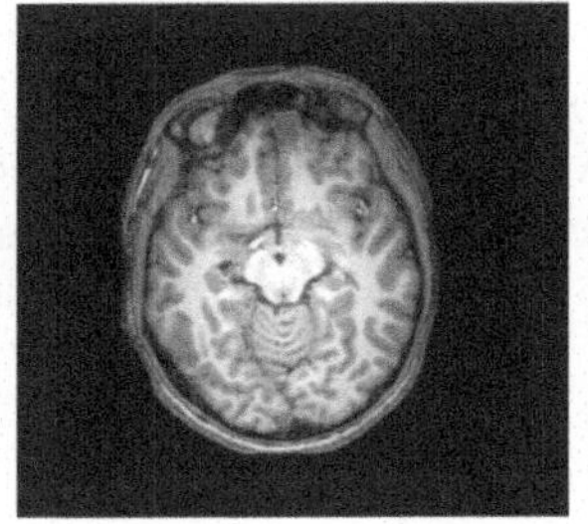
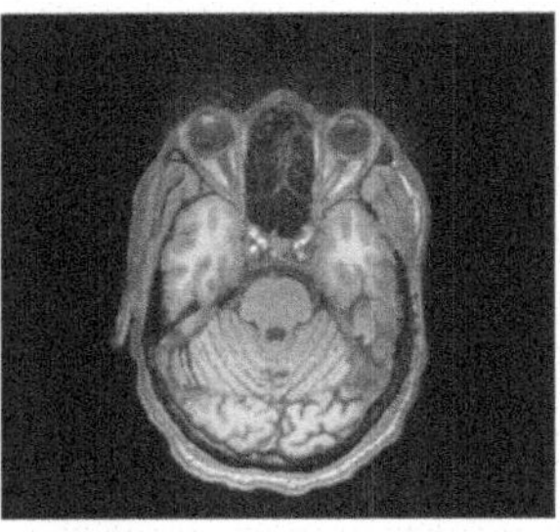

Fig. 1. Variability of msTBI cases in terms of location, affected anatomy, and size. Images are from the training set of the AIMS-TBI Challenge 2025.

Unlike lesions associated with stroke or tumors, which tend to be more localized, msTBI lesions can be focal or diffuse, unilateral or bilateral, and frequently span multiple tissue types (gray matter, white matter, and cerebrospinal fluid). This diversity complicates core neuroimaging tasks such as registration and normalization, and has been shown to induce systematic errors in cortical parcellation and morphometric analyses [6,16]. While lesion-aware preprocessing tools such as HD_Bet [12] and Virtual Brain Grafting (VBG) [22] have been developed, these often depend on manual lesion masks or extensive quality control, making them impractical for large datasets. Moreover, automated segmentation methods designed for other etiologies, such as stroke or tumors [24], do not generalize well to TBI cases.

In practice, many msTBI studies either ignore lesions altogether, exclude patients with large lesions, or rely on labor-intensive manual segmentation [1,4,17]. These approaches limit reproducibility and scalability, preventing researchers from adequately studying variability in lesion type, severity, and comorbidities across large cohorts. To move beyond small single-site investigations, the field requires automated segmentation methods trained on multi-site, multi-cohort MRI datasets. Existing TBI-specific approaches show promise, but often depend on multiple imaging modalities (e.g., T1, T2, FLAIR, GE, PD) [14] or focus exclusively on CT scans [13], which restricts their applicability.

The AIMS-TBI Segmentation Challenge was launched to address this gap by leveraging data from the ENIGMA TBI working group [25], including both pediatric and adult cohorts. Importantly, the challenge emphasizes the use of T1-weighted MRI only, as it is the most commonly available modality across sites and exhibits lower variability in acquisition protocols compared to modalities like diffusion MRI [5,15]. The inaugural challenge, hosted at MICCAI 2024, provided 764 scans split into training, validation, and test sets. Despite encouraging results, with the top-performing method achieving a Dice score of 0.61, the competition highlighted significant opportunities for improvement. Accurate lesion segmentation remains a prerequisite for advanced analyses such as parcellation, functional and structural connectivity, and fixel-based modeling, all of which have the potential to inform prognosis and treatment in msTBI.

Against this backdrop, we present our submission to the AIMS-TBI 2024 Challenge. In contrast to approaches relying on pretraining or multi-modal data, our work demonstrates how standard U-Net architectures, when combined with carefully designed postprocessing and ensembling strategies, can achieve competitive performance in a purely T1-weighted setting.

2 Methods

2.1 U-Net Training

We train all our models only on the 322 training volumes that include lesions, i.e., have a non-empty label. For the segmentation of moderate to severe traumatic brain injury (msTBI) lesions, we adopt an ensemble-based approach using multiple U-Net models [23]. Specifically, we train an ensemble of five U-Net networks through a 5-fold cross-validation strategy. This setup allows each model to learn slightly different features from the training data, increasing the robustness and generalizability of the predictions when combined in the ensemble. To complement this, we also train an additional U-Net model using the full training dataset without any folds. This model serves as a baseline to evaluate the benefits of cross-validation and ensemble averaging.

All six models employ the SW-FastEdit implementation of U-Net [9], which was originally developed for interactive click-based PET/CT lesion annotation [19,20] on the autoPET dataset [7,8]. In our study, we adapt the network for fully automated segmentation by removing the interactive click inputs [10] and modifying the pre-processing steps to accommodate T1-weighted MRI scans. This choice was motivated by SW-FastEdit's efficient handling of volumetric data and its proven performance in medical image segmentation tasks.

We train our models using a sliding window inference scheme with cubic patches of size $128 \times 128 \times 128$ voxels and an overlap of 25%. Gaussian weighting is applied to the overlapping regions, ensuring smoother aggregation of predictions. Gradients are averaged across overlapping patches during backpropagation to stabilize training. This approach allows the network to process large 3D images while maintaining manageable memory requirements.

Training is conducted for 300 epochs without any data augmentation. We normalize all MRI volumes using standard z-score normalization to reduce intensity variability across scans, which is critical when combining heterogeneous data. Optimization is performed using a combination of Dice Loss and cross-entropy loss, weighted equally to balance region-level and voxel-wise accuracy. A cosine annealing learning rate schedule is employed, starting from 1×10^{-4}, to facilitate convergence and prevent overfitting.

Our network backbone is the MONAI DynUNet[1], configured with five encoder-decoder levels. This results in a compact model, which is highly memory- and computationally efficient while still providing sufficient capacity to capture the heterogeneous msTBI lesions. A summary of all training parameters is provided in Table 1.

[1] https://docs.monai.io/en/0.7.0/_modules/monai/networks/nets/dynunet.html.

Overall, this training strategy balances efficiency, robustness, and accuracy, enabling our models to handle the complex and variable nature of msTBI lesions while remaining suitable for large-scale datasets.

Table 1. Detailed overview of the U-Net training configuration for msTBI lesion segmentation.

Hyperparameter	Configuration/Value
Network Architecture	MONAI DynUNet with 3 encoder-decoder levels
Total Trainable Parameters	∼31 million
Implementation Source	SW-FastEdit [9] adapted for T1-weighted MRI
Input Patch Dimensions	128 × 128 × 128 voxels
Sliding Window Overlap	25% between adjacent patches
Patch Weighting	Gaussian weighting in overlapping regions
Gradient Aggregation	Averaged across overlapping patches during backpropagation
Loss Function	Combination of Dice Loss and Cross-Entropy Loss (1:1 weighting)
Optimizer	Adam with initial learning rate 1×10^{-4}, cosine annealing schedule
Number of Training Epochs	300
Data Augmentation	Not applied (raw images only)
Intensity Normalization	Per-image z-score normalization
Training Mode	Fully automatic (non-interactive, no clicks) [10]

2.2 nnU-Net Training

In addition to the U-Net ensemble, we train a separate nnU-Net model [12] as part of our overall segmentation strategy. The nnU-Net framework is widely regarded as a robust baseline for medical image segmentation tasks, particularly when task-specific architectural tuning is limited. Its popularity stems from its strong out-of-the-box performance across diverse datasets, making it a reliable choice when minimal expert intervention is desired.

We train the nnU-Net model for 300 epochs using the full training dataset. Unlike our SW-FastEdit U-Nets, nnU-Net automatically applies a set of predetermined data augmentations, which are selected based on a set of internal rules and a dataset fingerprint that captures key properties such as image size, spacing, and intensity distribution [12]. These augmentations include rotations, scaling, flipping, and intensity perturbations. The purpose of using these automatic, dataset-informed augmentations is to encourage the network to learn features that are complementary to those captured by the U-Net ensemble. By introducing controlled variability in a principled manner, nnU-Net is likely to make segmentation errors that are partially independent from those of the other models, thereby increasing the potential benefit when combining predictions in an ensemble.

Other aspects of the nnU-Net training follow default design choices recommended by the framework, including dynamic patch sizing, automatic spacing resampling, and z-score normalization of each MRI volume. Including nnU-Net in our ensemble allows us to test whether architectural diversity and complementary errors can improve segmentation performance. As we show in the evaluation section, ensembling U-Net models with nnU-Net outperforms ensembles composed solely of U-Nets, highlighting the benefit of combining models with different inductive biases and data augmentation strategies (Fig. 2).

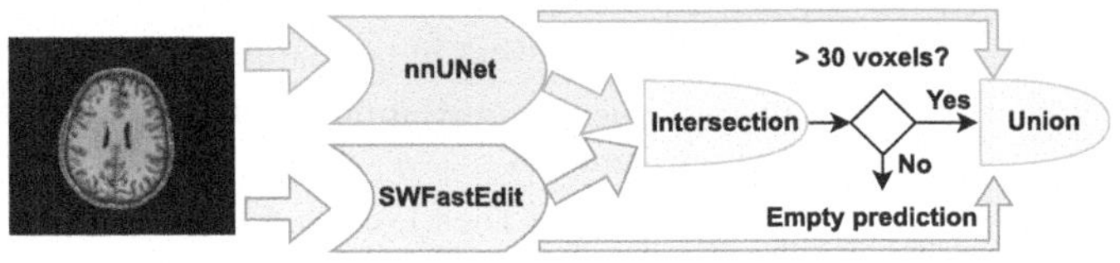

Fig. 2. Pipeline, summarizing our ensemble approach.

2.3 Post-processing Strategies

An important consideration in this challenge is the prevalence of negative cases: approximately 41% of the training volumes do not contain any lesions, and a similar distribution is observed in the validation and test sets. This has a direct impact on the evaluation metrics, as half of the final score depends on the Dice coefficient computed on empty labels (i.e., volumes without lesions), and is set to either 0 or 1. Consequently, accurately detecting whether a volume contains a lesion at all is critical, as false positives in otherwise healthy scans can drastically reduce the final ranking.

To address this challenge, we employ a straightforward yet effective post-processing step across all model predictions. Specifically, we remove small predicted lesion clusters that are likely the result of model uncertainty. Through empirical evaluation, we determined that discarding all predictions smaller than 30 voxels maximizes performance on the training set for volumes without lesions. These volumes were also never seen during model training, as we trained all models on lesion-only data. This threshold efficiently eliminates spurious predictions while retaining true lesions, thereby enhancing the Dice score on empty volumes and improving overall segmentation accuracy. The effect on the non-lesion and lesion-only volumes Dice scores can be seen in Table 2.

Table 2. Impact of post-processing thresholds on Dice scores for volumes with and without lesions from the training set. The results are tuned on our SW-FastEdit model trained on the full training set. †No post-processing.

Threshold (voxels)	0†	10	20	30	40
Dice Score - No Lesions	0.20	0.52	0.69	**0.74**	0.77
Dice Score - Only Lesions	0.82	0.82	0.81	**0.79**	0.53

2.4 Ensembling Strategies

To improve segmentation robustness and overall performance, we investigated several ensembling strategies using our six trained models (the five-fold cross-validated SW-FastEdit U-Nets plus the fully trained SW-FastEdit model). Specifically, we compared three common approaches for combining voxel-wise predictions:

- **Union:** A voxel is considered part of a lesion if *any* of the models predict it as a lesion. This strategy tends to maximize sensitivity at the cost of potentially more false positives.
- **Intersection:** A voxel is considered a lesion only if *all* models predict it as such. This is a conservative approach that reduces false positives but may miss smaller or uncertain lesions.
- **Majority Voting:** A voxel is labeled as a lesion if more than half of the models predict it as a lesion. This balances sensitivity and specificity by leveraging the consensus across models.

3 Results

3.1 Ensembling Tuning

Due to the limited number of submissions allowed for the validation and test sets in the challenge, we first evaluated the 3 ensembling strategies on the training data using our six models. This enabled us to assess their relative effectiveness and select the most promising approach for the final submission. The quantitative results of this evaluation are reported in Table 3.

We submitted both the six-model U-Net ensemble and the single model trained on the full dataset to the validation phase as Docker containers. This allowed us to evaluate which ensembling strategies perform best in practice. As shown in Table 3, while majority voting achieves the highest performance on the training data, it decreases substantially on positive volumes in the validation set, performing even worse than the single model in some cases.

However, two additional insights emerge from these experiments: (1) intersection ensembling acts as a strong filter for false positives, and (2) union ensembling preserves already well-segmented regions without discarding correct predictions. On their own, however, both strategies yield suboptimal results—intersection performs poorly on volumes containing lesions, while union struggles with volumes without lesions.

Table 3. Comparison of different ensembling strategies evaluated on training and validation sets. The validation scores (Dice) are taken from the official leaderboard.

Ensembling Strategy	Train		Validation	
	No Lesions	Only Lesions	No Lesions	Only Lesions
Union	0.03	0.75	N/A	N/A
Intersection	0.99	0.10	N/A	N/A
Majority	0.96	0.81	0.81	0.32
Single Model (SW-FastEdit)	0.74	0.79	0.40	0.36

3.2 Combining SW-FastEdit with nnUNet

Based on these insights, we adopted a two-stage ensembling strategy: first, we determine whether a lesion is present in the volume using intersection ensembling, and second, we combine the segmentation maps using union ensembling [11]. To further enhance diversity and reduce correlated errors, we combined the single full-dataset U-Net model with nnU-Net in the final ensemble. This setup produces complementary predictions, which are aggregated in a manner that improves both sensitivity and specificity.

Table 4 illustrates the effectiveness of this approach. The intersection Dice for volumes without lesions remains high, while the performance on lesion-containing volumes does not decrease, unlike the homogeneous U-Net ensemble shown in Table 3, where the Dice score for positive volumes dropped to 0.1. Furthermore, combining the predictions in a union ensembling step yields a Dice score of 0.92, demonstrating the benefit of leveraging complementary predictions across different model architectures.

Table 4. Dice scores on the training data for different models and ensembling strategies, reported separately for volumes without lesions and volumes containing lesions.

Model/Ensemble	No Lesions	Only Lesions
nnU-Net	0.27	0.55
SW-FastEdit	0.74	0.79
Intersection	**0.94**	0.70
Union	0.20	**0.92**

The results on the official validation and test leaderboards follow the same pattern, as shown in Table 5. For volumes without lesions, the SW-FastEdit model achieves moderate Dice scores (0.40 on validation), indicating some difficulty in avoiding false positives. The six-fold ensemble using majority voting improves performance on these volumes, raising the Dice to 0.81 on validation, but it performs worse on volumes containing lesions, with a Dice of 0.32.

The two-stage ensemble combining nnU-Net with SW-FastEdit achieves the best overall performance. It maintains a high Dice score on volumes without lesions (0.89) while also improving segmentation on lesion-containing volumes (0.48 on validation). These results demonstrate the advantage of combining models with different training schemes, as it provides complementary predictions and reduces errors compared to ensembles of similar models. Overall, the findings highlight the importance of model diversity and the two-stage approach for achieving robust performance in this challenge.

Table 5. Dice scores for models and ensembles. Bal. Acc.: Balanced Accuracy

Model/Ensemble	No Lesions	Only Lesions	Bal. Acc.	Set
SW-FastEdit	0.40	0.36	0.67	Validation
6-fold Ensemble (Majority)	0.81	0.32	0.80	
nnU-Net + SW-FastEdit 2-stage	**0.89**	**0.48**	**0.87**	
SW-FastEdit	N/A	N/A	N/A	Testing
6-fold Ensemble (Majority)	0.84	0.21	0.72	
nnU-Net + SW-FastEdit 2-stage	**0.89**	**0.33**	**0.75**	

4 Conclusion

In this work, we explored different strategies for the automatic segmentation of moderate to severe traumatic brain injury (msTBI) lesions using T1-weighted MRI scans. We trained an ensemble of SW-FastEdit U-Net models and a separate nnU-Net model, carefully evaluating various ensembling approaches, including majority voting, intersection, and union strategies. Our results show that model diversity and a two-stage ensembling approach—first detecting whether a lesion is present and then aggregating the segmentation maps—substantially improve performance compared to homogeneous ensembles or single models.

Post-processing played an important role, particularly for volumes without lesions, where filtering out small spurious predictions effectively reduced false positives and improved Dice scores. Across both training and validation data, the combination of complementary models led to the best balance between sensitivity and specificity. The two-stage ensemble, leveraging SW-FastEdit and nnU-Net, achieved high Dice scores on both lesion-containing and non-lesion volumes, confirming the importance of architectural diversity and thoughtful aggregation strategies in lesion segmentation tasks.

Overall, our study demonstrates that even without pretraining or highly complex architectures, careful model selection, ensembling, and post-processing can lead to substantial improvements in msTBI segmentation. These insights provide practical guidance for future work in automated lesion segmentation, particularly in multi-site or large-scale datasets where variability and heterogeneity pose significant challenges.

Acknowledgments. The present contribution is supported by the Helmholtz Association under the joint research school "HIDSS4Health – Helmholtz Information and Data Science School for Health. Parts of this work were performed on the HoreKa supercomputer, funded by the Ministry of Science, Research, and the Arts of Baden-Württemberg, and by the Federal Ministry of Education and Research.

References

1. Bennett, K.S., DeWitt, P.E., Harlaar, N., Bennett, T.D.: Seizures in children with severe traumatic brain injury. Pediatr. Crit. Care Med. **18**(1), 54–63 (2017). https://doi.org/10.1097/PCC.0000000000001040
2. Bullock, M.R., Chesnut, R., Ghajar, J., Gordon, D., Hartl, R., Newell, D.W., Servadei, F., Walters, B.C., Wilberger, J.E.: Guidelines for the surgical management of traumatic brain injury. Neurosurgery **58**(3 Suppl), S2–S62 (2006). https://doi.org/10.1227/01.NEU.0000208801.97194.E9
3. Covington, N.V., Duff, M.C.: Heterogeneity is a hallmark of traumatic brain injury, not a limitation: A new perspective on study design in rehabilitation research. Am. J. Speech Lang. Pathol. **30**(2S), 974–985 (2021)
4. Crawford, A.M., Yang, S., Hu, P., Li, Y., Lozanova, P., Scalea, T.M., Stein, D.M.: Concomitant chest trauma and traumatic brain injury, biomarkers correlate with worse outcomes. J. Trauma Acute Care Surg. **87**(1S Suppl 1), S146–S151 (2019). https://doi.org/10.1097/TA.0000000000002310
5. Dennis, E.L., et al.: Accelerated aging after traumatic brain injury: an enigma multi-cohort mega-analysis. bioRxiv p. 2023.10.16.562638 (2023). https://doi.org/10.1101/2023.10.16.562638
6. Diamond, B.R., et al.: Optimizing the accuracy of cortical volumetric analysis in traumatic brain injury. MethodsX **7**, 100994 (2020). https://doi.org/10.1016/j.mex.2020.100994
7. Gatidis, S., et al.: The autopet challenge: towards fully automated lesion segmentation in oncologic pet/ct imaging (2023)
8. Gatidis, S., et al.: Results from the autopet challenge on fully automated lesion segmentation in oncologic pet/ct imaging. Nature Mach. Intell. **6**(11), 1396–1405 (2024)
9. Hadlich, M., Marinov, Z., Kim, M., Nasca, E., Kleesiek, J., Stiefelhagen, R.: Sliding window fastedit: a framework for lesion annotation in whole-body pet images. In: 2024 IEEE International Symposium on Biomedical Imaging (ISBI), pp. 1–5. IEEE (2024)
10. Hadlich, M., Marinov, Z., Stiefelhagen, R.: Autopet challenge 2023: sliding window-based optimization of u-net. arXiv preprint arXiv:2309.12114 (2023)
11. Heiliger, L., et al.: Autopet challenge: combining nn-unet with swin unetr augmented by maximum intensity projection classifier. arXiv preprint arXiv:2209.01112 (2022)
12. Isensee, F., et al.: Automated brain extraction of multi-sequence mri using artificial neural networks. Hum. Brain Mapp. **40**(17), 4952–4964 (2019). https://doi.org/10.1002/hbm.24750
13. Jain, S., Van Vyvere, T., Terzopoulos, V., Sima, D.M., Roura, E., Maas, A., Wilms, G., Verheyden, J.: Automatic quantification of computed tomography features in acute traumatic brain injury. J. Neurotrauma **36**(11), 1794–1803 (2019). https://doi.org/10.1089/neu.2018.6034

14. Kamnitsas, K., et al.: Efficient multi-scale 3d cnn with fully connected crf for accurate brain lesion segmentation. Med. Image Anal. **36**, 61–78 (2017). https://doi.org/10.1016/j.media.2016.10.004
15. Keleher, F., et al.: Multimodal analysis of secondary cerebellar alterations after pediatric traumatic brain injury. bioRxiv p. 2022.12.24.22283926 (2022). https://doi.org/10.1101/2022.12.24.22283926
16. King, D.J., Novak, J., Shephard, A.J., Beare, R., Anderson, V.A., Wood, A.G.: Lesion induced error on automated measures of brain volume: Data from a pediatric traumatic brain injury cohort. Front. Neurosci. **14**, 491 (2020). https://doi.org/10.3389/fnins.2020.00491
17. Liesemer, K., Bratton, S.L., Zebrack, C.M., Brockmeyer, D., Statler, K.D.: Early post-traumatic seizures in moderate to severe pediatric traumatic brain injury: rates, risk factors, and clinical features. J. Neurotrauma **28**(5), 755–762 (2011). https://doi.org/10.1089/neu.2010.1611
18. Maas, A.I., Stocchetti, N., Bullock, R.: Moderate and severe traumatic brain injury in adults. Lancet Neurol. **7**(8), 728–741 (2008). https://doi.org/10.1016/S1474-4422(08)70164-9
19. Marinov, Z., Jäger, P.F., Egger, J., Kleesiek, J., Stiefelhagen, R.: Deep interactive segmentation of medical images: A systematic review and taxonomy. IEEE transactions on pattern analysis and machine intelligence (2024)
20. Marinov, Z., Stiefelhagen, R., Kleesiek, J.: Guiding the guidance: A comparative analysis of user guidance signals for interactive segmentation of volumetric images. In: International Conference on Medical Image Computing and Computer-Assisted Intervention, pp. 637–647. Springer (2023)
21. McKee, A.C., Daneshvar, D.H.: The neuropathology of traumatic brain injury. Handb. Clin. Neurol. **127**, 45–66 (2015). https://doi.org/10.1016/B978-0-444-52892-6.00004-0
22. Radwan, A.M., et al.: Virtual brain grafting: enabling whole brain parcellation in the presence of large lesions. Neuroimage **229**, 117731 (2021). https://doi.org/10.1016/j.neuroimage.2021.117731
23. Ronneberger, O., Fischer, P., Brox, T.: U-net: Convolutional networks for biomedical image segmentation. In: International Conference on Medical Image Computing and Computer-Assisted Intervention, pp. 234–241. Springer (2015)
24. Sanjuán, J., et al.: A review of automated brain lesion segmentation methods. Neuroinformatics **11**(2), 133–148 (2013). https://doi.org/10.1007/s12021-013-9172-9
25. Thompson, P.M., et al.: The enhancing neuroimaging genetics through meta-analysis consortium: 10 years of global collaborations in human brain mapping. Hum. Brain Mapp. **43**(1), 15–22 (2022). https://doi.org/10.1002/hbm.25672

nnU-Net and Synthetic Lesions for Automated Segmentation of Moderate-to-Severe Traumatic Brain Injury

Rachika E. Hamadache(✉), Clara Lisazo, Cansu Yalcin, Valeriia Abramova, Uma M. Lal-Trehan Estrada, Agustin Cartaya Lathulerie, Micaela Rivas Díaz, Adrià Casamitjana, Arnau Oliver, and Xavier Lladó

Research Institute of Computer Vision and Robotics (VICOROB), University of Girona, Girona, Spain
rachika.hamadache@udg.edu

Abstract. Moderate-to-Severe Traumatic Brain Injury (msTBI) is a major health concern caused by external forces that result in structural brain damage and can lead to life-threatening conditions. Accurate lesion segmentation remains highly challenging due to the heterogeneity of msTBI, limiting the effectiveness of conventional neuroimaging methods. The AIMS-TBI Segmentation Challenge 2025 was established to advance automated approaches for msTBI lesion segmentation using a large multi-site dataset of T1-weighted MRIs. This dataset included both cases with and without lesions, highlighting the importance of accurate lesion detection. In this work, we present our submission to the challenge, building on the nnU-Net framework and incorporating two enhancements: the augmentation of training data with blended synthetic small lesions and a multiclass strategy to improve small lesion detection. On the unseen test set, our method achieved promising performances, with an overall Dice score of 0.635 across all images.

Keywords: Traumatic Brain Injury (TBI) · MRI · Segmentation · nnU-Net

1 Introduction

Moderate-to-Severe Traumatic Brain Injury (msTBI) is a major health concern caused by external forces that rapidly move the brain within the skull, leading to neuropathological damage and dysfunction [1]. The initial impact results in primary injuries (such as haematoma, haemorrhage and contusion), which can subsequently induce secondary injuries (like gliosis and encephalomalacia) [2]. These may progress to life threatening conditions requiring acute surgical interventions. Compared to other common brain pathologies, such as stroke or multiple sclerosis, msTBI presents highly heterogeneous lesions that vary widely

S. Bakas et al. (Eds.): MICCAI 2025, LNCS 16377, pp. 292–300, 2026.
https://doi.org/10.1007/978-3-032-16370-7_26

in size, shape, number, and distribution across multiple brain regions and tissue types. These characteristics pose significant challenges for conventional neuroimaging processing methods, such as registration and brain parcellation, and often limit researchers with underperforming tools and time-consuming manual segmentation.

To address these challenges, the AIMS-TBI Segmentation Challenge 2025 aims to develop novel algorithms for the automatic and accurate detection and segmentation of 3D msTBI lesions, defined solely on T1-weighted MRI as structural damage, including: contusions, haemorrhage, haematoma, gliosis, encephalomalacia, white matter lesions, and surgical drainage tracts. The dataset comprises cases collected from 13 clinical sites, offering diverse representations and variability that better reflect real-world clinical scenarios, thereby facilitating the development of more robust and adaptable solutions with the potential to improve patient outcomes and treatment strategies.

In this work, we present an approach built on the well-known nnU-Net framework [3]. To improve the detection of small lesions, we explore two strategies: the augmentation of training data with synthetic small lesions blended into the images, and the use of the multi-size labeling (MSL) technique [4]. We trained two separate nnU-Net-based models (each consisting of five fold-specific models): a baseline model trained on real data for binary segmentation, and a multiclass model trained with MSL labels and synthetic lesions, whose predictions were subsequently binarized. During inference, ensemble predictions from both models were combined to produce the final segmentation mask. This approach yielded promising results, with improvements in the overall Dice score, reaching 0.635 in the final evaluation phase.

2 Methods

2.1 Dataset

The dataset contains a total of 875 T1-weighted MRIs, split into 552 for training (63%), 100 for validation (11%) and 223 for testing (26%) [2]. The data was collected from 13 different sites using both 1.5T and 3T scanners, with an approximately balanced distribution across the splits. Some cases contained no lesions, while others had corresponding segmentation masks. These masks were generated through a four-step process, starting with an automated segmentation and subsequently reviewed and edited in sequence by three expert raters (first, second, and final). To protect subject privacy, all data was defaced using *pydeface*. No further pre-processing was applied.

2.2 Method Description

Binary Segmentation As a baseline, we employed a 3D nnU-Net [3] for the binary lesion segmentation, training on the available data split into five folds. For each fold, the model was trained for 1000 epochs using the stochastic gradient descent (SGD) optimizer with an initial learning rate of $1e^{-2}$, a batch size of

2, and the default nnU-Net loss functions (Soft Dice and Cross Entropy). The initial results showed relatively good overall detection of true-negative cases, which is particularly important, given that false-positive lesion predictions would substantially compromise model performance.

Multiclass Segmentation. Given the large number of small lesions present in the dataset (Fig. 2) and the difficulty the model encounters in detecting and segmenting them, the next step was to augment the training set by blending additional small lesions into the images. The procedure, illustrated in Fig. 1, consisted of the following steps:

a. Extract all individual lesions within a predefined volume range (5-1500 voxels) and save them as 64×64×64 patches centered on the lesion.
b. Apply SynthSeg [5] to all lesion-containing images to extract brain tissues.
c. For each training image with lesions, generate a distorted (fluid-like) Perlin noise [6] mask matching the image dimensions, to later provide the lesion with texture before blending.
d. Randomly select up to 20 lesions from the saved patches and apply random elastic deformations to each one of them, using TorchIO's *RandomElasticDeformation()*' function.
e. If the deformed lesion volume remains within 10-2000 voxels, randomly choose a valid insertion location (that fits the bounding box of this lesion) within the appropriate tissue class previously generated with SynthSeg (excluding

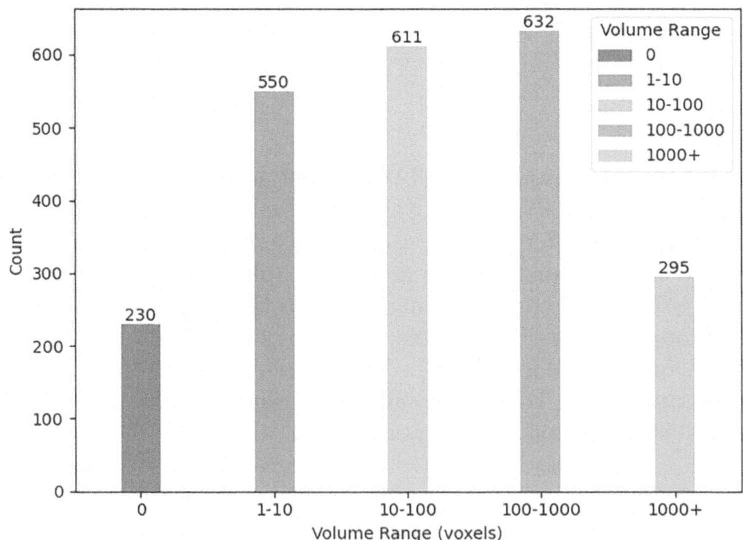

Fig. 1. Distribution of lesion counts across volume ranges in the training dataset.The first bar(volume=0)indicates the number of cases without lesions,while the remaining bars represent the total number of lesions with in each volume range.

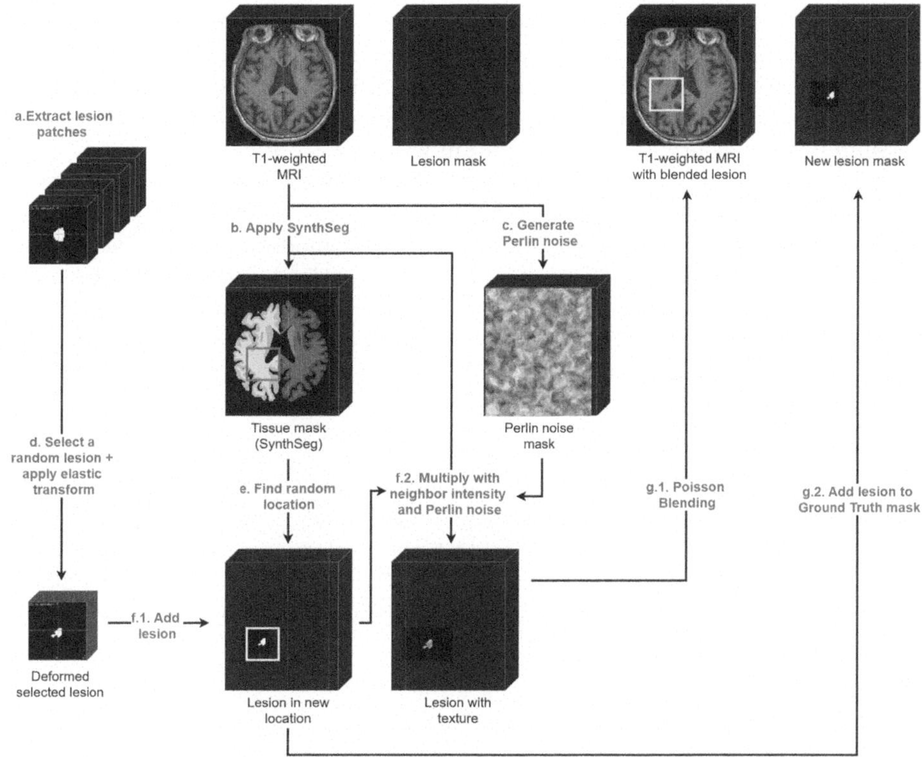

Fig. 2. Over view of the pipeline used to augment training data.

the ones already containing lesions, as well as the CSF region that is unlikely to have lesions).

f. Place the deformed lesion at the selected location within an empty mask of the same dimensions as the original image, then multiply it by both the distorted Perlin noise mask and the 70th percentile of the neighboring intensity values, estimated from the lesion's surrounding voxels in the T1-weighted image (obtained by expanding the lesion bounding box by 5 voxels when possible). This provides realistic texture and intensity for improved blending.
g. Finally, blend the lesion into the T1-weighted image using Poisson Blending [7] and add it to the ground-truth mask.

Steps (c–g) are applied to all training images containing lesions, with steps (e–g) repeated for each individual lesion selected (up to 20 per image).

In addition, inspired by [4] and in order to further emphasize small and challenging lesions, we applied the MSL strategy on both real and synthetic data. Lesions were divided into 3 subclasses based on their volume ranges: 1-100voxels, 100-2000voxels, and >2000 voxels. This division ensures that both the small lesions and the synthetically added ones (small- to medium-sized) are captured in the first two classes, which correspond to the most difficult lesions to segment. With the obtained data, we trained a 3D nnU-Net model for 1000 epochs for each of the five folds, using the stochastic gradient descent (SGD) optimizer with an initial learning rate of $1e^{-2}$, a batch size of 4, the default nnU-Net loss functions (Soft Dice and Cross Entropy) and maximum foreground oversampling to ensure all patches contain lesions.

In inference, in order to avoid predicting false lesions, and given the ability of the binary model to better discern true-negative cases, we use it as a condition, such that if the ensembled prediction of the binary model contains a lesion, the final mask was obtained by merging it with the binarized ensemble prediction of the multiclass model; otherwise, the output was kept empty, even if the multiclass model predicted a lesion. This strategy prevented performance degradation from false-positive detections.

2.3 Implementation Details

This work was implemented by adapting nnU-Net v2 (version 2.6.1), Pytorch 2.5.1 and CUDA 12.8. All experiments were conducted on two Nvidia A30 GPUs of 24Gb of memory each. In order to test the performance of our approaches in the AIMS-TBI Segmentation Challenge 2025 platform, Docker Engine 24.0.6 was used to build docker images and upload them on the Grand-Challenge online platform.

3 Results

3.1 Evaluation Metrics

To evaluate the performance of the proposed methods, both in terms of segmentation and detection, the following metrics were used:

Balanced Accuracy - BA:

$$BA = \frac{1}{2}\left(\frac{TP}{TP + FN} + \frac{TN}{TN + FP}\right) \tag{1}$$

where TP, FP, TN and FN denote the number of true-positives, false-positives, true-negatives and false-negatives, respectively.

Dice similarity coefficient - DSC (voxel-wise):

$$DSC = \frac{2TP}{2TP + FN + FP} \tag{2}$$

Absolute volume difference - AVD (voxel-wise):

$$AVD = |Predicted\ volume - Ground\ truth\ volume| \tag{3}$$

Absolute lesion count difference - Count (lesion-wise):

$$Count = |Total\ predicted\ lesions - Total\ ground\ truth\ lesions| \tag{4}$$

For the final challenge ranking, the average of balanced accuracy, Dice coefficient for lesion cases, Dice coefficient for non-lesion cases, and overall Dice (considering both lesion and non-lesion cases) was computed, and the mean rank across these metrics was used to determine the final position.

3.2 Cross-Validation

The cross-validation results are summarized in Table 1, with Dice scores and lesion-wise detection counts illustrated in Fig. 3. The binary (baseline) model demonstrated the ability to segment certain msTBI lesions while also correctly identifying lesion-free cases, achieving 206 true negatives out of 230 with a Dice score of 0.896. However, Fig. 3 shows that smaller lesions were frequently missed, with a low Dice score of 0.152, highlighting the need for further improvements.

Augmenting the training data with blended deformed lesions led to a slight increase in the overall Dice score, while the balanced accuracy (BA) remained unchanged due to the imposed condition.

In contrast, incorporating the MSL method produced consistent improvements in all metrics, including better detection of small lesions, as reflected on the right side of Fig. 3. Some qualitative results are provided in Fig. 4, where we can highlight the ability of the proposed approach to segment some small lesions compared to the general binary one.

Table 1. The resulting evaluation metrics on the cross-validation, validation and test sets of the AIMS-TBI Segmentation Challenge 2025, using different methods. The scores represent the mean and standard deviation (std) over all cases, when applicable. The best and second-best overall scores are shown in bold and underlined, respectively.

		DSC			AVD			Count			BA
		Lesion	No-lesion	Overall	Lesion	No-lesion	Overall	Lesion	No-lesion	Overall	
Cross- validation	Binary (baseline)	0.500± 0.318	0.896± 0.306	0.665± 0.369	2.355± 8.112	0.017± 0.071	1.381± 6.298	3.460± 5.717	0.152± 0.502	2.082± 4.670	**0.859**
	Binary with real and synthetic data	0.525± 0.306	0.896± 0.306	0.679± 0.357	1.982± 5.018	0.059± 0.370	1.181± 3.953	3.587± 5.365	0.343± 1.193	2.236± 4.463	**0.859**
	Multiclass (MSL) with real and synthetic data (proposed)	0.534± 0.305	0.896± 0.306	**0.684± 0.354**	1.951± 5.758	0.017± 0.071	**1.145± 4.497**	3.289± 5.235	0.152± 0.502	**1.982± 4.297**	**0.859**
Validation phase	Binary (baseline)	0.538± 0.310	0.957± 0.204	0.735± 0.338	3.652± 9.867	0.039± 0.238	1.954± 7.379	4.245± 5.435	0.128± 0.741	2.310± 4.476	**0.894**
	Binary with real and synthetic data	0.567± 0.309	0.957± 0.204	0.751± 0.328	2.901± 7.705	0.045± 0.262	**1.559± 5.768**	3.566± 4.348	0.191± 0.924	1.980± 3.632	**0.894**
	Multiclass (MSL) with real and synthetic data (proposed)	0.582± 0.302	0.957± 0.204	**0.758± 0.320**	3.057± 8.397	0.044± 0.248	1.641± 6.273	3.396± 4.054	0.149± 0.780	**1.870± 3.401**	**0.894**
Final phase	Multiclass (MSL) with real and synthetic data (proposed)	0.494± 0.318	0.919± 0.275	0.635± 0.364	18.279± 67.140	0.120± 0.773	12.253± 55.487	3.752± 8.050	0.351± 1.339	2.623± 6.809	0.855

3.3 Validation and Final Testing

For the evaluation on the hidden validation and test sets, all three methods were submitted to the validation phase, whereas only the final proposed approach was evaluated on the test set. The results, summarized in Table 1, are consistent with

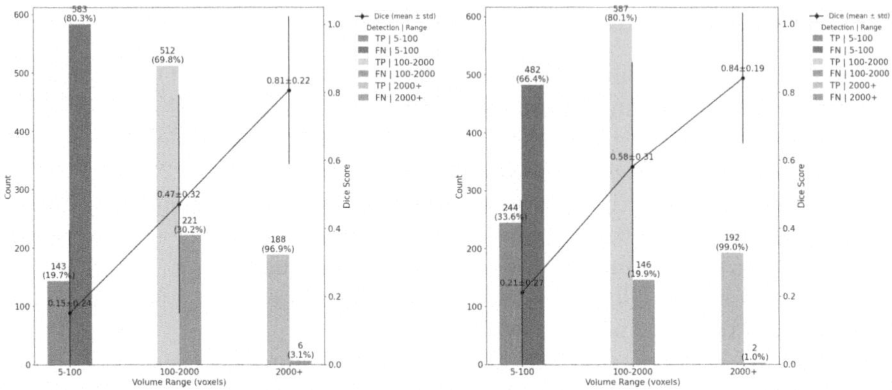

Fig. 3. Distribution of detected lesions (TP), missed lesions (FN), and Dice score (mean ± std) across lesion volume ranges for the binary segmentation model (left) and the proposed method (right).

the cross-validation findings. The proposed method improved upon the baseline, particularly in terms of lesion Dice. In the final test set, the approach achieved an overall Dice score of 0.635 and a balanced accuracy of 0.855, ranking among the top entries in the leaderboard.

4 Discussion

In this work, we described our approach used for the AIMS-TBI Segmentation Challenge 2025. Beyond the inherent challenges posed by the heterogeneity of msTBI lesions and the multi-centre nature of the dataset, one of the most critical difficulties revolved around missed lesions, particularly those of small sizes, as indicated by the number of false negatives among them.

Nonetheless, our targeted strategy addressing this issue still proved effective, such that expanding the training dataset with cases containing a larger number of small- to medium-sized lesions improved the overall predictions, with the validation set also showing reduced differences in both average lesion volume and lesion count. When combined with reframing the task as a multiclass problem, the ensemble of the two models further enhanced the overall performance, achieving better lesion detection with up to 33.6% and 80.1% TP rate for small lesions (5-100 voxels) and small/medium lesions (100-2000 voxels), respectively, compared to 19.7% and 69.8% using the baseline. This approach aligns with the clinical importance of lesion-wise detection, as accurately identifying small lesions can be crucial for patient prognosis and therapeutic decision-making in msTBI.

Furthermore, it is worth noting that the use of a further specialized model on small lesions only, with a dedicated classification model to exclude non-lesion cases rather than relying solely on the binary segmentation model, might further

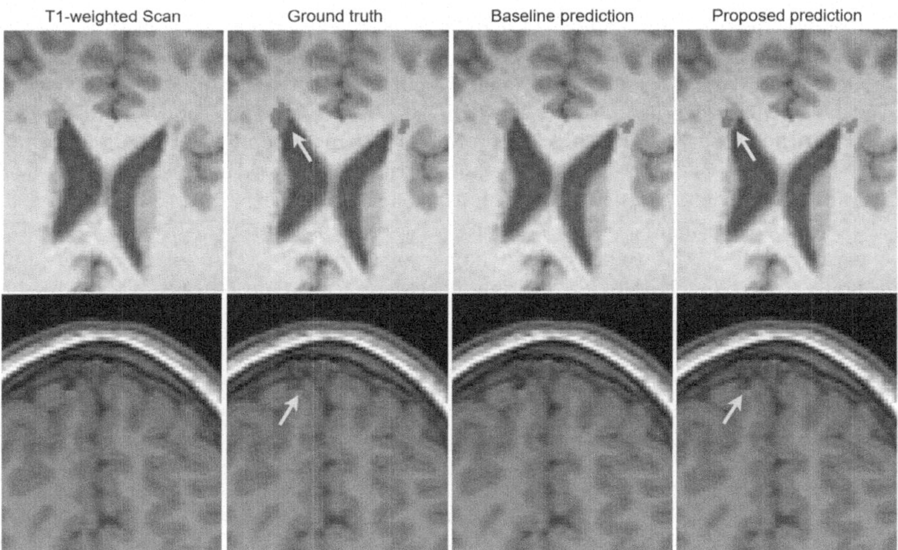

Fig. 4. Qualitative results for two cases, where the prediction masks are overlayed on the T1-weighted scan. Yellow arrows highlight lesions detected by the proposed method but missed by the baseline. (Color figure online)

enhance the performance by reducing false negatives and avoiding discarding potentially useful predictions.

Additional pre-processing steps, such as bias field correction, could also improve results by normalizing image intensities and mitigating the domain shift introduced by the multi-centre dataset. However, due to the time constraints of the challenge, this correction could not be applied and remains as a potential improvement for future work.

5 Conclusion

In this work, we described our approach for the AIMS-TBI Segmentation Challenge 2025. By augmenting the training data with additional small and medium-sized lesions and reframing the task as a multiclass segmentation problem, our method substantially reduced false negatives and improved both lesion-wise and volume-wise performance. These results align with the clinical need for accurate lesion-level detection, which is critical for patient prognosis and treatment planning. Finally, there remains room for improvements, such as using pre-processing steps like Bias Field Correction, that was removed here due to time constraints but that could mitigate domain shift issues present in the multi-centre nature of the data. Another step for the future would be to consider a classification model that could better discern true negative cases to avoid discarding potential useful predictions.

Acknowledgments. Rachika E. Hamadache holds an IFUdG2024 grant from Universitat de Girona. Clara Lisazo holds an FI grant from the Catalan Government with reference number 2024 FI-100103. Cansu Yalcin holds an FI grant from the Catalan Government with reference number 2023 FI-1 00096. Valeriia Abramova holds an FPI grant from the Ministerio de Ciencia, Innovación y Universidades with reference number PRE2021-099121. Uma M. Lal-Trehan Estrada holds an IFUdG2022 grant from Universitat de Girona. Agustin Cartaya Lathulerie hold an FPI grant from the Ministerio de Ciencia, Innovación y Universidades, with reference number PREP2023-001473. Micaela Rivas Díaz hold a DEXCOM Chair grant TSI-100932-2023-1. Adrià Casamitjana holds a POSTDOC-UdG2023 grant from Universitat de Girona. This work has been supported by PID2023-146187OB-I00 from the Ministerio de Ciencia, Innovación y Universidades and also by the ICREA Academia program.

References

1. Mckee, A.C., Daneshvar, D.H.: The neuropathology of traumatic brain injury. Handb Clin Neurol. 2015;127:45-66. https://doi.org/10.1016/B978-0-444-52892-6.00004-0. PMID: 25702209; PMCID: PMC4694720
2. Dennis, E., Tustison, N., Deutscher, E., Wilde, E., Pease, M., Bakas, S.: AIMS-TBI - Automated Identification of Moderate-Severe Traumatic Brain Injury Lesions. Zenodo (2025)
3. Isensee, F., Jaeger, P.F., Kohl, S.A.A., et al.: nnU-Net: a self-configuring method for deep learning-based biomedical image segmentation. Nat. Methods **18**, 203–211 (2021). https://doi.org/10.1038/s41592-020-01008-z
4. Shang, L., Lou, Z., Alexander, A.L., Prabhakaran, V., Sethares, W.A., Nair, V.A., Adluru, N.: Segmenting small stroke lesions with novel labeling strategies. In International Workshop on Machine Learning in Clinical Neuroimaging: 7, pp. 113–122. Springer, Cham (2024Oct)
5. Billot, B., et al.: SynthSeg: segmentation of brain MRI scans of any contrast and resolution without retraining. Med. Image Anal. **1**(86), 102789 (2023)
6. Perlin, K.: An image synthesizer. ACM Siggraph Computer Graphics. **19**(3), 287–96 (1985)
7. Huo, J., Ourselin, S., Sparks, R.: Self-supervised brain lesion generation for effective data augmentation of medical images. Neural Netw. **30**, 107629 (2025)

BLSegMamba: An Optimized SegMamba Framework for msTBI Lesion Segmentation in MRI

Yueyue Zhu, Xiaoyu Bai, Haotian Jiang, and Geng Chen(✉)

National Engineering Laboratory for Integrated Aero-Space-Ground-Ocean Big Data Application Technology, School of Computer Science and Engineering, Northwestern Polytechnical University, Xi'an, China
geng.chen@ieee.org

Abstract. Moderate-to-Severe Traumatic Brain Injury (msTBI) often leads to complex and highly heterogeneous structural damage in the brain. Lesions may be focal or diffuse and can involve multiple tissue types, including gray matter, white matter, and cerebrospinal fluid. They also exhibit considerable variability in size, shape, spatial distribution, and hemispheric symmetry. This high degree of heterogeneity greatly increases the difficulty of automatic segmentation based on unimodal T1-weighted MRI. To address this challenge, we propose a customized optimization of the SegMamba architecture. The resulting optimized version, Brain Lesion SegMamba (BLSegMamba), retains the core structural components of SegMamba while integrating a more robust data augmentation strategy and a loss function specifically designed for the segmentation of msTBI lesions. On the final test dataset of the AIMS-TBI Challenge, our BLSegMamba achieves the top overall ranking after weighted aggregation of all evaluation metrics. Our code is publicly available at https://github.com/YueyueZhu/BLSegMamba.

Keywords: msTBI · Segmentation · Mamba · U-net

1 Introduction

Moderate-to-Severe Traumatic Brain Injury (msTBI) often results in complex and highly heterogeneous structural damage to the brain. Lesions may be focal or diffuse, involving multiple tissue types such as gray matter, white matter, and cerebrospinal fluid, and exhibiting significant variation in size, shape, spatial distribution, and hemispheric symmetry. This high degree of heterogeneity is a hallmark of msTBI and greatly increases the complexity of neuroimaging analysis, particularly in automated processing pipelines.

Y. Zhu and X. Bai—Equal contribution.

This work was supported in part by the National Natural Science Foundation of China under Grant 62201465.

S. Bakas et al. (Eds.): MICCAI 2025, LNCS 16377, pp. 301–310, 2026.
https://doi.org/10.1007/978-3-032-16370-7_27

The irregular morphology and complex distribution of msTBI lesions not only increase the difficulty of lesion identification but also interfere with key downstream tasks such as image registration, brain parcellation, and functional connectivity modeling [1,8]. Although existing tools such as HD-BET [6] and Virtual Brain Grafting [11] partially alleviate these challenges, they often rely on manually annotated lesion masks, which are labor-intensive, time-consuming, and susceptible to subjectivity. In addition, many current automatic segmentation methods were originally developed for other brain pathologies such as stroke or tumors and often exhibit poor adaptability and limited generalization when applied directly to TBI data-particularly in scenarios where only T1-weighted MRI (T1w MRI) is available [3,7].

The AIMS-TBI 2025 Challenge aims to advance 3D lesion segmentation techniques based on single-modality T1w MRI. As the most widely used imaging sequence within the ENIGMA-TBI consortium, with relatively high consistency in imaging parameters, T1w MRI offers strong cross-site applicability and generalizability [13]. The challenge focuses on the accurate automatic segmentation of various TBI-induced structural lesions (e.g., contusions, hemorrhages, encephalomalacia, and gliosis), with the goal of providing a reliable structural foundation for subsequent tasks such as brain parcellation, and individualized outcome prediction, thereby improving clinical assessment and intervention strategies for msTBI patients.

To address the challenges of lesion heterogeneity, blurred boundaries, and class imbalance in msTBI lesion segmentation, SegMamba [14] was proposed. This network integrates Gated Spatial Convolution (GSC) and Tri-orientated Mamba (ToM) blocks, leveraging state space models for efficient long-range dependency modeling across scales. Although SegMamba has demonstrated state-of-the-art performance on 3D medical image segmentation tasks, its effectiveness on unimodal T1w MRI for msTBI remains unexplored.

To this end, we propose an optimized version, *Brain Lesion SegMamba* (BLSegMamba), tailored specifically for msTBI lesion segmentation. BLSegMamba preserves SegMamba's three core components and introduces the following targeted improvements:

1. We apply SegMamba to the multi-lesion segmentation task for msTBI and verify its effectiveness in brain injury scenarios.
2. We construct a diverse data augmentation pipeline using the batchgenerators library to improve generalization.
3. We design a weighted hybrid loss to simultaneously optimize overall classification, foreground overlap, and hard-to-segment regions, mitigating class imbalance.
4. The proposed BLSegMamba is comprehensively validated on the challenge dataset, demonstrating high segmentation accuracy and stability.

2 Method

2.1 Overview of BLSegMamba

The task of automatic multi-lesion segmentation for msTBI based on unimodal T1w MRI presents significant challenges, including considerable lesion morphological variation and blurred boundaries. In this study, we customize and enhance the publicly available SegMamba architecture. Originally designed for medical image segmentation, we first reproduce the baseline model to ensure functional correctness, and then introduce improvements tailored to the structural lesion characteristics of msTBI.

As illustrated in Fig. 1, BLSegMamba is a single-modality processing architecture centered on the Tri-oriented Mamba Block (TMB). The framework first performs down-sampling and feature extraction through the left-side Down-Sampling and TMB. After multiple processing stages, the features are fed into the right-side U-net Encoder Blocks (UEBs) and U-net Decoder Blocks (UDBs). The UEB is responsible for further feature extraction, while the UDB achieves feature fusion and up-sampling, and the final output is generated through the Seg-Head.

The improvements focus on three main aspects: (1) A preprocessing pipeline to augment training data, aiming to improve generalization under conditions of limited data and high noise. (2) A weighted loss to mitigate class imbalance and improve segmentation performance. (3) To retain the original model architecture, we integrate these changes into an optimized version, which we refer to as BLSegMamba.

2.2 BLSegMamba Architecture Recall

SegMamba is an efficient architecture tailored for 3D medical image segmentation. Built upon the linear-complexity Mamba module, GSC and U-net architecture [12].

Gated Spatial Convolution. To enhance local spatial structural information, SegMamba introduces a GSC module before the ToM block. GSC employs two parallel convolutional branches to extract features: one branch uses a $3 \times 3 \times 3$ kernel to capture contextual information, while the other applies a $1 \times 1 \times 1$ convolution for channel-wise feature fusion. The outputs of the two branches are added element-wise and passed through an activation function, thereby forming a spatial gating mechanism. [9], and the result is fused with the original input through a residual connection. The operation is defined as:

$$\mathrm{GSC}(z) = z + \sigma(\mathrm{Conv1}(\mathrm{Conv3}(\mathrm{Conv3}(z)) + \mathrm{Conv1}(z))), \quad (1)$$

where Conv1 and Conv3 denote the $1 \times 1 \times 1$ and $3 \times 3 \times 3$ convolutional modules, respectively, and σ denotes the ReLU activation function.

This module enhances spatial feature representations while preserving the original input features, thereby improving the global modeling performance of the subsequent ToM module.

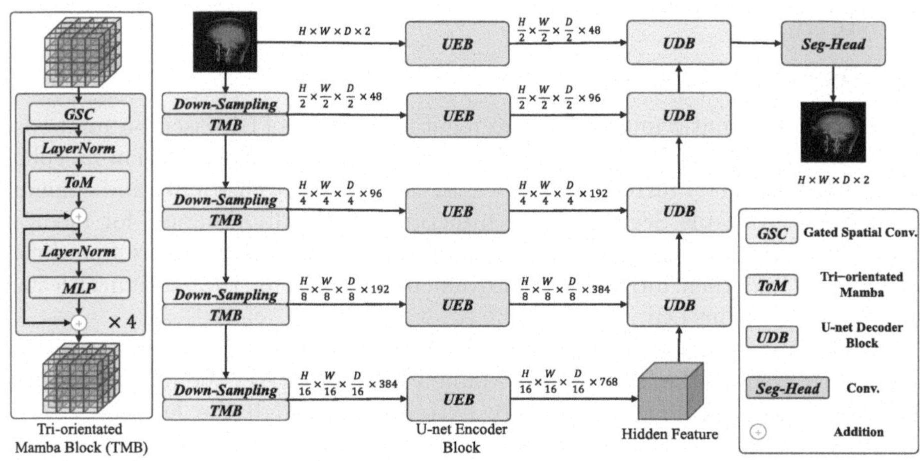

Fig. 1. Overall architecture of BLSegMamba, comprising four Tri-orientated Mamba Blocks, a U-net encoder, and a U-net decoder.

Tri-orientated Mamba. To overcome the limitation that the original Mamba [2] supports only unidirectional modeling, the model designs a ToM module. This module flattens 3D features along three orthogonal directions-depth (D), height (H), and width (W)-and models global dependencies in each direction separately. Given an input feature $z \in \mathbb{R}^{C\times D\times H\times W}$, the ToM module computes:

$$\mathrm{ToM}(z) = \mathrm{Mamba}(z_f) + \mathrm{Mamba}(z_r) + \mathrm{Mamba}(z_s), \tag{2}$$

where z_f, z_r, and z_s are the flattened sequences along the forward (depth), reverse (height), and slice-wise (width) axes, respectively.

U-net Architecture. The model also adopts a U-Net architecture; unlike the standard U-Net, it employs four TMB modules to obtain multi-scale features, which are then fed into the UEBs for further feature extraction and subsequently passed to the UDBs for decoding to produce the final segmentation.

2.3 Data-Level Optimization: Augmentation Strategy

To mitigate overfitting and improve the generalization ability of the model for msTBI lesion segmentation, we constructed a data augmentation pipeline based on the `batchgenerators` [5] framework, mainly including the following aspects:

Spatial Transformations. To enhance geometric diversity, we apply 3D spatial transformations to the input patches. Each patch undergoes spatial augmentation with a probability of 0.2, including random rotations around the x, y, and z axes with angles uniformly sampled from $\pm 30°$, as well as isotropic scaling with scale factors sampled from 0.7 to 1.4. The rotation is applied independently to each axis with a probability of 1.0.

Intensity-level Augmentation. To improve the model's robustness against common noise and artifacts in T1w MRI, intensity perturbations are incorporated. These include adding Gaussian noise with a probability of 0.1; applying Gaussian blur with σ sampled from [0.5, 1.0], with a probability of 0.2 per sample and 0.5 per channel; brightness and contrast adjustments each with a probability of 0.15; gamma correction applied in two modes within the range [0.7, 1.5], with a probability of 0.1 for the histogram-normalized mode and 0.3 for the non-normalized mode.

Mirror Flipping. To introduce leftâĂŞright anatomical symmetry, random mirror flipping is performed along the axial, coronal, and sagittal planes (axes 0, 1, and 2).

2.4 Hybrid Loss Function

In this study, we design a hybrid loss function for msTBI lesion segmentation to comprehensively optimize overall segmentation performance. The final training loss is defined as a weighted combination of three individual losses:

$$L = \lambda_1 L_{\mathrm{CE}} + \lambda_2 L_{\mathrm{Dice}} + \lambda_3 L_{\mathrm{Focal}}, \tag{3}$$

where L_{CE}, L_{Dice}, and L_{Focal} denote the cross-entropy loss, Dice loss, and focal loss, respectively, with the weighting coefficients specified as $\lambda_1 = 0.3$, $\lambda_2 = 0.4$, and $\lambda_3 = 0.3$. This combination ensures stable training while simultaneously improving foreground overlap and emphasizing hard-to-segment regions, leading to better overall segmentation performance. The contributions of the three losses are detailed below:

Cross-Entropy (CE) Loss. The CE loss measures the discrepancy between predicted probabilities and ground truth (GT) labels:

$$L_{\mathrm{CE}} = -\frac{1}{N}\sum_{i=1}^{N}\left[y_i \log(p_i) + (1 - y_i)\log(1 - p_i)\right], \tag{4}$$

where p_i denotes the predicted probability, and $y_i \in \{0, 1\}$ is the GT label. CE loss provides stable training but may be biased toward the majority class in highly imbalanced scenarios.

Dice Loss. The Dice loss directly optimizes the overlap between predicted segmentation and GT:

$$\mathrm{Dice} = \frac{2|P \cap G| + \epsilon}{|P| + |G| + \epsilon}, \quad L_{\mathrm{Dice}} = 1 - \mathrm{Dice}, \tag{5}$$

where P and G represent the sets of predicted and GT foreground voxels, respectively, and ϵ is a small constant for numerical stability. Dice loss is robust to class imbalance and effectively improves the segmentation of small targets.

Focal Loss. The focal loss extends cross-entropy by down-weighting easy samples and focusing on hard examples:

$$L_{\text{Focal}} = -\alpha(1 - p_i)^{\gamma} \log(p_i), \tag{6}$$

where γ is the focusing parameter, and α balances class weights. Focal loss improves sensitivity to small lesions and boundary regions.

3 Experiments

3.1 Experimental Settings

Datasets. This study was conducted on the dataset provided by the AIMS-TBI 2025 Challenge. The task focuses on automatic multi-lesion segmentation of the brain in msTBI patients using unimodal T1w MRI images. The dataset consists of 551 subjects, each with original images and corresponding annotations. Among them, 321 subjects are lesion-positive, with lesions present in the segmentation masks, while 230 subjects are lesion-negative, with no lesions annotated in the segmentation masks.

Preprocessing. The dataset is preprocessed to ensure consistent spatial resolution, and we randomly split the officially released training data into training and validation sets at a $9:1$ ratio. All images and labels are re-sampled to an isotropic voxel spacing of size $1.0 \times 1.0 \times 1.0$ mm^3. During both training and inference, we randomly extract 3D patches of size $64 \times 64 \times 64$ from the preprocessed volumes.

Implementation Details. The model is implemented using PyTorch. During training, we use Stochastic Gradient Descent (SGD) as the optimizer with a learning rate of 0.01, momentum of 0.99, weight decay of 3×10^{-5}, and Nesterov acceleration enabled. A polynomial learning rate decay is employed to gradually reduce the learning rate over training epochs. The model is trained for 1,000 epochs, with 250 iterations per epoch. The batch size is set to 24. All experiments are conducted on NVIDIA GTX 3090 GPUs with 24GB memory.

3.2 Results

Ablation Study on Loss Functions and Hyperparameters. We evaluate the segmentation performance of our proposed method on the validation set of the msTBI multi-lesion segmentation task using single-modal T1-weighted MRI. The evaluation includes Dice Similarity Coefficient (DSC) and 95th percentile Hausdorff Distance (HD95) for both lesion and background regions.

As summarized in Table 1, our method attains a maximum lesion Dice of 0.8003 (HD95 = 8.98 mm), together with near-perfect background segmentation (Dice $\approx$ 0.9999). Compared with the coarse-patch baseline ($128 \times 128 \times 128$, Dice = 0.6617, HD95 = 19.81 mm), the best configuration ($64 \times 64 \times 64$, batch size = 24, with hybrid loss) yields a relative Dice improvement of about 20.95%

Table 1. Segmentation results under different patch sizes, batch sizes, and loss settings. The HD95 for the background class is always 0 due to the absence of boundary discrepancies, and is thus denoted as "-" to indicate non-informativeness.

Patch Size	Batch Size	Hybrid Loss	Lesion		Background	
			Dice	HD95	Dice	HD95
$128 \times 128 \times 128$	2	✗	0.6617	19.81	0.9999	-
$64 \times 64 \times 64$	16	✗	0.6079	22.23	0.9999	-
$64 \times 64 \times 64$	20	✗	0.6444	19.34	0.9999	-
$64 \times 64 \times 64$	24	✗	0.6849	15.93	0.9999	-
$64 \times 64 \times 64$	20	✓	0.7775	11.51	0.9999	-
$64 \times 64 \times 64$	24	✓	0.8003	8.98	0.9999	-

and reduces HD95 by 10.83 mm (a 54.67% decrease), indicating substantially improved lesion overlap and much tighter boundary localization.

Examining the $64 \times 64 \times 64$ experiments without the hybrid loss reveals a clear batch-size effect: increasing the batch size from 16 to 20 and then to 24 raises lesion Dice from 0.6079 to 0.6444 and 0.6849, respectively (each step produces roughly a 6% relative gain). Introducing the hybrid loss produces a much larger boost: at batch size 20, Dice increases from 0.6444 to 0.7775 ($\approx$ 20.65% relative gain) and at batch size 24, from 0.6849 to 0.8003 ($\approx$ 16.85% relative gain). The hybrid loss also substantially improves boundary accuracy: HD95 falls from 19.34 to 11.51 mm at batch 20 ($\approx$ 40.5% reduction) and from 15.93 to 8.98 mm at batch 24 ($\approx$ 43.6% reduction).

Taken together, these results indicate three main points: (1) using a smaller patch size (64^3) with larger effective batch sizes yields more stable training and better lesion overlap than the larger 128^3 patch in our setting; (2) the hybrid loss substantially improves both region overlap and boundary fidelity, especially when combined with sufficiently large batch sizes; and (3) background regions are consistently and robustly identified (Dice $\approx$ 0.9999), so improvements are concentrated on lesion delineation. Overall, the best configuration ($64 \times 64 \times 64$, batch $=$ 24, hybrid loss) achieves the most accurate and stable segmentation across multiple lesion regions, making it the recommended setting for subsequent experiments or clinical validation efforts. During the challenge's final testing phase, our model achieves Dice coefficients of 0.4904 for lesion segmentation and 0.9324 for background segmentation.

Visualization Analysis. To qualitatively evaluate segmentation performance, we visualize the results on a representative subject randomly selected from our internally held-out validation set (9 : 1 split of the official training data). Since the GT for the official validation set is not publicly available, this internal validation subset allows for direct visual comparison.

As illustrated in the visualization results in Fig. 2, the brain lesion regions predicted by our method exhibit a high degree of consistency with the GT across

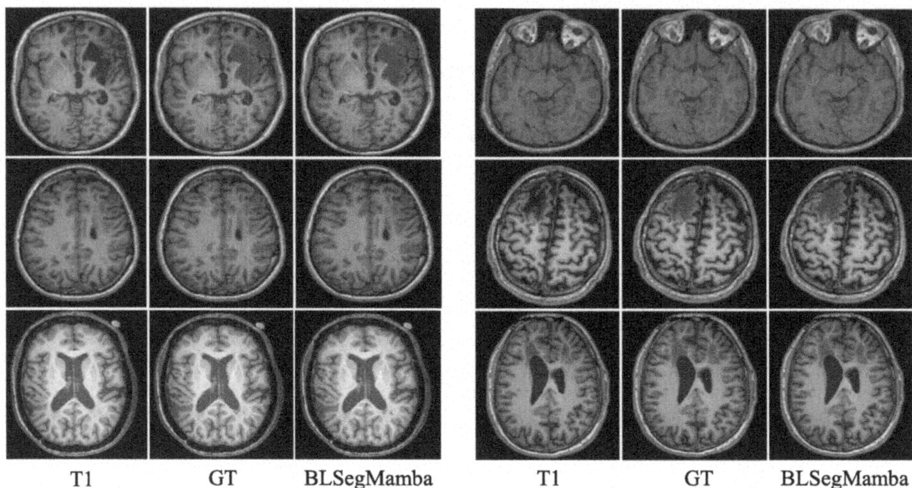

Fig. 2. Visual comparison between GT and BLSegMamba predictions on a subject from the internal validation set.

multiple anatomical planes. In views along different axes-such as axial, coronal, and sagittal-the model clearly and accurately segments the lesion areas, with sharp boundaries that align well with the GT. These results robustly demonstrate the effectiveness and reliability of our approach in the task of brain lesion segmentation. Furthermore, the visual comparisons underscore the strong generalization capability of the method across various anatomical sections, consistently maintaining high segmentation accuracy. Overall, the proposed method not only achieves superior quantitative performance but also offers highly interpretable visual results, providing a reliable tool for brain injury diagnosis and analysis.

4 Discussion

We tried several other models [4, 10, 15] for msTBI segmentation, but found that SegMamba performed better.

Our study demonstrates that the proposed method achieves robust msTBI lesion segmentation under challenging imaging conditions through multi-scale feature modeling, appropriate data augmentation, and training configurations. The results in Table 1 highlight several key factors contributing to its superior performance. First, smaller patches combined with larger batch sizes capture fine-grained spatial information, leading to more stable optimization and more precise lesion delineation. Second, the hybrid loss, which combines cross-entropy, Dice, and Focal losses, simultaneously optimizes overall classification accuracy, foreground overlap, and hard-to-segment regions, resulting in significant improvements in Dice and HD95, particularly for irregularly shaped lesions with fuzzy boundaries. Overall, the combination of multi-scale features, appropriate training strategies, and the hybrid loss enables the model to excel in lesion identification and boundary delineation. Despite limited computational resources, the method clearly demonstrates advantages for complex and heterogeneous lesions. Future work will explore larger-scale experiments and additional augmentation strategies to further validate its generalizability.

5 Conclusion

In this work, we explore the applicability of SegMamba for the task of multi-lesion segmentation in msTBI patients using unimodal T1w MRI. To address the challenges posed by the irregular morphology and complex distribution of msTBI lesions, we improve the original model by proposing a series of practical optimizations, including a comprehensive data augmentation strategy based on the batchgenerators framework and an optimized loss function. Experimental results demonstrate that the optimized model, BLSegMamba, achieves accurate and stable performance in msTBI lesion segmentation, laying a solid foundation for effectively advancing clinical assessment and intervention for msTBI patients.

References

1. Diamond, B.R.: Optimizing the accuracy of cortical volumetric analysis in traumatic brain injury. MethodsX **7**, 100994 (2020)
2. Gu, A., Dao, T.: Mamba: Linear-time sequence modeling with selective state spaces. In: First Conference on Language Modeling (2024)
3. Henschel, L.: Fastsurfer-a fast and accurate deep learning based neuroimaging pipeline. Neuroimage **219**, 117012 (2020)
4. Huang, S.: Tissue segmentation of thick-slice fetal brain MR scans with guidance from high-quality isotropic volumes. IEEE Trans. Biomed. Eng. **71**(4), 1404–1415 (2023)
5. Isensee, F.: batchgenerators–a python framework for data augmentation. Zenodo **3632567**, 3 (2020)
6. Isensee, F.: Automated brain extraction of multisequence MRI using artificial neural networks. Hum. Brain Mapp. **40**(17), 4952–4964 (2019)
7. Jain, S.: Automatic quantification of computed tomography features in acute traumatic brain injury. J. Neurotrauma **36**(11), 1794–1803 (2019)
8. King, D.J.: Lesion induced error on automated measures of brain volume: data from a pediatric traumatic brain injury cohort. Front. Neurosci. **14**, 491478 (2020)
9. Liu, H., Dai, Z., So, D., Le, Q.V.: Pay attention to MLPs. Adv. Neural. Inf. Process. Syst. **34**, 9204–9215 (2021)
10. Ni, Y., et al.: DA-Tran: multiphase liver tumor segmentation with a domain-adaptive transformer network. Pattern Recogn. **149**, 110233 (2024)
11. Radwan, A.M.: Virtual brain grafting: enabling whole brain parcellation in the presence of large lesions. Neuroimage **229**, 117731 (2021)
12. Ronneberger, O., Fischer, P., Brox, T.: U-Net: Convolutional networks for biomedical image segmentation. In: International Conference on Medical image computing and computer-assisted intervention, pp. 234–241. Springer (2015)

13. Thompson, P.M.: Enigma and global neuroscience: a decade of large-scale studies of the brain in health and disease across more than 40 countries. Transl. Psychiatry **10**(1), 100 (2020)
14. Xing, Z., Ye, T., Yang, Y., Liu, G., Zhu, L.: SegMamba: Long-range sequential modeling mamba for 3D medical image segmentation. In: International Conference on Medical Image Computing and Computer-Assisted Intervention, pp. 578–588 (2024)
15. Zhu, Y., et al.: Hybrid graph mamba: unlocking non-euclidean potential for accurate polyp segmentation. In: Medical Image Computing and Computer Assisted Intervention – MICCAI 2025, pp. 277–286. Springer Nature Switzerland, Cham (2026)

Hybrid Traumatic Brain Injury Lesion Segmentation Using Voxel-Based V-NET Model and Connected Component Filtering

Balázs Zavadil(✉), András Lenkovics, Bálint Szabó, Ákos Szlávecz, and Balázs Benyó

Department of Control Engineering and Information Technology, Budapest University of Technology and Economics, 1111 Műegyetem rkp. 3., Budapest, Hungary
{zavadilb,lenkovics.andras}@edu.bme.hu,
{bszabo,szlavecz,bbenyo}@iit.bme.hu
https://www.iit.bme.hu/

Abstract. This paper presents a novel segmentation method aiming at Hybrid Traumatic Brain Injury Lesion Segmentation. The proposed model was submitted to the MICCAI's Automated Identification of Moderate-Severe TBI Lesions 2025 (AIMS-TBI25) on behalf of the team "SüSü". The proposed segmentation algorithm comprises a custom V-NET model and filtering based on connected component features. The neural network model was trained using 553 annotated T1-weighted MRI images provided by the challenge organizers. The dataset was split into 455 training and 97 validation images. The learning process was controlled by early stopping to avoid overfitting. Preprocessing normalized intensities to $[0, 1]$ per image and padded smaller scans to $256 \times 256 \times 256$ voxels. The proposed method couples a 3D VNET-based segmentation network with a lightweight connected component filter that removes small predictions; the voxel number threshold is selected on the validation set via a simple sweep. Training used BCEWithLogitsLoss, Adam optimizer, and Instance Normalization (superior to BatchNorm at batch size 1), with augmentation (flips, $\pm 30^\circ$ rotations, and random resized crops). Models were trained on the Komondor HPC (A100, < 40 GB VRAM) and evaluated under a 16 GB VRAM constraint.

In the hidden test set (n=223), our submission was ranked 14th on the leaderboard, corresponding to 9th place among unique teams. A deployment oversight caused the algorithm to return empty masks for 31 scans whose size exceeded 256 in at least one dimension; for transparency, we report results on all test scans (mean Dice 0.496) and on the subset where the model actually produced predictions (n=192, mean Dice 0.571). Despite its simplicity, the connected component filter in the post-processing pipeline yielded an average Dice improvement of 0.098 on the entire test dataset and 0.114 on the filtered dataset compared to raw model predictions.

S. Bakas et al. (Eds.): MICCAI 2025, LNCS 16377, pp. 311–321, 2026.
https://doi.org/10.1007/978-3-032-16370-7_28

Keywords: Traumatic brain injury · MRI · Lesion segmentation · 3D CNN · VNET · Connected component analysis

1 Introduction

Traumatic brain injury (TBI) is a major cause of long-term neurological disability, with moderate-to-severe cases (msTBI) often resulting from external forces such as traffic accidents, falls, or sports-related impacts. These injuries cause the brain to move rapidly in the skull, triggering a cascade of structural changes in the brain. A defining characteristic of msTBI is the high degree of lesion heterogeneity [1]: patients can present with lesions that differ widely in size, location, laterality, and tissue involvement, spanning gray matter, white matter, and cerebrospinal fluid. Unlike stroke, tumors, or multiple sclerosis - conditions that have shaped most existing brain lesion segmentation tools - msTBI lesions are uniquely variable, both focal and diffuse, and can occur across homologous regions in both hemispheres.

Automatic lesion segmentation is needed because current approaches are either unreliable (ignoring lesions), restrictive (excluding patients with large lesions), or impractical (manual segmentation, which is time-consuming and feasible only in small studies). These limitations prevent large-scale, multi-site research and reduce the ability to study how injury type, severity, and accompanying complications affect outcomes. Existing TBI-specific algorithms are also limited, as they require multiple imaging modalities [2] or only work with CT [3], reducing their applicability across large MRI datasets.

The Automated Identification of Mod-Sev TBI Lesions Challenge (AIMS-TBI25) [4], organized as part of the MICCAI 2025 challenges, directly addresses this gap by supporting the development of algorithms capable of accurately segmenting msTBI lesions from T1-weighted MRI scans.

T1-weighted imaging is both widely available and consistent across sites, making it an ideal modality for large-scale, multi-cohort analyses. The ultimate goal is to create robust tools that enable reliable lesion segmentation at scale, thereby supporting downstream analyses such as brain parcellation, connectomics, and prediction of clinical outcomes.

This paper presents a novel segmentation method developed for AIMS-TBI25, submitted under the team name SüSü. Our team consists of students and faculty members from the Budapest University of Technology and Economics.

2 Methods and Data

2.1 Data

Dataset. The dataset provided by the challenge organizers contained a total of 553 annotated T1-weighted MRI images. Each T1-weighted image was accompanied by a lesion mask: masks contained lesion annotations when present, and were empty when no visible lesions were detected. For network training, the dataset was divided into a training and a validation set, 455 randomly selected images were used for training, and 97 were used for validation. In the training iterations, early stopping logic was applied, to avoid overfitting.

Additionally, the algorithm was evaluated on a test dataset that was not available to challenge participants through the grand-challenge.org website. The metrics deciding the leaderboard positions were calculated automatically by the platform and combined classical image comparison metrics like Dice coefficient, Balanced Accuracy and F1 score.

2.2 Data Preprocessing

The dataset consisted of raw T1-weighted MRI images. An analysis on the relative intensity distribution within each image revealed that, after normalization, the voxel intensities followed a Gaussian distribution across the entire dataset.

Therefore, a preprocessing step was introduced: normalize all intensity voxels to the $[0, 1]$ range based on the minimum and maximum values of the image they are in. This makes the images more uniform and comparable to each other.

Additionally, the dimensions of the images were not uniform. Since the vast majority of images were $256 \times 256x256$, we chose this as the input shape for the neural network. As this was the largest shape in the dataset available to us, all images that were smaller were padded on the edges with 0 intensity voxels.

After normalization and padding, the transformed images were saved to `.mha` formats so they can be compressed and read quicker than the `.nii.gz` originals. The conversions were performed using the SimpleITK [5] library.

2.3 Methods

Network Architecture. To assess baseline performance, we compared UNET [6] and VNET [7] based models with different input configurations and architectural depths. Dice coefficient across the entire validation dataset was used to compare the performance of our models.

As shown in Table 1, both UNET variants achieved relatively low Dice scores, while VNET consistently outperformed them, particularly when combined with a connected component (CC) filter to remove small predictions that contain less than a certain amount of voxels. These results motivated our decision to adopt a VNET-based architecture with CC filtering as the foundation for our proposed hybrid method.

Figure 1 shows a schematic representation of the entire data processing workflow, while Fig. 2 details the inner architecture of the neural network used for binary segmentation.

Figure 2 outlines the VNET-based architecture that was chosen for the binary segmentation. The input to this model are the preprocessed (normalized, padded) images and the output is a binary mask with the same dimensions as the input.

As a result of being limited by the amount of hardware VRAM, during training, the loss was calculated for a batch size of just one. This made it possible to train the model with a peak VRAM usage of less than 40GB (making it possible

Table 1. Mean Dice coefficients for different segmentation architectures. The UNET channel sizes show how many slices were considered by the model on each level at once. The numbers in square brackets denote the channel sizes on each level of the VNET model. All metrics were calculated on the validation dataset.

Architecture	Dice coeff.
3-channel UNET	0.354
5-channel UNET	0.322
VNET (raw) [16, 32, 64, 128, 256, 512, 1024]	0.526
VNET + CC Filter [16, 32, 64, 128, 256, 512, 1024]	0.561
VNET + CC Filter [32, 64, 128, 256, 512, 1024]	0.566

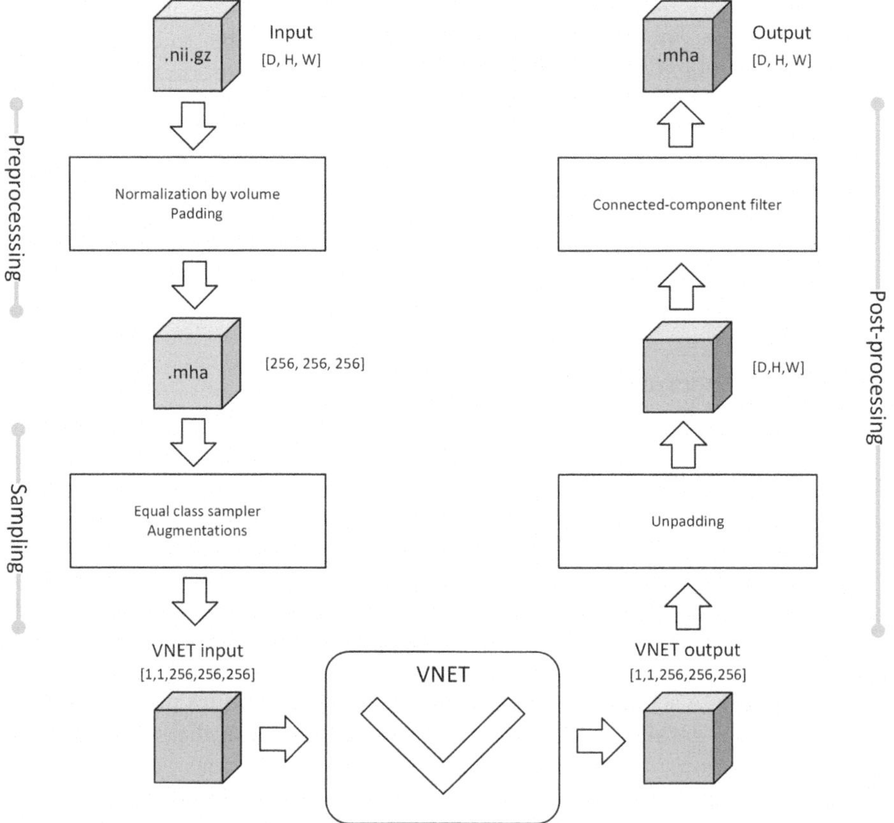

Fig. 1. Overview of the preprocessing, sampling, VNET inference and post-processing pipeline. Tensor shapes are given as [Depth, Height, Width]. For the VNET input and output, two additional leading dimensions denote batch size and number of channels, yielding [Batch size, Channel, Depth, Height, Width].

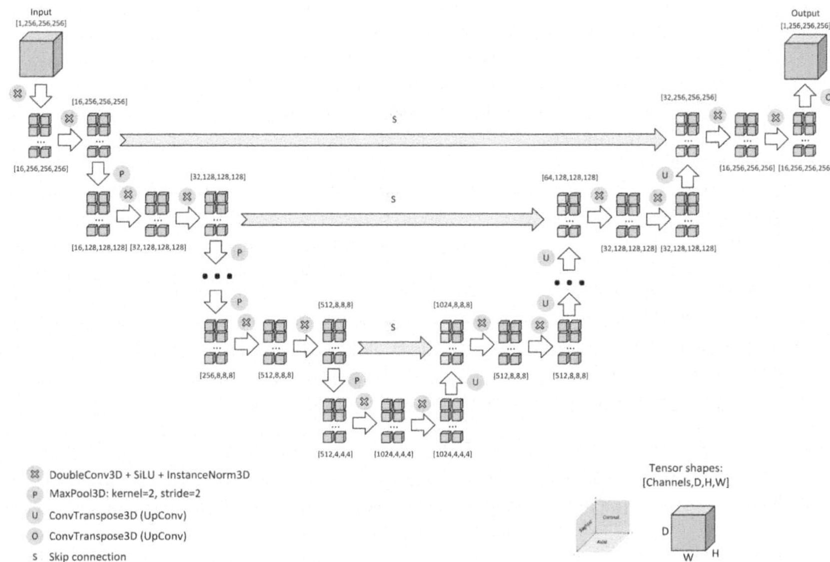

Fig. 2. The proposed VNET-based CNN implementation used for binary segmentation. The tensor shapes are denoted as [Channels, Depth, Width, Height] on the chart. Due to hardware (VRAM) limitations, the batch size is 1 in each case.

to train using an NVIDIA A100 GPU on the Komondor HPC). Additionally, to meet the submission criteria given by the grand challenge organizers, the model would have to use less than 16GB of VRAM (NVIDIA T4 GPU).

After experimenting with different architectures, a model with inner features of [16, 32, 64, 128, 256, 512, 1024] (denoting channels on each level of the VNET) was used. Although, as shown on Table 1, the model with [32, 64, 128, 256, 512, 1024] channels (marginally) outperformed the one we chose, this model used 21724MiB of VRAM during evaluation, which was more than what was available (16GB) on the challenge submission platform.

Please note that even though on Fig. 2 the tensor shape is denoted as $[C, H, D, W]$, in the proposed implementation it is $[B, C, H, D, W]$, but $B = 1$ (batch size) for all instances due to the hardware limitations outlined above.

Data Augmentation and Sampling. The training process incorporated image level balanced sampling to address class imbalance. For data augmentation, we applied the following transformations provided by the Albumentations library [8]:

- **HorizontalFlip** (left-right) with a $p = 0.5$ chance.
- **Rotate** with a $p = 0.5$ chance.
  - Range: $\pm 30°$ around the craniocaudal axis.
- **RandomResizedCrop** (axial slice-wise) with a $p = 0.9$ chance.
  - Scale randomly in the range of $[0.7, 1.0]$ times the original area.

- Jitter the aspect ratio randomly in the range of $[0.9, 1.1]$.
- Finally, crop to: 256×256 for uniform tensor shape.

Loss Function and Optimizer. As a loss function, we used the `BCEWithLogitsLoss` function from the PyTorch [9] library. This loss combines a Sigmoid layer and Binary Cross Entropy.

As the optimizer, the PyTorch implementation of Adam [10] was used.

As mentioned earlier, the proposed model was trained with a batch size of 1 motivated by hardware constraints. Previous research has indicated, that for smaller batch sizes, the widely used Batch Normalization (BatchNorm) is outperformed by Instance Normalization (InstanceNorm). In particular, Kolarik et al. demonstrated that with limited batch sizes, InstanceNorm can improve performance in neural networks for 3D image segmentation [11]. After training two models with the two normalization strategies, it was found that InstanceNorm yielded better results in terms of the Dice coefficient, in line with our findings.

Early Stopping Logic. During training, after each epoch validation and training loss were calculated. As long as validation loss decreases, the model still has useful information to extract from the training dataset. Therefore, an early stopping logic was implemented, where if the validation loss does not improve for 10 epochs, the training would stop and the model with the best validation loss would be evaluated on.

Additionally, as running deep 3D convolutional neural networks is computationally intensive, after each epoch, the model and the optimizer state were saved. With these checkpoints, in case the training stopped for unforeseen reasons or due to running out of the allocated time frame in high-performance computing environments, the training could be resumed later.

Post-processing. Based on connected component analysis of the output masks of the model, we found that there were a large number of false positive predictions among small lesions. This indicated that our algorithm alone was not sufficient. To address this issue, we complemented the VNET with an explicit feature-model-based approach, a simple connected component filter. Although we initially intended to incorporate additional explicit features, in the end we only implemented this post-processing step.

After analyzing the sizes of the predicted masks, we found that 80% of all predicted connected components were below 334 voxels in size.

To counteract this issue, we introduced a filter that would remove all connected components that had less than a certain amount of voxels. The threshold X was calculated the following way using the validation dataset:

1. The model was run on the validation dataset, producing binary segmentation masks as its output.
2. We defined $s = 334/100$ as a step in the filter threshold.

3. After this, we ran a loop for 100 iterations.
4. At each iteration indexed by i, we applied the filter with a threshold of $X_i = \lfloor i \cdot s \rfloor$
5. During each iteration we calculated the average Dice coefficient for all images using the filter with threshold X_i.
6. The X_i with the highest Dice coefficient was selected as X.

Figure 3 shows the Dice coefficients calculated during 100 iterations. The threshold at each iteration i (horizontal axis) was $X_i = \lfloor i \cdot s \rfloor$, yielding roughly evenly distributed filters between 0 and 334. The vertical axis shows the average Dice coefficient for all images, after the connected component filter with the threshold X_i is applied to the model output.

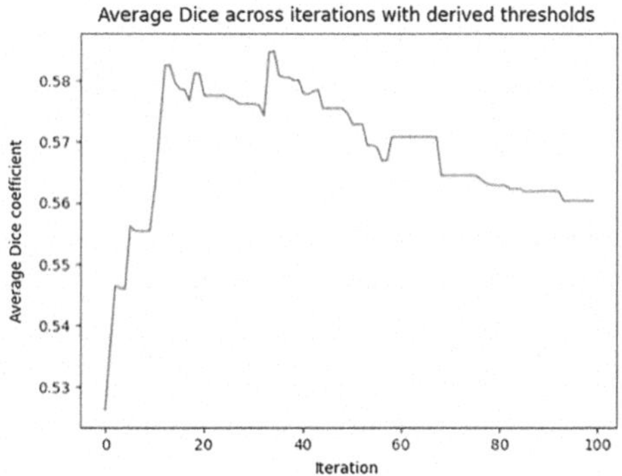

Fig. 3. Average Dice coefficients across 100 connected-component filter thresholds on the validation dataset. The horizontal axis indicates the applied threshold $X_i = \lfloor i \cdot s \rfloor$, distributed between 0 and 334; the vertical axis shows the mean Dice coefficient over all images after filtering.

Additionally, since the images were not uniform in terms of shape, the padding process during preprocessing was inversely applied at the end of post-processing.

Limitations. The connected component filter in our pipeline was tuned to remove predictions smaller than 117 voxels, the threshold that yielded the highest Dice score on the validation dataset. While this step effectively reduced false positives, it likely also removed true lesions below the chosen size. Given the high heterogeneity of msTBI, including the presence of small and diffuse abnormalities, this approach may have sacrificed sensitivity in favor of specificity. Future work should therefore explore more adaptive post-processing strategies that preserve small but clinically relevant lesions.

Implementation. The experiments were carried out on NVIDIA GPUs using CUDA for parallel computation. PyTorch was used as the main deep learning framework for building and training the models. Data augmentation was performed with the Albumentations library. The GPU and AI partitions of the Komondor HPC were used for training and evaluating the proposed models.

3 Results

Based on the metrics provided by the challenge organizers, in the hidden test dataset, the proposed algorithm was deployed on a total of 223 images. Model performance was evaluated based on segmentation accuracy. We placed 14th on the leaderboard, corresponding to 9th place among unique teams.

In the training and validation dataset, there were only images where the width, height and depth were all ≤ 256 voxels. However, in the hidden test dataset, there were 31 images that had more than this in at least 1 dimension. Due to a technical mistake in the proposed model's implementation, for these images, the proposed model was not used, and the algorithm returned an empty mask each time.

To give an accurate picture of the proposed model performance, we will show raw statistics on all images (based on which our leaderboard position was decided) and statistics on only the ones where the proposed model actually performed segmentation. A histogram of Dice coefficients can be seen on Fig. 4.

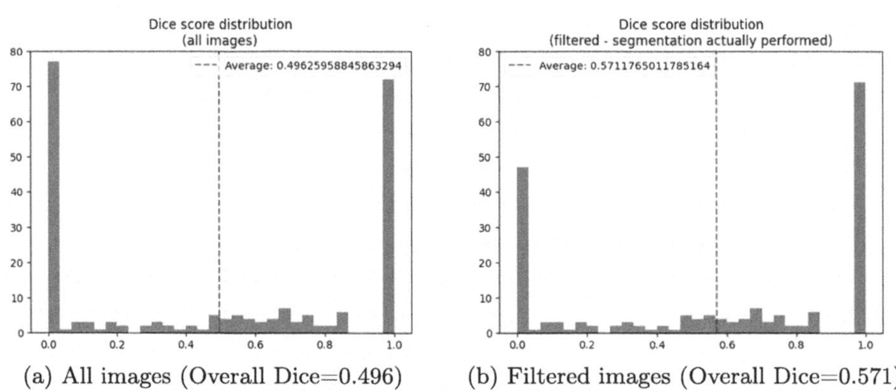

(a) All images (Overall Dice=0.496) (b) Filtered images (Overall Dice=0.571)

Fig. 4. Dice coefficient distributions on all images (a) and on images, where segmentation was actually performed using the proposed model (b). The difference is due to a technical mistake in the proposed model's implementation: the algorithm would return empty masks for all images with a shape larger than 256 in any dimension. Such images were only present in the hidden test dataset.

Table 2 shows the calculated Dice coefficients with and without the connected component filter on the validation and hidden test datasets, using the $X =$

117 threshold for the connected component filter. This yielded an average Dice improvement of 0.098 on the entire test dataset and 0.114 on the filtered dataset compared to raw model predictions. We also saw an improvement of 0.088 and 0.072 in terms of balanced accuracy.

Table 2. Quantitative evaluation of raw VNET outputs and connected component–filtered predictions on the full hidden test set and on the subset of images actually segmented by the algorithm (filtered hidden dataset).

Dataset (n)	Dice	Bal. Acc.	Sens.	Spec.
Hidden DS (n=223), raw output	0.398	0.667	0.685	0.649
Hidden DS (n=223), CC filter	0.496	0.755	0.537	0.973
Filt. hidden DS (n=192), raw output	0.457	0.750	0.857	0.644
Filt. hidden DS (n=192), CC filter	0.571	0.822	0.672	0.973

4 Discussion

A novel VNET-based architecture combined with component-based filtering was proposed for hybrid traumatic brain injury lesion segmentation. Due to a deployment oversight, our submission produced empty masks for 31 scans larger than 256 voxels in at least one dimension, resulting in an overall Dice of 0.496—the score used for leaderboard ranking and corresponding to 9th place among unique participants of the AIMS-TBI25 challenge. When considering only the cases where the algorithm actually performed segmentation, the Dice increased to 0.571, highlighting the method's potential under correct deployment.

The combination of a 3D VNET-based architecture with a simple connected component (CC) filter yielded a consistent boost in segmentation accuracy compared to raw model outputs.

The CC filter was set to remove components smaller than 117 voxels, corresponding to the optimal threshold numerically derived from the validation dataset. While this significantly reduced false positives, it likely also removed true lesions below this size. As msTBI lesions are highly heterogeneous, including small and diffuse abnormalities, the filter may have sacrificed sensitivity in exchange for specificity. This reduction in sensitivity could in turn degrade clinical performance, as small but clinically relevant lesions might be missed. This trade-off highlights the need for more sophisticated post-processing using additional features of the identified connected components.

A major technical limitation in our submission was the failure to handle test images with dimensions exceeding 256 in at least one axis, resulting in empty predictions for 31 cases. A robust improvement would be to include an automated preprocessing step that detects and resamples any input volume to a shape of $256 \times 256 \times 256$ prior to inference. After inference, the segmentation output could then be resampled back to the original image space to ensure consistency with the input data.

The AIMS-TBI25 challenge was important both as a benchmark for developing and comparing lesion segmentation methods, and from a clinical perspective, as it promotes robust lesion detection from widely available T1-weighted MRI. The methods developed will enable large-scale studies of msTBI cases and will support applications such as parcellation, connectomics, and outcome prediction.

5 Conclusion

A VNET-based segmentation pipeline with connected component filtering was proposed for msTBI lesion detection in the AIMS-TBI25 challenge. Despite a deployment oversight that caused empty predictions on oversized scans, the method ranked 9th among unique teams and achieved strong performance when segmentation was correctly applied. The model reached an overall Dice of 0.571 (n=192) on cases it segmented, compared to 0.496 (n=223) when all, including 31 oversized volumes were also considered. While the size-based filter effectively reduced false positives, it also risked discarding small but clinically important lesions. However, the proposed solution enables further development opportunities to improve the sensitivity and better meet the clinical requirements. Future work will aim to make the preprocessing more robust and explore post-processing strategies that preserve sensitivity to small lesions.

Acknowledgments. We acknowledge the Digital Government Development and Project Management Ltd. for awarding us access to the Komondor HPC facility based in Hungary.

References

1. Covington, N.V., Duff, M.C.: Heterogeneity is a hallmark of traumatic brain injury, not a limitation: a new perspective on study design in rehabilitation research. Am. J. Speech Lang. Pathol. **30**(2S), 974–985 (2021)
2. K., Kamnitsas, et al.: Efficient multi-scale 3D CNN with fully connected CRF for accurate brain lesion segmentation. Med. Image Anal. **36**, 61–78 (2017)
3. Jain, S., et al.: Automatic quantification of computed tomography features in acute traumatic brain injury. J. Neurotrauma **36**(11), 1794–1803 (2019)
4. Aims-tbi25 grand challenge. Accessed 23 Sep 2025
5. Lowekamp, B.C., Chen, D.T., Ibanez, L., Blezek, D.: The design of simpleitk. Front. Neuroinform. **7**, 45 (2013)
6. Ronneberger, O., Fischer, P., Brox, T.: U-Net: Convolutional networks for biomedical image segmentation. CoRR, abs/1505.04597 (2015)
7. Milletari, F., Navab, N., Ahmadi, S.: Fully convolutional neural networks for volumetric medical image segmentation, V-net (2016)
8. Khvedchenya, E., Iglovikov, V.I., Buslaev, A., Parinov, A., Kalinin, A.A.: Albumentations: fast and flexible image augmentations. ArXiv e-prints (2018)

9. Paszke, A.: PyTorch: an imperative style, high-performance deep learning library. Curran Associates Inc., Red Hook, NY, USA (2019)
10. Kingma, D.P., Adam, J.B.: A method for stochastic optimization (2017)
11. Kolarik, M., Burget, R., Riha, K.: Comparing normalization methods for limited batch size segmentation neural networks. In: 2020 43rd International Conference on Telecommunications and Signal Processing (TSP), pp. 677–680. IEEE (2020)

Lesion Segmentation in Moderate to Severe Traumatic Brain Injury: An NnU-Net Based Approach with Adaptive Normalization in the AIMS-TBI 2025 Challenge

Inhwa Son[1], Gaeun Lee[1], Sohyeon Sim[1], and Kwang-Hyun Uhm[1,2(✉)]

[1] Gachon University, Seongnam, Republic of Korea
{inhwa1127,tong0430aa,thgus0101,khuhm}@gachon.ac.kr
[2] MEDAI, Seoul, Republic of Korea

Abstract. The segmentation of lesions in Moderate to Severe Traumatic Brain Injury (msTBI) from T1-weighted MRI presents a significant clinical challenge due to the profound heterogeneity of lesion characteristics in terms of size, shape, and location. To address this, the AIMS-TBI 2025 Challenge was organized to promote the development of robust and accurate segmentation algorithms. In this paper, we present our deep learning-based solution. Our methodology employs the nnU-Net framework with an adaptive intensity normalization strategy confined to the brain parenchyma, effectively reducing inter-subject variability and mitigating artifacts from non-brain structures. Upon final evaluation on the held-out test set, our method demonstrated highly competitive performance on the official leaderboard, achieving an Overall Dice Coefficient of 0.6305. The model obtained a Dice score of 0.4805 for lesion segmentation and 0.9324 for non-lesion tissue. While the lesion Dice reflects the difficulty of detecting highly heterogeneous lesions, the high non-lesion Dice primarily indicates the model's strong ability to correctly identify non-lesion voxels, demonstrating good specificity in differentiating lesion from non-lesion regions. These results demonstrate that incorporating anatomically constrained normalization within the nnU-Net pipeline is a powerful and effective strategy for tackling the complexities of msTBI lesion segmentation.

Keywords: Moderate to Severe Traumatic Brain Injury · Magnetic Resonance Imaging · Lesion Segmentation · Adaptive Normalization · Brain Parenchyma

1 Introduction

Traumatic brain injury (TBI) is a leading cause of mortality and long-term disability worldwide, arising from external mechanical forces such as traffic accidents, falls, or sports-related impacts. In moderate to severe TBI (msTBI), the

S. Bakas et al. (Eds.): MICCAI 2025, LNCS 16377, pp. 322–329, 2026.
https://doi.org/10.1007/978-3-032-16370-7_29

rapid acceleration and deceleration of the brain within the skull induces both primary injuries (e.g., hematomas, hemorrhages, contusions) and secondary injuries (e.g., gliosis, encephalomalacia), which may necessitate urgent surgical intervention. These injuries produce diverse structural deformations in the brain, and each patient typically presents with a unique combination of lesion patterns. Such heterogeneity—spanning lesion size, number, laterality, and tissue involvement across gray matter, white matter, and cerebrospinal fluid—is widely recognized as a hallmark of msTBI.

This extreme heterogeneity introduces substantial challenges for neuroimaging analysis. Lesions in msTBI differ fundamentally from other pathologies such as stroke or tumors, as they may be focal or diffuse and frequently extend across multiple tissue types or bilateral regions. These complex patterns complicate image registration, normalization, and downstream parcellation, often leading to both local and global errors in brain analysis. While lesion compensation methods have been proposed—such as brain extraction or lesion inpainting—most approaches require labor-intensive manual segmentation, which is impractical in large-scale studies. Automated lesion segmentation tools developed for other etiologies have also shown limited performance in TBI, reflecting the need for specialized solutions.

In the absence of accurate automated tools, researchers have resorted to strategies such as ignoring lesions, excluding patients with large injuries, or relying on manual segmentation. These workarounds either reduce reliability, restrict generalizability, or limit statistical power for subgroup analyses. As a result, progress in understanding how factors such as lesion type, severity, or comorbid conditions influence patient outcomes has been constrained. To address these barriers, robust and scalable algorithms for msTBI lesion segmentation are urgently needed. In recent years, deep learning methods have been increasingly applied to medical image analysis and have shown rapid progress, offering state-of-the-art performance across a wide range of tasks [3–7]. This makes deep learning a particularly promising approach for addressing the unique challenges of lesion segmentation in msTBI.

The Automated Imaging for Moderate-to-Severe TBI (AIMS-TBI) Challenge was established to accelerate progress in this area. Leveraging multi-site data from the ENIGMA Consortium, the challenge focuses specifically on T1-weighted MRI—the most widely available modality across clinical cohorts—thereby enhancing applicability in large-scale, multi-institutional research. The inaugural AIMS-TBI Challenge, held at MICCAI 2024, demonstrated the feasibility of this task, with top-performing methods achieving a Dice score of 0.61. However, these results also underscored significant room for improvement, motivating subsequent editions with larger datasets and more diverse cohorts.

Building upon this foundation, the 2025 AIMS-TBI Challenge provides an expanded dataset and continues to benchmark lesion segmentation algorithms under realistic, multi-cohort conditions. Accurate automated segmentation of msTBI lesions will not only streamline neuroimaging workflows but also enable advanced analyses such as parcellation, functional and structural connectivity, and outcome prediction, ultimately contributing to improved clinical understanding and patient care. In this work, we present our solution to the AIMS-TBI 2025 Challenge, which leverages the nnU-Net framework enhanced with an adaptive intensity normalization strategy confined to the brain parenchyma. By incorporating anatomically constrained normalization into the preprocessing pipeline, our method reduces inter-subject variability and mitigates artifacts from non-brain structures, leading to more robust lesion segmentation performance on heterogeneous multi-site MRI data.

2 Method

2.1 Dataset

We utilized the dataset provided by the AIMS-TBI 2025 Challenge [1], which consists of multi-site T1-weighted (T1w) MRI scans of patients with moderate to severe traumatic brain injury (msTBI). The data were aggregated from 13 international sites participating in the ENIGMA Pediatric and Adult msTBI working groups, covering subjects aged 5âĂŞ85 years (64% male), with enrichment for adolescent cases to reflect epidemiological trends. Imaging was performed on 1.5T and 3T scanners from multiple manufacturers (GE, Siemens, Philips). Most scans had isotropic 1 mm^3 voxel resolution, though acquisition parameters varied within standard ranges.

A total of 875 MRI scans were included, split into 500 training (57%), 100 validation (11%), and 275 test (32%) cases. A case was defined as one T1w MRI scan from a particular patient. While the majority of patients contributed a single scan, some contributed longitudinal scans (up to four time points); in these cases, all longitudinal scans were assigned to the same split (training, validation, or test) to prevent data leakage. The test set was designed to reflect real-world heterogeneity in age, sex, scanner, and lesion distribution.

Lesions encompassed a wide spectrum of injury-related pathologies, including contusions, hematomas, hemorrhages, encephalomalacia, gliosis, white matter lesions, and surgical drainage tracts. Reference lesion annotations were generated through a four-step process: (i) initial automated segmentation using a U-Net pretrained on the ATLAS v2.0 dataset, (ii) manual review and edits by a trained rater, (iii) secondary review by another rater, and (iv) final approval by an expert annotator. In total, seven primary and five expert annotators contributed to the labeling, following a standardized protocol. Annotation was performed in ITK-SNAP, and all raters underwent training with feedback to ensure consistency. Each image was reviewed by at least three annotators sequentially, minimizing missed lesions and boundary errors.

No lesions were excluded based on size; even very small lesions (e.g., < 10 voxels) were retained during both training and evaluation. To protect privacy, all MRI scans were defaced using `pydeface`, and identifying metadata were removed. Only age (rounded to the nearest year) and time since injury (in weeks) were provided as demographic information.

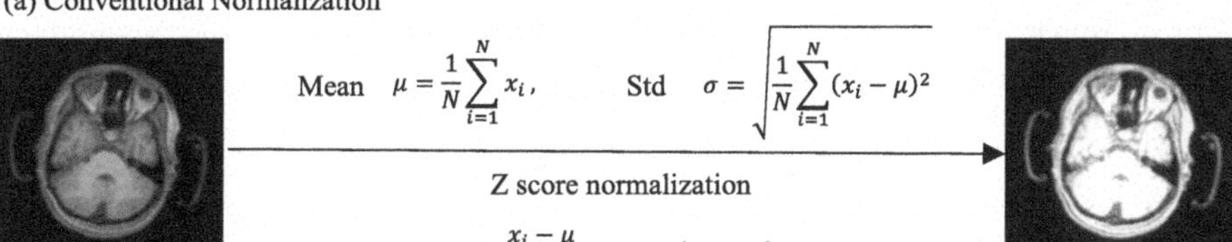

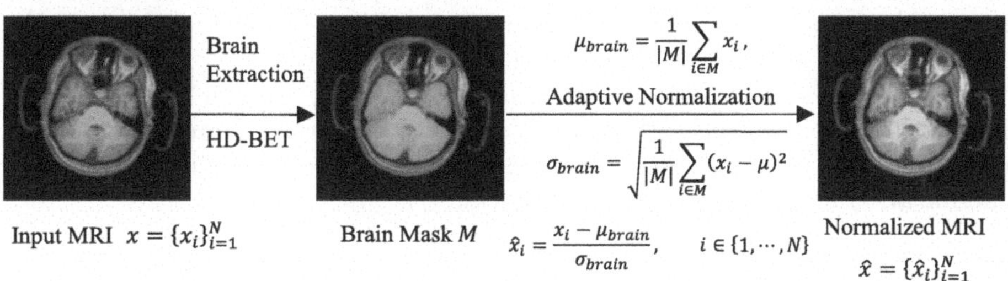

Fig. 1. Comparison of normalization strategies within the nnU-Net framework. (a) Conventional normalization computes mean and standard deviation over all voxels, leading to potential variability from non-brain regions. (b) The proposed anatomically constrained adaptive normalization restricts computation to brain parenchyma voxels using a brain mask, thereby reducing inter-subject variance and improving robustness.

2.2 Preprocessing

A key component of our method is an *adaptive intensity normalization strategy* tailored to the heterogeneity of msTBI. In conventional preprocessing pipelines, normalization statistics (mean and standard deviation) are calculated over the entire image volume, including skull and background regions. This often results in substantial inter-subject variability, as skull brightness and non-brain tissues introduce inconsistencies across scans. Such variability can obscure lesion-specific signal characteristics and reduce the effectiveness of subsequent learning. As illustrated in Fig. 1, our approach differs from conventional normalization by restricting the computation of normalization statistics to the brain parenchyma.

To mitigate this issue, we extracted the *brain parenchyma mask* from each MRI scan. Normalization parameters were then computed exclusively within this intracranial region, and voxel intensities were normalized using these brain-specific statistics. Formally, given an input MRI $x = \{x_i\}_{i=1}^{N}$ with N voxels and a binary brain mask M, we defined the masked mean and variance as

$$\mu_{\text{brain}} = \frac{1}{|M|}\sum_{i \in M} x_i, \quad \sigma_{\text{brain}} = \sqrt{\frac{1}{|M|}\sum_{i \in M}(x_i - \mu_{\text{brain}})^2}, \tag{1}$$

where μ_{brain} and σ_{brain} denote the mean and standard deviation computed within the brain mask M, and $|M|$ is the number of voxels inside the mask. Normalized intensities were then obtained as

$$\hat{x}_i = \frac{x_i - \mu_{\text{brain}}}{\sigma_{\text{brain}}}, \quad i = 1, \ldots, N, \tag{2}$$

By confining normalization to brain tissue, this strategy reduces variance across subjects caused by non-brain structures, leading to more stable intensity distributions and allowing the segmentation model to better focus on pathological regions. All MRI volumes were further resampled to isotropic 1 mm^3 resolution and cropped or padded to standardized sizes as specified by the nnU-Net framework.

We applied extensive data augmentation, including random rotations, scaling, flipping, intensity perturbations, elastic deformations, gamma corrections, and Gaussian noise, to enhance robustness to site-specific variability and improve generalization across heterogeneous cohorts.

2.3 Model Architecture

We adopted the *Residual Encoder Large (resencL)* variant of the nnU-Net [2] framework. This configuration employs residual blocks in the encoder path to improve feature representation and gradient flow, while maintaining the standard U-shaped architecture with skip connections and deep supervision. The large variant increases model capacity, making it suitable for capturing the heterogeneous and complex lesion patterns characteristic of msTBI.

2.4 Training and Inference

The network was trained end-to-end using a hybrid loss function combining *Dice loss* and *cross-entropy loss*, balancing overlap-based and voxel-wise optimization objectives. Optimization employed stochastic gradient descent with momentum, an initial learning rate of 0.01, and a polynomial decay schedule. Training was performed for 1000 epochs with extensive online data augmentation. In inference, *test-time augmentation (TTA)* was applied by mirroring images along different spatial axes, and predictions were averaged across augmentations.

3 Results

3.1 Evaluation Metrics

The final evaluation was conducted on the hidden test set of the AIMS-TBI 2025 Challenge using four official metrics: (1) the mean position across all criteria, (2) the Dice coefficient for lesion segmentation, (3) the Dice coefficient for non-lesion tissue, and (4) the overall Dice coefficient, computed as the average of lesion and non-lesion Dice scores. This multi-metric evaluation ensured that algorithms were not only accurate in lesion segmentation but also reliable in preserving non-lesion regions.

Table 1. Performance comparison across variants during preliminary development and final test leaderboard. Results highlight the effect of extensive data augmentation (DA5) and adaptive normalization (Adaptive Norm.).

Method	Balanced Acc.	Dice (les.)	Dice (no les.)	Overall
Preliminary Development Results (leaderboard)				
Base (ResEnc L)	0.8713	0.5514	0.8936	0.7123
DA5 (extensive augmentation)	0.8725	0.5428	**0.9149**	0.7177
Adaptive Normalization	0.8537	0.5450	**0.9149**	**0.7189**
DA5 + Adaptive Norm.	**0.8808**	**0.5550**	0.8936	0.7141
Final Test Results (leaderboard)				
DA5 (extensive augmentation)	0.8587	**0.4820**	0.9054	0.6225
DA5 + Adaptive Norm.	**0.8622**	0.4805	**0.9324**	**0.6305**

3.2 Effect of Adaptive Normalization and Data Augmentation

Table 1 summarizes the performance across different variants during both the preliminary development phase (Phase 1) and the final test leaderboard. The baseline model ("Base") corresponds to ResEnc L without additional normalization or augmentation. Comparisons with "DA5" (extensive augmentation) and "Adaptive Norm." (adaptive normalization) allow us to directly assess the contribution of each component.

During Phase 1, both DA5 and Adaptive Norm. independently improved robustness, particularly in terms of no-lesion Dice. Their combination ("DA5 + Adaptive Norm.") achieved the highest overall score (0.8808), highlighting complementary benefits. These outcomes demonstrate that the proposed Adaptive Norm. provides measurable gains over no-normalization or augmentation-only strategies.

Final test results further confirm this trend: "DA5 + Adaptive Norm." achieved the best overall Dice (0.6305), outperforming augmentation-only (0.6225). This consistency across development and test phases indicates that Adaptive Norm. enhances generalization, especially when combined with strong data augmentation.

3.3 Leaderboard Results

Table 2 summarizes the performance of the top-ranking methods on the final test leaderboard. Our approach achieved a mean position of 5.5, with a lesion Dice of 0.4805, a non-lesion Dice of 0.9324, and an overall Dice of 0.6305. These results demonstrate that our adaptive normalization strategy, combined with the residual encoder large variant of nnU-Net, yields a balanced trade-off between lesion segmentation and preservation of non-lesion tissue.

Table 2. Final test leaderboard results of the AIMS-TBI 2025 Challenge. Five metrics were reported: mean position, score, Dice for lesions, Dice for non-lesion tissue, and overall Dice.

Team	Pos.	Balanced Acc.	Dice (Les.)	Dice (No Les.)	Overall
iMedIA_2025	3.5	**0.8924**	0.4904	**0.9324**	**0.6371**
AIMHI-MEDAI (ours)	5.5	0.8622	0.4805	**0.9324**	0.6305
NIC-VICOROB	6.0	0.8554	0.4941	0.9189	0.6351
SpaceCY	8.3	0.8383	**0.5149**	0.8243	0.6176
jianghaotian0001	8.3	0.8585	0.5013	0.8243	0.6085

3.4 Performance Analysis

Compared to other submissions, our method maintained highly competitive performance on both lesion and non-lesion Dice coefficients. Although the lesion Dice (0.4805) was modest relative to some teams, the strong non-lesion Dice (0.9324) contributed to a well-balanced overall Dice of 0.6305, placing our method among the top systems. These results validate the effectiveness of our anatomically constrained normalization strategy in reducing inter-subject intensity variance and improving robustness across heterogeneous multi-site MRI data.

Interestingly, while some methods achieved higher lesion Dice, this often came at the cost of reduced non-lesion accuracy, leading to more false positives or over-segmentation. In contrast, our approach prioritized robust representation of healthy tissue while maintaining reasonable lesion segmentation accuracy, yielding a well-balanced overall performance. This trade-off suggests that future improvements may come from enhancing sensitivity to small or diffuse lesions without sacrificing non-lesion fidelity.

4 Conclusion

In this study, we presented a deep learning-based solution to the AIMS-TBI 2025 Challenge for lesion segmentation in moderate to severe TBI. Our method built upon the nnU-Net framework and introduced an adaptive normalization strategy restricted to the brain parenchyma, reducing inter-subject variance and improving robustness. By employing the residual encoder large (resencL) variant, and extensive data augmentation, our approach achieved strong performance on the official test leaderboard, with a balanced trade-off between lesion and non-lesion segmentation.

These findings highlight the importance of anatomically informed preprocessing for robust lesion segmentation in heterogeneous clinical populations. In future work, we aim to further enhance lesion sensitivity, particularly for small and diffuse injuries, by incorporating multi-scale feature representations and integrating complementary MRI modalities. While our current analysis did not specifically examine performance variations across lesion size or anatomical location, we recognize this as an important direction for future investigation. Ultimately, accurate and automated lesion segmentation will facilitate advanced neuroimaging analyses and contribute to improved clinical understanding and prognostic modeling in msTBI.

References

1. Dennis, E., et al.: AIMS-TBI - automated identification of moderate- severe traumatic brain injury lesions (2025). https://doi.org/10.5281/zenodo.15084120
2. Isensee, F., Jaeger, P.F., S.K.e.a.: nnU-Net: a self-configuring method for deep learning-based biomedical image segmentation. Nat. Methods **18**, 203—-211 (2021)
3. Uhm, K.H., Cho, H., Hong, S.H., Jung, S.W.: An anisotropic cross-view texture transfer with multi-reference non-local attention for CT slice interpolation. IEEE Trans. Med. Imaging 1 (2025). https://doi.org/10.1109/TMI.2025.3596957
4. Uhm, K.H., et al.: Exploring 3D U-Net training configurations and post-processing strategies for the MICCAI 2023 kidney and tumor segmentation challenge. In: Kidney and Kidney Tumor Segmentation, pp. 8–13. Springer Nature Switzerland (2024)
5. Uhm, K.H., Jung, S.W., Choi, M.H., Hong, S.H., Ko, S.J.: A unified multi-phase CT synthesis and classification framework for kidney cancer diagnosis with incomplete data. IEEE J. Biomed. Health Inform. **26**(12), 6093–6104 (2022)
6. Uhm, K.H., Jung, S.W., Hong, S.H., Ko, S.J.: Lesion-aware cross-phase attention network for renal tumor subtype classification on multi-phase CT scans. Comput. Biol. Med. **178**, 108746 (2024)
7. Uhm, K.H., et al.: Deep learning for end-to-end kidney cancer diagnosis on multi-phase abdominal computed tomography. NPJ Precis. Onc. **5**(54) (2021)

NeuroNetMix: A 3D Encoder-Decoder with Quasiseparable Mixing for Robust Lesion Segmentation in Traumatic Brain Injury

Moona Mazher[1], Steven A. Niederer[2], and Abdul Qayyum[2](✉)

[1] Centre for Medical Image Computing, Department of Computer Science, University College London, London, UK

[2] National Heart and Lung Institute, Faculty of Medicine, Imperial College London, London, UK

a.qayyum@imperial.ac.uk

Abstract. Moderate to severe traumatic brain injury (msTBI) results in complex and heterogeneous brain lesions, posing significant challenges for neuroimaging analysis. These lesions vary widely in size, number, and tissue distribution, complicating processes such as image registration and parcellation. Traditional segmentation tools often require multiple imaging modalities or manual intervention, limiting their effectiveness for msTBI. To address these challenges, we propose NeuroNetMix, a 3D encoder-decoder framework specifically designed for T1-weighted MRI, the most widely available scan type in the ENIGMA TBI consortium. NeuroNetMix integrates bidirectional quasiseparable mixing at its bottleneck to capture both local lesion detail and long-range spatial dependencies, enhancing volumetric continuity and segmentation accuracy. The encoder extracts hierarchical volumetric features while preserving small and irregular lesions via skip connections, and the decoder reconstructs high-resolution segmentation maps. Evaluations demonstrate that NeuroNetMix outperforms existing methods, including xLSTM and 3D Mamba UNet, achieving state-of-the-art performance on both validation and testing datasets. By providing reliable and precise lesion maps, NeuroNetMix facilitates improved downstream analyses such as brain parcellation and connectomics, supporting more accurate prognostic assessment and treatment planning for msTBI patients.

Keywords: Bidirectional Quasiseparable Mixing · State-Space Models · Brain Lesion Segmentation · Moderate to Severe Traumatic Brain Injury (msTBI) · xLSTM

1 Introduction

Moderate to severe traumatic brain injury (msTBI) results from external forces, such as traffic accidents, falls, or sports injuries, causing rapid movement of the brain within the skull. This movement initiates complex pathophysiological processes and multiple primary, secondary, and surgery-related mechanisms that can induce structural deformations in the brain. Each msTBI patient exhibits a unique combination of these changes,

S. Bakas et al. (Eds.): MICCAI 2025, LNCS 16377, pp. 330–340, 2026.
https://doi.org/10.1007/978-3-032-16370-7_30

resulting in highly heterogeneous lesions—a hallmark of msTBI [1]. Unlike other common brain pathologies (e.g., stroke, multiple sclerosis, brain tumors), msTBI lesions can be both focal and diffuse, varying widely in size, number, and laterality. They may span multiple tissue types (gray matter, white matter, cerebrospinal fluid) and even occur in homologous regions of both hemispheres. Such variability complicates image registration, normalization, and brain parcellation, potentially introducing both local and global errors [2].

Existing neuroimaging tools, including HD_Bet [3], VBG [4], and FastSurfer, often rely on time-consuming manual lesion masks and quality assessment steps. Methods designed for other lesion etiologies (e.g., stroke or tumors [5]) generally perform poorly on TBI data. TBI-specific algorithms exist but may require multiple MRI modalities (T1, T2, FLAIR, GE, PD) [6] or are limited to CT images [7], which complicates large-scale, multi-site studies and introduces variability across scans. To address these challenges, we focus on accurate lesion identification using only T1-weighted MRI is most commonly available modality in the ENIGMA TBI consortium. Reliable lesion segmentation in medical imaging is critical for downstream analyses such as parcellation, functional connectivity, connectomics, and fixel-based studies, and has the potential to improve prognostication and long-term outcomes for msTBI patients. In recent years, numerous segmentation models have been developed for medical image analysis [8–17], demonstrating the potential of deep learning to accurately delineate complex anatomical structures and lesions.

To address these challenges, we propose NeuroNetMix, a 3D encoder-decoder framework that integrates bidirectional quasiseparable mixing at its bottleneck to capture both local lesion detail and long-range spatial dependencies. The encoder extracts hierarchical volumetric features while preserving small and irregular lesion information via skip connections, and the decoder reconstructs high-resolution segmentation maps. At the bottleneck, NeuroNetMix treats the 3D feature volume as a sequence, applying causal and anti-causal mixing using semiseparable state-space models (SSMs) [18] to efficiently aggregate global contextual information. This combination of local convolutional feature extraction with global sequence-based context modeling enhances volumetric continuity and segmentation accuracy, outperforming existing methods such as xLSTM [19] and 3D UNet. NeuroNetMix thus provides reliable lesion maps for clinical assessment and supports improved prognostication and treatment planning in msTBI.

2 Proposed Method

In this section, we describe the dataset used for training and evaluation, followed by the architecture and implementation details of the proposed NeuroNetMix framework.

2.1 Dataset

We used the 2025 AIMS-TBI challenge dataset, comprising T1-weighted MRI scans from 552 subjects with moderate-to-severe traumatic brain injury (msTBI). High-quality manual lesion annotations are provided for supervised learning and validation. The dataset captures heterogeneous lesions varying in size, location, and tissue type, including both focal and diffuse injuries.

2.2 Model

1. **NeuroNetMix: Proposed Model for 3D TBI Lesion Segmentation**

Accurate segmentation of traumatic brain injury (TBI) lesions is crucial for diagnosis, prognosis, and treatment planning. The proposed NeuroNetMix is illustrated in Figure 1. NeuroNetMix is a 3D encoder-decoder framework enhanced with bidirectional quasiseparable mixing to capture both local lesion details and long-range spatial dependencies. Traditional CNNs (e.g., xLSTM, 3D UNet) capture local features well but often miss global context; NeuroNetMix addresses this by integrating sequence-based global feature mixing at the bottleneck.

2. **Encoder–Decoder Framework**

NeuroNetMix employs a classical 3D encoder-decoder design optimized for volumetric brain MRI:

- Encoder: Hierarchical 3D convolutional blocks with batch normalization and non-linear activation, downsampling via strided convolutions. Skip connections preserve fine anatomical details.
- Decoder: Mirrors the encoder with 3D transposed convolutions and skip connections, reconstructing high-resolution segmentation maps.

3. **NeuroNetMix Mixing at the Bottleneck**

The NeuroNetMix mixing layer performs bidirectional quasiseparable operations to model long-range spatial dependencies. The encoder employs convolutional layers to extract rich local spatial features while progressively reducing spatial resolution. The decoder then uses upsampling layers to restore spatial details and generate the final segmentation output. Crucially, at the network's bottleneck, we integrate the NeuroNetMix layer, which implements bidirectional quasiseparable mixing. A bidirectional quasiseparable mixing is specifically designed to handle sequences derived from volumetric spatial data such as 3D medical images. Given an input volume of shape (B, C, H, W, D), the spatial dimensions (H, W, D) are flattened into a sequence length S=H $\times$ W $\times$ D. This transformation allows the model to process the volume as a sequence of spatial positions, facilitating the application of sequential mixing operations that aggregate information across the entire spatial domain.

Additionally, a self-connection term applies learnable diagonal parameters to each position's features, preserving local information and stabilizing the mixing process. Mathematically, this operation corresponds to a quasiseparable mixing matrix M structured as follows: the diagonal entries represent self-connection weights, the lower triangular part encodes causal mixing weights for past positions, and the upper triangular part encodes anti-causal mixing weights for future positions. The quasiseparable structure implies a low-rank representation that enables efficient computation without explicitly forming a large dense matrix [20]. The equation below describes how the output at each sequence position i is computed by combining three components.

For each batch b, position i:

$$Y_{b,i} = \sum_{j<i} A_i b_j X_{b,j} + \sum_{j>i} A'_i b'_j X_{b,j} + \delta_i X_{b,i}$$

Where A_i, b_j: causal parameters, A'_i, b'_j: anti-causal parameters and δ_i: diagonal/self-connection

The matrix M shown for sequence length 16 illustrates how the bidirectional mixing operates. Its diagonal elements δ_i represent self-connection weights that preserve local information at each position i. This structured matrix efficiently captures dependencies in both directions while maintaining a sparse, low-rank form for fast computation.

$$M = \begin{bmatrix} \delta_1 & A'_1b'_2 & A'_1b'_3 & \cdots & A'_1b'_{16} \\ A_2b_1 & \delta_2 & A'_2b'_3 & \cdots & A'_2b'_{16} \\ A_3b_1 & A_3b_2 & \delta_3 & \cdots & A'_3b'_{16} \\ \vdots & \vdots & \vdots & \ddots & \vdots \\ A_{16}b_1 & A_{16}b_2 & A_{16}b_3 & \cdots & \delta_{16} \end{bmatrix}$$

Where,

Diagonal: δ_i for $i = 1, \ldots, 16$
Lower triangle: A_ib_j for $i > j$
Upper triangle: $A'_ib'_j$ for $i < j$
Lower triangle (below diagonal): Each entry M_{ij} for $i > j$ mixes information from past positions using parameters A_i and b_j (causal direction).
Upper triangle (above diagonal): Each entry M_{ij} for $i < j$ mixes information from future positions using parameters A'_i and b'_j (anti-causal direction).
Diagonal: Each M_{ii} is a self-connection parameter δ_i.

4. **Multi-Scale Feature Fusion**

After mixing, the sequence is reshaped to 3D. Multi-scale skip connections from the encoder refine both small lesions and larger structural patterns, improving segmentation of heterogeneous TBI lesions.

- Local + Global Feature Integration: Convolutional encoders capture local texture, while NeuroNetMix mixing captures long-range spatial dependencies.
- Efficient Global Context Modeling: Bidirectional SSMs with quasiseparable matrices efficiently propagate voxel-level information without large dense matrices.

3 Results

3.1 Validation Phase Performance

The NeuroNetMix model was evaluated on the validation dataset to compare against the baseline xLSTM and 3D Mamba models. The comparative performance is summarized in Table 1.

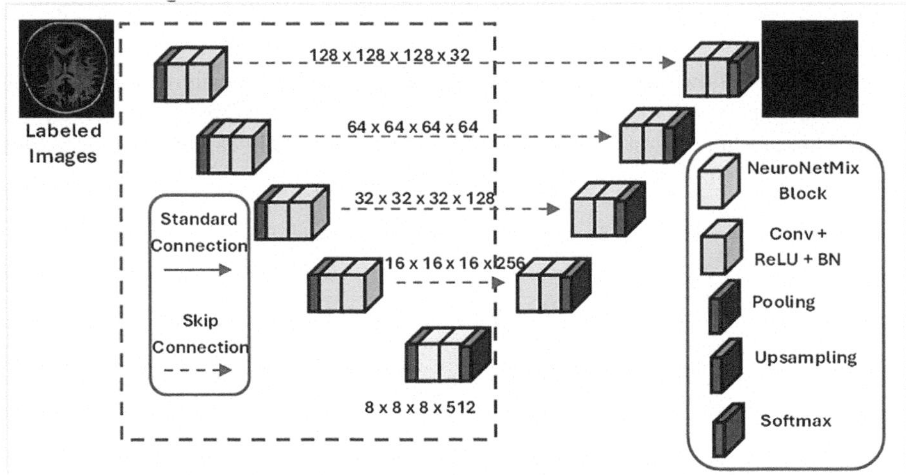

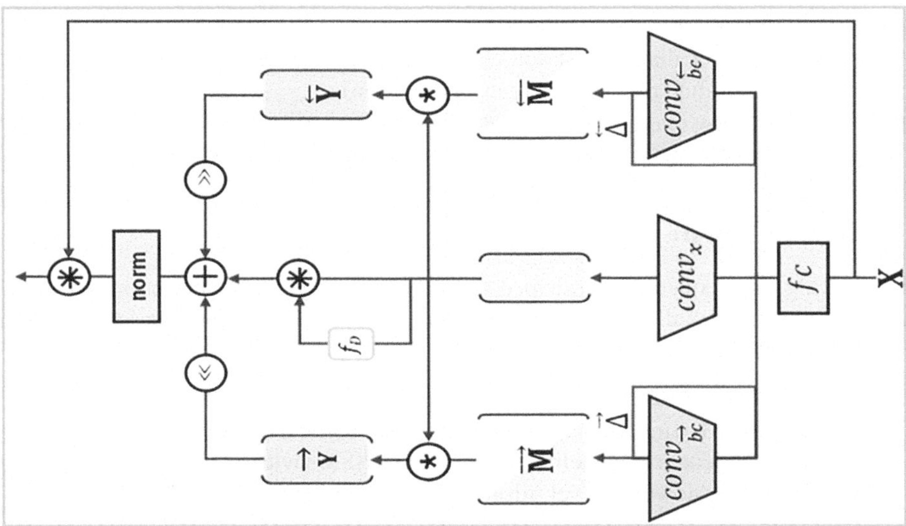

Fig. 1. Architectural framework of NeuroNetMix designed for segmentation of complex and heterogeneous brain lesions in moderate-to-severe traumatic brain injury (msTBI).

Table 1. Comparative Validation Performance

Metric	NeuroNetMix (Proposed)	3D xLSTM	3D Mamba
Sensitivity	0.943	0.925	0.906
Specificity	0.830	0.851	0.851
Balanced Accuracy	0.887	0.888	0.878
True Positives (TP)	50	49	48
True Negatives (TN)	39	40	40
False Positives (FP)	8	7	7
False Negatives (FN)	3	4	5
Lesion Detection Rate (mean)	0.522	0.531	0.491
Lesion Dice (mean)	0.597	0.596	0.565
Overall Dice (mean)	0.716	0.706	0.699
Lesion F1-score (mean)	0.568	0.541	0.526
Overall F1-score (mean)	0.691	0.687	0.679
Lesion Absolute Lesion Diff.	3.34	3.81	3.74
Overall Absolute Lesion Diff.	1.89	2.13	2.14

NeuroNetMix achieved the highest lesion and overall Dice, as well as superior lesion-wise and overall F1-scores, demonstrating robust voxel- and lesion-level performance. Its high sensitivity (0.943) and low false negatives (3) indicate reliable detection of clinically relevant lesions. The bidirectional quasiseparable mixing integrates local lesion features with global brain context, effectively handling heterogeneous TBI patterns. xLSTM performed well in specificity and balanced accuracy but was slightly lower in lesion detection and F1, while 3D Mamba underperformed in lesion-level metrics.

3.2 Test Phase Performance

The generalization of NeuroNetMix was evaluated on the unseen test set. The results are summarized in Table 2.

Table 2. NeuroNetMix Test Phase Performance

Metric	Test Score
Sensitivity	0.893
Specificity	0.716
Balanced Accuracy	0.804
True Positives (TP)	133
True Negatives (TN)	53
False Positives (FP)	21
False Negatives (FN)	16

(*continued*)

Table 2. (*continued*)

Metric	Test Score
Lesion Detection Rate (mean)	0.515
Lesion Dice (mean)	0.491
Overall Dice (mean)	0.566
Lesion F1-score (mean)	0.545
Overall F1-score (mean)	0.602
Lesion Absolute Lesion Diff.	3.37
Overall Absolute Lesion Diff.	2.43

On the test set, NeuroNetMix maintained strong sensitivity (0.893) and F1-score (0.602), with a slight decrease in lesion Dice (0.491), reflecting some under-segmentation of large or irregular lesions. For NO-lesion cases, Dice and F1 were 0.716, indicating reliable discrimination. Overall, NeuroNetMix generalized well, consistently outperforming xLSTM and 3D Mamba in key metrics. Its bidirectional quasiseparable mixing effectively models long-range spatial dependencies, balancing voxel-level accuracy with lesion-level detection and count reliability, making it suitable for automated, clinically robust TBI segmentation.

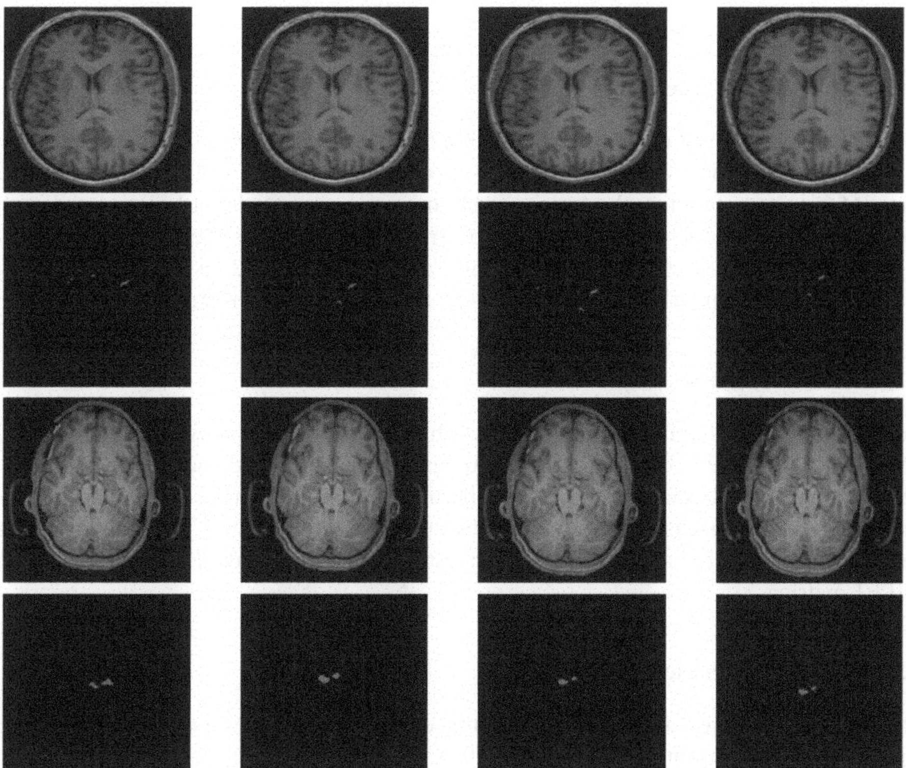

Fig. 2. Segmentation results for validation subjects 20 and 63. The first column shows the ground truth (GT) images with lesion masks. The second column presents predictions from the proposed NeuroNetMix model, the third column shows predictions from xLSTM, and the fourth column shows predictions from 3D Mamba. Each subject is displayed with an axial slice overlaid with the mask (top row) and a 3D reconstruction of the predicted lesions (bottom row).

Figure 2 shows segmentation results for two validation subjects (20 and 63) using NeuroNetMix, xLSTM, and 3D Mamba. For each subject, the first row displays an axial slice with lesion masks, and the second row shows a 3D reconstruction. For Subject 20, small, scattered cortical and subcortical lesions are captured almost entirely by NeuroNetMix with accurate shapes and locations. xLSTM detects most lesions but misses smaller ones and underestimates volumes, while 3D Mamba produces sparser, less accurate segmentations. For Subject 63, elongated cortical lesions are effectively captured by NeuroNetMix with smooth 3D continuity. xLSTM undersegments some regions and occasionally produces disconnected lesions, and 3D Mamba shows fragmented segmentations. Overall, NeuroNetMix outperforms the other models in detecting small, scattered, and elongated lesions, preserving 3D continuity, and achieving precise voxel-level overlap, providing more reliable lesion maps for clinical assessment and volumetric measurement.

4 Discussion

4.1 Segmentation Accuracy

NeuroNetMix achieved the highest validation accuracy (lesion Dice 0.597, overall Dice 0.716) and maintained strong generalization on the test set (lesion Dice 0.491, overall Dice 0.566). Its bidirectional quasiseparable mixing integrates local lesion detail with global context, enabling robust detection of irregular TBI lesions. Sensitivity remained high (0.943 validation, 0.893 test) with low false negatives, and lesion counts closely matched ground truth. xLSTM and 3D Mamba showed lower performance.

4.2 Lesion Detection

NeuroNetMix excelled in lesion detection, achieving the highest sensitivity (0.943) and fewest false negatives (3) in validation, with lesion-wise F1 0.568 and overall F1 0.691. Lesion counts closely matched ground truth (difference 3.34). On the test set, sensitivity was 0.893 and lesion-wise F1 0.545, with absolute lesion difference 3.37, showing strong generalization. xLSTM and 3D Mamba consistently underperformed in lesion detection and F1 metrics.

4.3 Role of State Space Models

The model's state space architecture efficiently captures long-range spatial dependencies, with bidirectional mixing enhancing voxel-level and lesion-level segmentation beyond standard LSTM or CNN approaches.

4.4 Clinical Implications

NeuroNetMix's high sensitivity and accurate lesion counts support reliable TBI assessment and treatment planning. Baselines lack global context modeling or require refinement for clinical reliability.

4.5 Limitations and Future Work

NeuroNetMix has limitations. Evaluation was limited to the TBI challenge dataset, which may not reflect real-world variability. Only structural MRI was used; multimodal integration (e.g., DTI, fMRI, CT) could improve robustness. The complex state space architecture increases training demands, limiting accessibility. Future work will explore multimodal fusion, self-supervised pretraining, and interpretability methods to enhance generalization and clinical relevance.

5 Conclusion

Accurate segmentation of moderate-to-severe traumatic brain injury (msTBI) lesions is critical for clinical assessment, prognosis, and treatment planning. In this work, we introduced NeuroNetMix, a 3D encoder-decoder framework that integrates bidirectional quasiseparable mixing to capture both local lesion details and long-range spatial dependencies. Our model effectively addresses the challenges posed by the heterogeneous and diffuse nature of msTBI lesions, outperforming existing methods such as xLSTM and 3D umamba UNet in both validation and test datasets. NeuroNetMix preserves volumetric continuity, accurately delineates small and irregular lesions, and produces reliable segmentation maps that can be integrated into downstream analyses, including brain parcellation, connectomics, and fixel-based studies. These results demonstrate that NeuroNetMix not only advances automated lesion segmentation in msTBI but also has the potential to improve clinical decision-making and long-term outcome prediction for patients with traumatic brain injury.

References

1. Covington, J.E., Duff, M.: msTBI: a dataset for multi-site traumatic brain injury detection and classification from MRI. In: Proceedings of the International Conference on Medical Imaging with Deep Learning (MIDL 2021) (2021)
2. Diamond, J.M., Ko, A.R., Schultz, J.E.: A multi-site study of traumatic brain injury using advanced MRI techniques. J. Neurotrauma. **37**(5), 765–775 (2020). https://doi.org/10.1089/neu.2019.6611
3. Isensee, F., Jaeger, P.F., Kohl, S.A.A., Petersen, J., Maier-Hein, K.H.: Automated brain extraction of MRI data: the HD-BET approach. In: Medical Image Computing and Computer-Assisted Intervention – MICCAI 2019, pp. 1–10. Springer (2019). https://doi.org/10.1007/978-3-030-32245-8_1
4. Radwan, N., Kayhan, A., Demir, A.: An ensemble deep learning framework for brain tumor segmentation from multi-modal MRI. In: Proceedings of the International Conference on Medical Image Computing and Computer-Assisted Intervention (MICCAI 2021), pp. 203–212. Springer (2021). https://doi.org/10.1007/978-3-030-87243-4_22
5. Henschel, R., Maier-Hein, L.: A comprehensive evaluation of deep learning for tumor segmentation in brain MRI. In: Proceedings of the International Conference on Medical Image Computing and Computer-Assisted Intervention (MICCAI 2020), pp. 111–120. Springer (2020). https://doi.org/10.1007/978-3-030-59709-5_14
6. Kamnitsas, K., Castillo, C., A: Efficient multi-scale 3D CNN with dense skip connections for brain tumor segmentation. In: Proceedings of the International Conference on Medical Image Computing and Computer-Assisted Intervention (MICCAI 2017), pp. 464–472. Springer (2017). https://doi.org/10.1007/978-3-319-66179-7_52
7. Jain, V., K. B: 3D U-Net for brain tumor segmentation. In: Proceedings of the International Conference On Medical Image Computing and Computer-Assisted Intervention (MICCAI 2019), pp. 1–9. Springer (2019). https://doi.org/10.1007/978-3-030-32245-8_23
8. Mazher, M., et al.: Self-supervised spatial–temporal transformer fusion based federated framework for 4D cardiovascular image segmentation. Inf. Fusion. **106**, 102256 (2024)
9. Wang, K., et al.: Extreme Cardiac MRI Analysis under Respiratory Motion: Results of the CMRxMotion Challenge. arXiv preprint arXiv, 2507.19165 (2025)

10. Yang, K., et al.: Benchmarking the cow with the topcow challenge: topology-aware anatomical segmentation of the circle of Willis for cta and mra. ArXiv, arXiv-2312 (2024)
11. de la Rosa, E., et al.: Isles' 24: improving final infarct prediction in ischemic stroke using multimodal imaging and clinical data (2024). arXiv preprint arXiv, 2408.10966
12. Payette, K., et al.: Multi-center fetal brain tissue annotation (feta) challenge 2022 results. IEEE Trans. Med. Imaging. (2024)
13. Imran, M., et al.: Multi-class segmentation of aortic branches and zones in computed tomography angiography: The aortaseg24 challenge. arXiv preprint arXiv, 2502.05330 (2025)
14. Qayyum, A., et al.: Transforming heart chamber imaging: self-supervised learning for whole heart reconstruction and segmentation. arXiv preprint arXiv, 2406.06643 (2024)
15. Nan, Y., et al.: Hunting imaging biomarkers in pulmonary fibrosis: benchmarks of the AIIB23 challenge. Med. Image Anal. **97**, 103253 (2024)
16. de la Rosa, E., et al.: A robust ensemble algorithm for ischemic stroke lesion segmentation: Generalizability and clinical utility beyond the isles challenge. arXiv preprint arXiv, 2403.19425 (2024)
17. de la Rosa, E., et al.: DeepISLES: a clinically validated ischemic stroke segmentation model from the ISLES'22 challenge. Nat. Commun. **16**(1), 7357 (2025)
18. Zhu, L., et al.: Vision mamba: Efficient visual representation learning with bidirectional state space model. arXiv preprint arXiv, 2401.09417 (2024)
19. Mazher, M., Qayyum, A., Niederer, S.A.: Effective approach based on student-teacher self-supervised deep learning for multi-class bi-atrial segmentation challenge. In: International Workshop on Statistical Atlases and Computational Models of the Heart, pp. 132–139. Springer Nature Switzerland, Cham (2024)
20. Hwang, S., Lahoti, A., Puduppully, R., Dao, T., Gu, A.: Hydra: bidirectional state space models through generalized matrix mixers. Adv. Neural Inf. Proces. Syst. **37**, 110876–110908 (2024)

Traumatic Brain Injury Segmentation Using an Ensemble of Encoder-Decoder Models

Ghanshyam Dhamat and Vaanathi Sundaresan(✉)

Department of Computational and Data Sciences, Indian Institute of Science, Bengaluru, Karnataka 560012, India
vaanathi@iisc.ac.in

Abstract. The identification and segmentation of moderate-severe traumatic brain injury (TBI) lesions pose a significant challenge in neuroimaging. This difficulty arises from the extreme heterogeneity of these lesions, which vary in size, number, and laterality, thereby complicating downstream image processing tasks such as image registration and brain parcellation, reducing the analytical accuracy. Thus, developing methods for highly accurate segmentation of TBI lesions is essential for reliable neuroimaging analysis. This study aims to develop an effective automated segmentation pipeline to automatically detect and segment TBI lesions in T1-weighted MRI scans. We evaluate multiple approaches to achieve accurate segmentation of the TBI lesions. The core of our pipeline leverages various architectures within the nnUNet framework for initial segmentation, complemented by post-processing strategies to enhance evaluation metrics. Our final submission to the challenge achieved an accuracy of 0.8451, Dice score values of 0.4711 and 0.8514 for images with and without visible lesions, respectively, with an overall Dice score of 0.5973, ranking among the top-6 methods in the AIMS-TBI 2025 challenge. The Python implementation of our pipeline is publicly available.

Keywords: Traumatic Brain Injury · Medical Image Segmentation · Deep Learning

1 Introduction

Traumatic brain injuries (TBI) occur when external forces cause brain movement within the skull, resulting in biological and functional alterations [4]. These injuries lead to heterogeneous lesions, a key characteristic of moderate-severe (MS)-TBI. These lesions can be focal or diffuse, varying in size and number, affecting different brain tissues, and potentially appearing in similar regions on both sides. Figure 1 illustrates the heterogeneity in MS-TBI lesion characteristics across different subjects. If these lesions are overlooked during image processing tasks like registration or brain parcellation, it can lead to significant errors in analytical outcomes [4]. Although manual segmentation of MS-TBI lesions is

S. Bakas et al. (Eds.): MICCAI 2025, LNCS 16377, pp. 341–349, 2026.
https://doi.org/10.1007/978-3-032-16370-7_31

considered the gold standard, it is time-consuming, subjective, and shows high variability between raters. This drives research towards automated methods for identifying and delineating lesions. Automated segmentation speeds up the process and can provide additional information to clinicians.

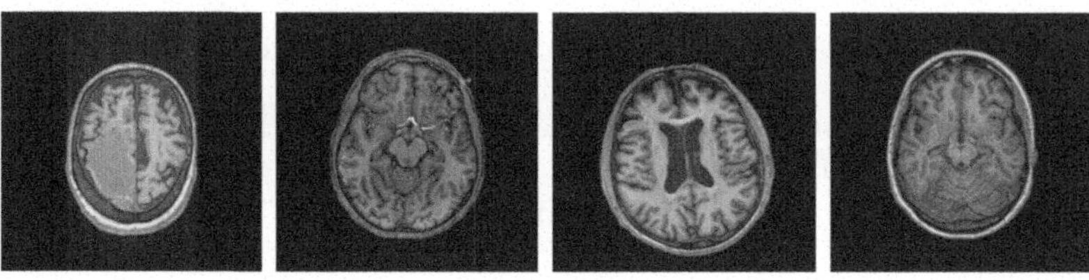

Fig. 1. Heterogeneity in the appearance of traumatic brain injury lesions on T1-weighted MRI (images overlaid with manual annotations of TBI lesions in yellow). (Color figure online)

The AIMS-TBI 2025 challenge aims to develop automated algorithms that effectively detect and segment lesions while addressing the heterogeneous nature of MS-TBI lesions. The challenge focuses on T1-weighted MRI as they are most commonly used by the ENIGMA TBI consortium and show less parameter variation compared to other MRI modalities [4].
In this work, we investigate various approaches, including ensemble networks, based on the nnUNet framework to train segmentation models. These approaches incorporate variations in encoder-decoder architectures and classifier-based post-processing strategies to enhance accuracy. We also experiment with radiomics-based features for improving TBI lesion segmentation. Evaluation on heterogeneous AIMS-TBI challenges data shows the effectiveness of ensemble models in accurate TBI lesion segmentation.

2 Method

We explore automated pipelines to identify and segment TBI lesions. The process begins with preprocessing applied to all volumes. We investigate settings of the encoder-decoder model and their ensemble, combined with a radiomics feature-based classifier. The components are detailed below.

Data preprocessing: Before training, we apply bias field correction using ANTsPyx library in python [10] to mitigate low-frequency intensity inhomogeneities in the MRI volumes.

2.1 Traumatic Brain Injury Initial Candidate Segmentation

We build the pipelines based on the widely used nnUNet framework [7,8], with configurations to achieve optimal performance while handling all preliminary steps involving resampling, normalization, and tight cropping.

UNET (integrated with nnUNet framework). We initially use a 3D UNet [9] integrated within the nnUNet framework. The UNet architecture is a convolutional neural network with an encoder-decoder structure, interconnected with skip connections which combine texture (from encoder) with localization features (in the decoder). Each stage consists of double convolution operations, enhancing the network's ability to learn hierarchical features for segmentation.

UNETPP (integrated with nnUNET framework). As an improvisation to the vanilla UNet, the UNet++ architecture [11] integrates nested, dense skip pathways, as shown in Fig. 2, designed to capture finer-grained details in complex structures.

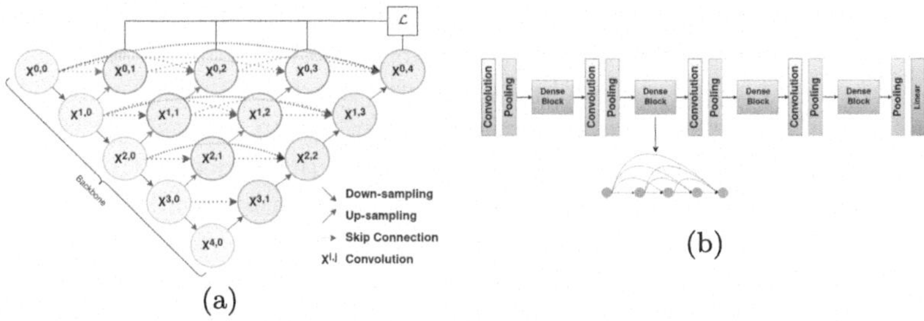

Fig. 2. (a) UNET++ architecture with nested skip connections and (b) DenseNet architecture with dense block where each layer uses feature map from preceding layers.

2.2 2D Classification of Slices with Visible Lesions Vs Without Lesions

As a post-processing strategy for removal of false positives (FPs), we classify slices with segmented regions as slices with visible lesions vs without lesion using DenseNet architecture [6] on 2D slices from 3D volumes. The DenseNet architecture contains dense blocks within which each layer connects to every subsequent layer, facilitating feature reuse and improving information flow. These dense blocks are placed between transition layers that change feature map size. Classification was performed only on slices where the segmentation model predicted a potential lesion. To cut down on minor false positives in cases without a lesion, we restricted the use of 2D classifiers to subjects whose segmented lesion volume was less than 2000 mm^3.

2.3 Radiomics-Based Classifier for Refining Segmentation

To further refine the segmentation model's output, we use a radiomics-based classifier to remove false positive voxels. We extract voxel-based radiomics features capturing intensity, shape, and texture information using Python's PyRadiomics library [5]. Among various classifiers explored (using Scikit-learn package), including SVM [3] and Random forest [1], XGBoost [2] is selected since it offered 71% accuracy (outperformed others by at least 11%). Due to computational constraints, we limit the processing to lesions with a volume < 1000 voxels and use the top 25 important features for training XGBoost.

The various components explained above are utilized into ensembles explained as different settings in experiments (Sect. 3.2).

3 Experimental Setup

3.1 Dataset Overview

The AIMS-TBI 2025 challenge dataset [4] includes 875 T1-weighted MRI scans, divided into 552 training, 100 validation, and 223 unseen test cases, with balanced distribution across sets. The scans were collected from 13 sites using 1.5T and 3T scanners. The dataset includes patients aged 5–85 years, with 64% male subjects. Lesions were segmented through a three-step process for high-quality ground truth annotations. All MRI images were pre-processed by defacing to protect patient privacy [4]. Of the 552 training samples available, we kept 24 cases for testing and used the remainder for training and validation (with training:validation=90:10). Among the 24 samples, 5 were from subjects with no visible lesions, and the rest were from those with lesions. Training phase results are reported on the 24 testing samples, while the final evaluation phase results are reported on 223 unseen test cases, after submission for an in-house evaluation by organizers.

3.2 Experiments

We explore the following settings trained using the parameters specified in Sect. 3.3: **Setting 1: (Baseline U-Net):** The baseline 3D UNet is trained using the default nnUNet pipeline with 5-fold cross-validation on the 528 training cases, and tested locally on 24 held-out samples. We generate predictions by averaging the probability maps from 5 folds. **Setting 2 (UNETPP):** We trained the UNET++ architecture integrated within the nnUNet framework on 528 training samples. **Setting 3 (UNET + slice-based classifier):** To reduce false positives, 2D slice-based visible lesion vs no lesion classification is trained using DenseNet (sec. 2.2). To mitigate class imbalance, we exclude the first 45 slices from each volume in the axial direction (starting from the neck) where lesions were negligible, and ensure an equal number of positive and negative slices per batch. The model was trained on slices from 390 volumes and validated on 80. If the classifier predicted "no visible lesion" on more than 50% of the slices containing segmentation, those predictions were removed. **Setting 4 (UNETPP + slice-based classifier):** This setting combined the UNET++ segmentation model with the same DenseNet-based classification approach from Setting 3. **Setting 5 (UNET + slice-based classifier + radiomics classifier):** To evaluate the cumulative effect of postprocessing steps on segmentation accuracy and FP reduction, in this setting, the UNET segmentation was first refined by the slice-based classifier and then further refined at the voxel level by the radiomics-based XGBoost classifier (sec. 2.3). **Setting 6 (UNETPP + slice-based classifier + radiomics classifier):** Similar to setting 5, this setting is built upon setting 4 by adding a second stage of voxel-level radiomics-based XGBoost classifier. **Setting 7 (UNET + UNETPP):** We evaluate an ensemble approach to leverage the strengths of both UNet and UNET++ by averaging the probability maps from the 5-fold UNet ensemble (Setting 1) and the single-fold UNET++ model (Setting 2).

3.3 Implementation Details

Experiments are conducted on an Intel i9-10980XE CPU, 128 GB RAM, and two NVIDIA RTX A6000 GPUs (each with 48 GB memory) using Python 3.10 and PyTorch 2.8. For training segmentation models, we use a combination of Dice loss and cross-entropy loss. We trained for 1000 epochs, with a batch size of 2, an initial learning rate of $1e^{-2}$ with a linear decay scheduler. For nnUNet training, we use a patch size of $128 \times 160 \times 112$ voxels. Data augmentations include flipping, intensity rescaling ($\gamma \in (0.7, 1.5)$) and rotation ($\theta \in (-180^o, 180^o)$).

3.4 Performance Metrics and Statistical Evaluation

We use Dice Similarity Coefficient (DSC) and subject-level accuracy for the evaluation of TBI segmentation. To provide a comprehensive assessment, three DSC metrics were determined as part of the challenge: mean DSC value calculated only for subjects with visible lesion (**DSC-Lesion**), for subjects with no visible lesion (**DSC-no-Lesion**) and finally for all subjects (**Overall DSC**). To determine the statistical significance of the results, we perform two-tailed paired t-tests between the best settings and the baseline setting 1 in the training phase, and between the settings in the final evaluation phase.

4 Results and Discussion

Table 1 shows the segmentation performance for our experimental settings, and Fig. 3 shows the visual results.On the local test set, the baseline UNET model (setting 1) established a strong benchmark with a DSC-Lesion of 0.7 ± 0.11. It was particularly reliable in correctly identifying subjects with no visible lesions; however, it tended to merge distinct, adjacent lesions, thus yielding a lower DSC than that of setting 2. Setting 2 with the UNETPP model achieved the best DSC-Lesion (0.72 ± 0.095), however, it suffered on subjects with no visible lesion. This indicates that UNETPP, designed to capture finer details, was overly sensitive to image noise, which resulted in small FPs as shown in Fig. 3 (also setting 4 involving UNETPP). The setting 7 successfully balanced these characteristics, showcased in Fig. 3 setting 7 for columns 2 and 4. Overall, setting 7 maintains competitive scores in both cases with and without a lesion. The introduction of post-processing stages yielded mixed results - while the 2D slice-based classifier proved effective in increasing DSC on subjects with no visible lesion, it led to a reduction in DSC for subjects with lesions in both setting 3 and setting 4, with a statistically significant decrease in setting 3 ($0.68 \pm 0.12, p = 0.003$). DenseNet architecture was opted for the classifier due to its parameter efficiency and strong feature propagation. By conditionally applying this classifier only to cases with small predicted volumes, we created a fast and effective filter against minor FPs without affecting larger, more confident segmentations. We explored the radiomics-based classifier to refine the segmentation by removing FPs at the voxel level. However, from Table 1, we can see that the DSC-lesion values reduced for setting 6 (0.687 ± 0.13) and significantly for setting 5 ($0.673 \pm 0.13, p < 0.0001$). The reduction in performance suggests that radiomics features could not sufficiently discriminate lesions from FPs, especially for small TBI lesions. For instance, any FPs likely arose from image artifacts whose low-level texture and shape features, captured by radiomics, were indistinguishable from those of small, true lesions. Furthermore, the computational constraint limited the application of radiomics to lesions < 1000 voxels, and hence, the classifier could not leverage potentially more discriminative features of FPs from larger lesions.

For the final challenge submission, we selected two of our models: the robust UNET + 2D classifier pipeline (setting 3) and UNET + UNETPP ensemble (setting 7). The former represented a stable, well-vetted approach, while the latter was chosen to leverage the diverse feature extraction capabilities of two distinct architectures. On the unseen test data, the ensemble approach (UNET + UNETPP) proved superior, outperforming the post-processing pipeline in setting 3 across all key metrics, achieving a significantly higher overall Dice of 0.59 compared to 0.56 (p-value = 0.013) and an increased accuracy from 0.8 to 0.84 (p-value = 0.004).

Table 1. Comparison of segmentation performance across various settings, for training and final evaluation phases. Statistical significance is assessed for the best settings with respect to the baseline setting 1 using a two-tailed paired t-test,with * indicating significant improvement with p-value < 0.05.

Phase	Exp. Setting	Accuracy	DSC-Lesion	DSC-no-Lesion	Overall DSC
Training	Setting 1	1.00	0.70 ± 0.11	1.00 ± 0.0	0.77 ± 0.16
phase: local	Setting 2	0.916	0.72 ± 0.095	0.60 ± 0.48	0.697 ± 0.24
test data	Setting 3	1.00	$(0.68 \pm 0.12)^*$	1.00 ± 0.0	$(0.75 \pm 0.17)^*$
created	Setting 4	1.00	0.695 ± 0.12	1.00 ± 0.0	0.76 ± 0.16
from the	Setting 5	1.00	$(0.673 \pm 0.13)^*$	1.00 ± 0.0	$(0.74 \pm 0.17)^*$
training	Setting 6	1.00	0.687 ± 0.13	1.00 ± 0.0	0.75 ± 0.17
data	Setting 7	1.00	0.698 ± 0.11	1.00 ± 0.0	0.76 ± 0.16
Final phase:	Setting 3	0.80	0.41 ± 0.34	0.86 ± 0.34	0.56 ± 0.40
Test data	Setting 7	$(0.84)^*$	$(0.47 \pm 0.31)^*$	0.85 ± 0.36	$(0.59 \pm 0.37)^*$

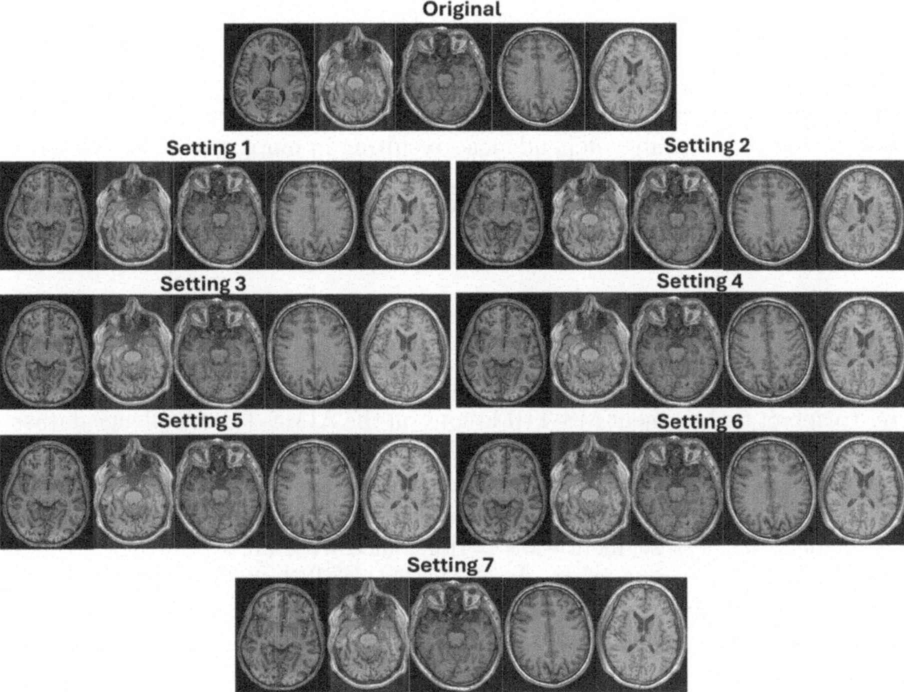

Fig. 3. Comparison of results from various ensemble settings, with each setting shown for five sample subjects (left to right). Predicted lesions are shown in green while the ground-truth TBI lesions are shown in red. Results indicate better performance with settings 3 and 7. (Color figure online)

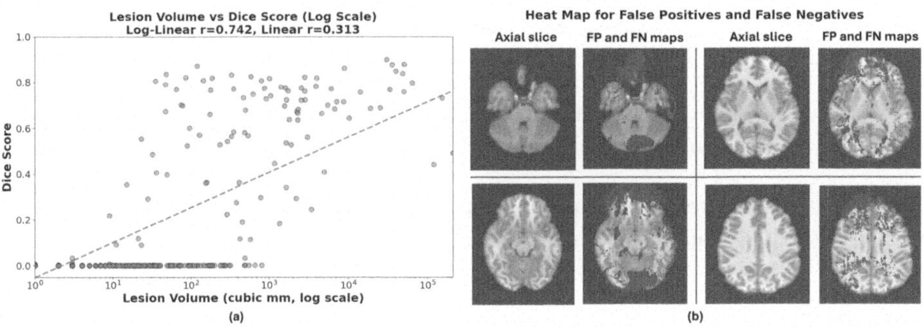

Fig. 4. (a) Relationship of lesion size (cubic mm) in log scale vs Dice score on local test set, (b) Heatmap for false positive (red) and false negative (blue) in local test set. (Color figure online)

Figure 4 shows that, while our model is mainly overlooking small lesions with volume less than 100 mm^3, a few large ones are also getting missed due to the lack of representative training instances. The log-linear Pearson coefficient of 0.734 shows an overall positive correlation of the Dice score with lesion size.

The future directions include: (1) use of transformer-based architecture, as they have been shown to provide better results across various tasks due to their ability to model long-range dependencies resulting in more global understanding of the image context, (2) self-supervised pretraining of the segmentation model on a large corpus of unlabeled brain MRIs to learn richer and more robust representations and fine-tuning them to improve segmentation results.

5 Conclusions

In this study, we compare various ensemble settings of encoder-decoder architectures to detect and segment MS-TBI lesions on the AIMS-TBI Challenge dataset. Our pipelines are built based on the nnUNet framework, and we also investigate the effect of a classification-based post-processing strategy and the ensemble of networks. Our results on the final evaluation indicate that the ensemble models provided the best segmentation performance with an overall DSC of 0.59, ranking among the top-6 methods in the AIMS-TBI 2025 challenge, including subjects with and without lesion, which is significantly better than other settings. While the postprocessing strategy involving 2D slice-based classification eliminated false positives, there is still scope for improvement in terms of accurate identification of small TBI lesions. Future directions include exploring transformer-based architectures and self-supervised preprocessing techniques for better performance. The python code for our pipelines has been made available at https://github.com/ghanshyamdhamat/aims_tbi_2025.git.

Acknowledgments. This work was supported by DBT Wellcome Trust India Alliance Fellowship [IA/E/22/1/506763], the Council of Scientific and Industrial Research (CSIR) under its ASPIRE program [25WS(013)/2023–24/EMR-II/ASPIRE], the Science and Engineering Research Board Start-up Research Grant [SRG/2023/001406], Siemens Healthineers-CDS Collaborative Laboratory of Artificial Intelligence in Precision Medicine, India and Pratiksha Trust, Bangalore, India [FG/PTCH-23-1004].

Disclosure of Interests. The authors have no competing interests to declare that are relevant to the content of this article.

References

1. Breiman, L.: Random forests Mach. learn. **45**(1), 5–32 (2001). https://doi.org/10.1023/A:1010933404324
2. Chen, T., Guestrin, C.: Xgboost: a scalable tree boosting system. In: Proceedings of the 22nd ACM SIGKDD International Conference on Knowledge Discovery and Data Mining, pp. 785–794. KDD '16, ACM (Aug 2016. https://doi.org/10.1145/2939672.2939785, http://dx.doi.org/10.1145/2939672.2939785
3. Cortes, C., Vapnik, V.: Support-vector networks. Mach. Learn. **20**, 273–297 (1995).https://doi.org/10.1007/BF00994018

4. Dennis, E., et al.: Aims-tbi - automated identification of moderate- severe traumatic brain injury lesions (2025). https://doi.org/10.5281/zenodo.15084120, https://doi.org/10.5281/zenodo.15084120
5. van Griethuysen, J.J.M., et al.: Computational radiomics system to decode the radiographic phenotype. Can. Res. **77**(21), e104–e107 (2017). https://doi.org/10.1158/0008-5472.CAN-17-0339
6. Huang, G., Liu, Z., van der Maaten, L., Weinberger, K.Q.: Densely connected convolutional networks (2018). https://arxiv.org/abs/1608.06993
7. Isensee, F., Jaeger, P.F., Kohl, S.A.A., Petersen, J., Maier-Hein, K.H.: NNU-net: self-adapting framework for u-net-based medical image segmentation (2018). https://github.com/MIC-DKFZ/nnUNet, Accessed 04 Sep 2025
8. Isensee F., Jaeger P. F., K.S.A.P.J..M.H.K.H.: NNU-net: a self-configuring method for deep learning-based biomedical image segmentation. Nature Methods (2021)
9. Ronneberger, O., Fischer, P., Brox, T.: U-net: convolutional networks for biomedical image segmentation (2015). https://arxiv.org/abs/1505.04597
10. Tustison, N.J., et al.: The antsx ecosystem for quantitative biological and medical imaging. Sci. Rep. **11**, 9068 (2021). https://doi.org/10.1038/s41598-021-87564-6
11. Zhou, Z., Siddiquee, M.M.R., Nima, T., Liang, J.: Unet++: redesigning skip connections to exploit multiscale features in image segmentation. IEEE Transactions on Medical Imaging (2019)

DeaMNet: A Dual-Encoder Network with Hybrid Morphology-Aware Loss for Precise TBI Lesion Segmentation

Hee Kuk[1], Zeeshan Abbas[2,3](✉), and Seung Won Lee[1,2,3,4,5](✉)

[1] Department of Metabiohealth, Institute for Cross-disciplinary Studies, Sungkyunkwan University, Suwon, Republic of Korea
gmldi990519@gmail.com

[2] Department of Precision Medicine, Sungkyunkwan University School of Medicine, Sungkyunkwan University, Suwon, Republic of Korea

[3] Department of Artificial Intelligence, Sungkyunkwan University, Suwon, Republic of Korea
zabbas@jbnu.ac.kr

[4] Personalized Cancer Immunotherapy Research Center, Sungkyunkwan University School of Medicine, Sungkyunkwan University, Suwon, Republic of Korea

[5] Department of Family Medicine, Kangbuk Samsung Hospital, Sungkyunkwan University School of Medicine, 29 Saemunan-ro, Seoul 03181, Jongno-gu, Republic of Korea
swleemd@g.skku.edu

Abstract. The precise, automated segmentation of lesions in moderate-to-severe traumatic brain injury (msTBI) is a formidable clinical challenge, hindered by their minute size, erratic shapes, and diverse appearances. This paper introduces DeaMNet, a novel dual-encoder network with a hybrid morphology-aware loss, designed for the MICCAI 2025 AIMS-TBI Challenge. The novelty of DeaMNet lies in its synergistic combination of three key innovations: (1) a dual-encoder architecture that simultaneously extracts deep semantic features and lightweight spatial details, (2) multi-level skip connections that effectively fuse hierarchical features into the decoder, and (3) a hybrid morphology-aware loss function that addresses severe class imbalance and boundary ambiguity. DeaMNet leverages a powerful ResNet backbone in parallel with a lightweight MobileNetV2 backbone to comprehensively learn both the complex high-level patterns and the fine-grained boundary characteristics of TBI lesions. The proposed hybrid loss, which combines Dice, contrast-weighted Binary Cross-Entropy (BCE), and Boundary Loss, guides the model to focus on irregular and ambiguous lesion boundaries. DeaMNet significantly outperforms the standard DeepLabV3+ baseline and other common segmentation models, demonstrating this synergistic approach is a key strategy for maximizing performance in complex TBI MRI analysis.

Keywords: Traumatic Brain Injury · Medical Image Segmentation · DeepLabV3+ · Dual-Encoder · Hybrid Loss Function · AIMS-TBI Challenge

S. Bakas et al. (Eds.): MICCAI 2025, LNCS 16377, pp. 350–358, 2026.
https://doi.org/10.1007/978-3-032-16370-7_32

1 Introduction

Traumatic Brain Injury (TBI) is a major global health crisis, causing substantial mortality and disability for over 50 million people annually [1,2]. Mitigating the cascade of secondary injuries (e.g., hypoxia, edema) is a key goal of acute care, making the accurate segmentation of brain lesions essential for patient management [3,4]. While automated segmentation is a critical task, it remains a formidable challenge [5]. To accelerate progress, the AIMS-TBI Challenge at MICCAI 2025 calls for robust algorithms to segment lesions from T1-weighted (T1w) MRI [2].

The difficulty stems from the intrinsic properties of TBI lesions. Their high heterogeneity, being focal or diffuse, with varying sizes and spanning multiple tissue types (GM, WM, CSF), complicates standard analyses [6,7]. Standard models like U-Net [8] tend to lose fine-grained details, while foundation models like SAM [9] often fail to capture their subtle local contrast and irregular morphology. Critically, TBI segmentation faces a dual-imbalance problem: region-based losses (e.g., Dice) address class imbalance (lesion vs. background) but fail to resolve the "difficulty imbalance" by treating challenging boundary pixels and simple interior pixels equally [10,11].

To overcome these challenges, we propose **DeaMNet**, a framework synergizing architectural and loss-function innovations. Our contributions are:

1. **A Novel Dual-Encoder Architecture:** DeaMNet integrates a deep ResNet for robust high-level semantic features and a lightweight MobileNetV2 for preserving critical low-level boundary information, creating a rich, combined feature representation.
2. **Hierarchical Feature Fusion via Multi-level Skip Connections:** A sophisticated fusion strategy intelligently integrates feature maps from multiple encoder stages into the decoder for superior boundary reconstruction.
3. **A Hybrid, Morphology-Aware Loss Function:** A composite loss tackles the dual-imbalance problem by combining three components: Dice Loss for regional stability, contrast-weighted BCE for edges, and a Boundary Loss [10] for contour accuracy.

For the AIMS-TBI 2025 Challenge, we show that this purpose-built design allows DeaMNet to achieve high performance in TBI lesion segmentation.

2 Proposed Method: DeaMNet

DeaMNet is an encoder-decoder framework architecturally derived from DeepLabV3+ [12]. Its novelty lies in a purpose-built design integrating a dual-branch encoder, a multi-skip decoder, and a hybrid morphology-aware loss function. The overall data processing pipeline is illustrated in Fig. 1, and a detailed schematic of the DeaMNet architecture is shown in Fig. 2.

DeaMNet is applied to 2D axial slices extracted from 3D MRI volumes. Each slice undergoes a two-step preprocessing phase consisting of N4ITK bias field

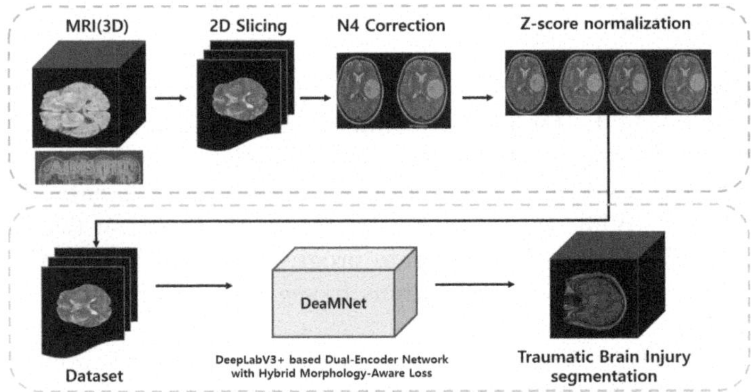

Fig. 1. Overview of the data processing pipeline for TBI lesion segmentation.

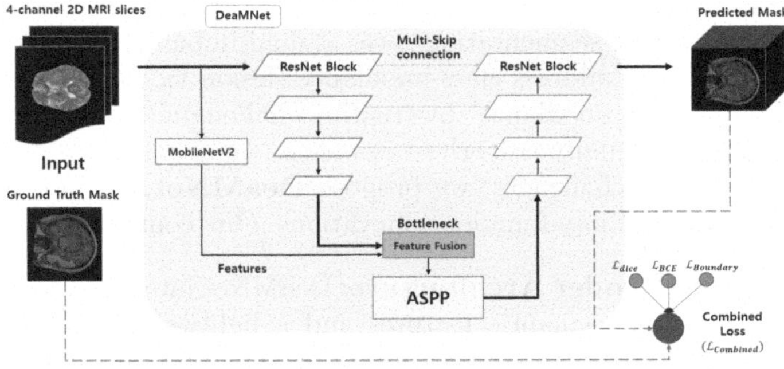

Fig. 2. Detailed architecture of the proposed DeaMNet.

correction and z-score normalization before being fed into the network. As illustrated in Fig. 2, the core of DeaMNet is its dual-encoder and multi-skip decoder structure.

2.1 Dual-Branch Encoder for Multi-faceted Feature Extraction

To overcome the trade-off in standard single-pathway encoders between capturing semantic features and preserving spatial detail, DeaMNet employs two parallel backbones with complementary strengths:

- **Primary Branch (ResNet-50):** A deep ResNet-50 backbone [13] serves as the primary extractor, learning complex, high-level semantic representations for understanding the global context of TBI lesions.
- **Auxiliary Branch (MobileNetV2):** A lightweight MobileNetV2 backbone runs in parallel to efficiently capture fine-grained, low-level features like edges and textures. This is critical for preserving the boundary details of small lesions at a low computational cost.

Features from the deepest layers of both branches are fused and processed by an Atrous Spatial Pyramid Pooling (ASPP) module, yielding a comprehensive feature representation.

2.2 Multi-skip Decoder for High-Fidelity Boundary Reconstruction

The decoder progressively upsamples multi-scale context from the ASPP module. At each upsampling stage, multi-level skip connections source feature maps from the early layers (layer1, layer2, layer3) of the ResNet-50 backbone. These skip connections are processed through projection layers before being concatenated with the decoder features. This strategy provides the decoder with a rich, multi-scale information stream, enabling it to reconstruct intricate lesion boundaries with high precision.

2.3 Hybrid Morphology-Aware Loss Function

To address severe class imbalance and morphological complexity, we designed a composite loss function (L_{Seg}) that combines three synergistic components:

$$L_{Seg} = w_1 L_{Dice} + w_2 L_{wBCE} + w_3 L_{Boundary} \tag{1}$$

where weights w_1, w_2, w_3 were empirically set to 1.0, 1.0, and 0.5 to balance each term's contribution based on preliminary experiments.

- **Dice Loss (L_{Dice}):** Maximizes the overlap between the prediction and ground truth, providing robustness against class imbalance [11].

$$L_{Dice} = 1 - \frac{2 \times |P \cap G| + \epsilon}{|P| + |G| + \epsilon} \tag{2}$$

  where P denotes the predicted mask, G is the ground-truth mask, and ϵ is a smoothing factor.
- **Contrast-Weighted BCE (L_{wBCE}):** A novel adaptation of BCE loss that tackles "difficulty imbalance" by using a Sobel-filtered contrast map from the input image as a pixel-wise weight, forcing the model to focus on challenging lesion boundaries.
- **Boundary Loss ($L_{Boundary}$):** An explicit contour-based loss that penalizes shape inaccuracies by minimizing the distance between predicted and true boundaries, providing a strong geometric gradient for learning irregular shapes [10].

This hybrid loss ensures regional correctness (Dice), sharpens focus on difficult edges (L_{wBCE}), and refines the exact contour shape (Boundary Loss), leading to a more accurate segmentation.

3 Experiments and Results

3.1 Dataset and Preprocessing

This study used the official AIMS-TBI Challenge dataset from the ENIGMA Consortium. To prevent data leakage, we performed a patient-level 8:2 split on the 553 available patients, assigning 442 to training and 111 to testing. No external validation dataset was provided by the organizers for offline development. Our preprocessing pipeline consisted of N4ITK bias field correction [14], z-score normalization of non-zero voxels within a brain mask, and axial 2D slice extraction.

3.2 Implementation and Evaluation

DeaMNet was implemented in PyTorch and trained for 500 epochs using an Adam optimizer (learning rate of 1e-4). To validate our design, we performed an extensive ablation study and benchmarked the model's initial efficiency against baselines like U-Net and MedSAM over 20 epochs. For a comprehensive view of overall performance, a holistic, patient-level 3D bias analysis was also conducted. All models were evaluated using the Dice Similarity Coefficient (DSC) and Intersection over Union (IoU).

3.3 Results

Quantitative Analysis. As shown in Table 1, after a brief 20-epoch training period, our DeaMNet already demonstrates a clear performance advantage. This initial result highlights its architectural efficiency. For this comparison, foundation models (SAM, MedSAM, MobileSAM) were adapted for this fully automatic task by fine-tuning only their mask decoders using tight bounding boxes derived from the ground-truth masks as prompts.

Table 1. Comparison of TBI lesion segmentation performance against baseline and foundation models (20 epochs).

Model	DSC	IoU
U-Net [8]	0.2862	0.2189
SAM [9]	0.3206	0.2353
MedSAM [15]	0.3714	0.2584
MobileSAM [16]	0.3939	0.2743
DeaMNet (Ours)	**0.4976**	**0.4049**

Next, to analyze the contribution of each of DeaMNet's components at full convergence, we conducted an extensive ablation study over 500 epochs (Table 2).

Our proposed model, DeaMNet (Ours), achieved the highest scores, establishing a strong benchmark. The most significant performance drop was observed when replacing our hybrid loss with a standard Dice Loss, confirming that our morphology-aware loss function is essential. The removal of the MobileNetV2 branch or the multi-skip connections also led to notable decreases in performance, validating our dual-encoder and feature fusion strategies.

Table 2. Ablation study of DeaMNet components (500 epochs). The performance drop in DSC (ΔDSC) is calculated relative to our final model.

Model Variant	DSC	IoU	Test Loss	ΔDSC
DeepLabV3+ (Baseline)	0.6200	0.5127	0.2178	-0.0395
DeaMNet (w/ AdamW optimizer)	0.6330	0.5270	0.2236	-0.0265
DeaMNet (w/ Dice Loss only)	0.5832	0.4890	0.2095	-0.0763
DeaMNet (w/o MobileNetV2 branch)	0.6423	0.5357	0.2114	-0.0172
DeaMNet (w/o Multi-skip connections)	0.5133	0.4207	0.2632	-0.1462
DeaMNet (Ours, w/ Adam optimizer)	**0.6595**	**0.5505**	**0.2066**	**Baseline**

Qualitative Analysis. Figure 3 presents a qualitative assessment of DeaMNet's performance across a variety of challenging TBI lesion types found in the test set. The selected cases highlight the model's robustness in handling significant variations in lesion size, shape, and distribution. These results visually confirm the quantitative findings, demonstrating DeaMNet's ability to generate precise and reliable segmentation masks under difficult conditions.

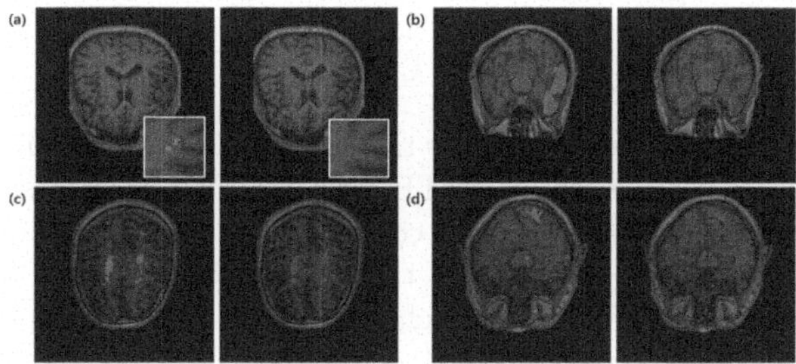

Fig. 3. Qualitative segmentation results of DeaMNet. Each case shows the original T1w MRI, ground-truth mask (green), and prediction (blue). The examples highlight the model' s proficiency with: (a) very small, subtle lesions; (b) large, contiguous lesions; (c) lesions with complex and irregular boundaries; and (d) multiple, spatially distributed lesions of varying sizes.(Color figure online)

Performance Bias Analysis. A patient-level 3D bias analysis of the full dataset (Fig. 4) confirms the model's robustness. Most patients achieved a 3D Dice score above 0.90, demonstrating consistently high performance across varying lesion volumes (marker size) and spatial locations (position).

This strong patient-level performance contextualizes the lower overall Dice score of 0.6595 from the ablation study (Table 2). The discrepancy is due to metric granularity: the high 3D Dice score is driven by performance on the total lesion burden, where large volumes dominate. In contrast, the lower overall score is averaged down by a subset of extremely small 'micro-lesions' (e.g., $\leq$8 pixels) with substantially lower segmentation accuracy. This suggests the model is highly effective but has a performance threshold for the most minute lesions.

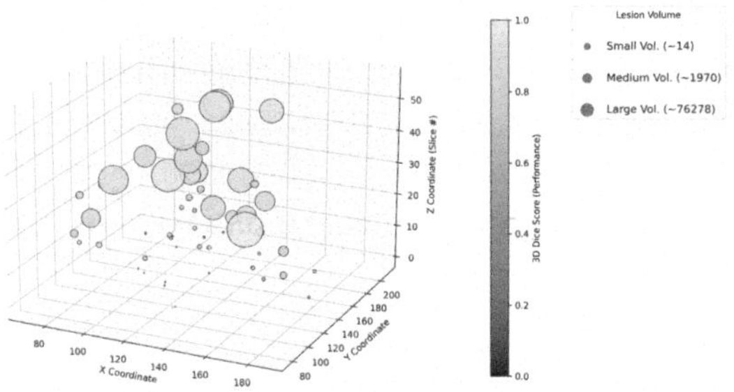

Fig. 4. 3D bias analysis of DeaMNet on the full dataset. Each marker represents a patient. The marker's position is the 3D lesion centroid, its size corresponds to the total lesion volume, and its color indicates the 3D Dice score. The results show consistently high performance across different lesion sizes and locations

4 Discussion

The success of DeaMNet stems from its targeted design, which directly addresses the core challenges of segmenting msTBI lesions. The ablation study provides clear evidence for the efficacy of each component, confirming that the synergy between the dual-encoder design and the hybrid loss was the primary driver of performance. This targeted approach provides a clear advantage over more generic models like U-Net or MedSAM, which lack the specific inductive biases required for this challenging task.

Our study's limitations include its 2D, single-modality approach and a clear performance threshold for 'micro-lesions' ($\leq$8 pixels), where segmentation accuracy was substantially lower. Future work should therefore focus on extending DeaMNet to a 3D architecture to better leverage volumetric context, which may help distinguish these extremely small lesions from noise. Furthermore, integrating information from other MRI sequences could enhance segmentation accuracy, particularly for these subtle pathological features.

5 Conclusion

In this paper, we introduced DeaMNet, a specialized dual-encoder network that significantly improves the accuracy of msTBI lesion segmentation. By synergistically combining a dual-branch feature extractor, multi-level skip connections, and a novel hybrid loss function tailored for complex lesion morphologies, DeaMNet produces highly precise segmentations that outperform strong baseline and foundation models. This work offers a robust solution for the AIMS-TBI 2025 Challenge and provides a generalizable framework for other challenging medical imaging tasks.

References

1. Mikolic, A.: Treatment, outcome and prediction after mild traumatic brain injury. Doctoral Thesis, Erasmus University Rotterdam (2022)
2. Olsen, A., et al.: Toward a global and reproducible science for brain imaging in neurotrauma: the ENIGMA adult moderate/severe traumatic brain injury working group. Brain Imaging Behav. **15**, 526–554 (2021)
3. Kim, J.E., Park, J.C., Kang, H.S., Oh, C.W.: Controversies in acute care of patients with severe traumatic brain injury. Brain NeuroRehabilitation **1**(2), 136–142 (2008)
4. Maas, A.I., Stocchetti, N., Bullock, R.: Moderate and severe traumatic brain injury in adults. Lancet Neurol. **7**(8), 728–741 (2008)
5. Bhalodiya, J.M., Lim Choi Keung, S.N., Arvanitis, T.N.: Magnetic resonance image-based brain tumour segmentation methods: a systematic review. Digital Health **8**, 20552076221074122 (2022)
6. Diamond, B.R., et al.: Optimizing the accuracy of cortical volumetric analysis in traumatic brain injury. MethodsX **7**, 100994 (2020)
7. Radwan, A.M., et al.: Virtual brain grafting: Enabling whole brain parcellation in the presence of large lesions. NeuroImage **229**, 117731 (2021)
8. Ronneberger, O., Fischer, P., Brox, T.: U-Net: convolutional networks for biomedical image segmentation. In: Navab, N., Hornegger, J., Wells, W.M., Frangi, A.F. (eds.) MICCAI 2015. LNCS, vol. 9351, pp. 234–241. Springer, Cham (2015). https://doi.org/10.1007/978-3-319-24574-4_28
9. Kirillov, A., et al.: Segment anything. In: Proceedings of the IEEE/CVF International Conference on Computer Vision (ICCV), pp. 3899–3910 (2023)
10. Kervadec, H., et al.: Boundary loss for highly unbalanced segmentation. In: Proceedings of Machine Learning Research, vol. 102, pp. 285–296. PMLR (2019)
11. Yeung, M., Sala, E., Schönlieb, C.B., Rundo, L.: Unified focal loss: generalising dice and cross entropy-based losses to handle class imbalanced medical image segmentation. Comput. Med. Imaging Graph. **95**, 102026 (2022)
12. Chen, L.C., Zhu, Y., Papandreou, G., Schroff, F., Adam, H.: Encoder-decoder with atrous separable convolution for semantic image segmentation. In: Proceedings of the European conference on computer vision (ECCV), pp. 801–818 (2018)
13. He, K., Zhang, X., Ren, S., Sun, J.: Deep residual learning for image recognition. In: Proceedings of the IEEE conference on computer vision and pattern recognition, pp. 770–778 (2016)
14. Tustison, N.J., et al.: N4ITK: improved N3 bias correction. IEEE Trans. Med. Imaging **29**(6), 1310–1320 (2010)

15. Ma, J.: Segment anything in medical images. Nat. Commun. **15**, 654 (2024)
16. Zhang, C., et al.: Faster segment anything: towards lightweight SAM for mobile applications. arXiv preprint arXiv:2306.14289 (2023)

Author Index

S. Bakas et al. (Eds.): MICCAI 2025, LNCS 16377, pp. 359–360, 2026.
https://doi.org/10.1007/978-3-032-16370-7

The manufacturer's authorised representative in the EU is Springer Nature Customer Service Centre GmbH, Europaplatz 3, 69115 Heidelberg, Germany. If you have any concerns regarding our products, please contact ProductSafety@springernature.com

Printed and bound by CPI Group (UK) Ltd, Croydon, CR0 4YY
07/07/2026
02160917-0012